SUPPORTING SUCKING SKILLS IN BREASTFEEDING INFANTS

Catherine Watson Genna, BS, IBCLC
Woodhaven, NY

JONES AND BARTLETT PUBLISHERS

Sudbury, Massachusetts

BOSTON   TORONTO   LONDON   SINGAPORE

World Headquarters

Jones and Bartlett Publishers
40 Tall Pine Drive
Sudbury, MA 01776
978-443-5000
info@jbpub.com
www.jbpub.com

Jones and Bartlett Publishers
Canada
6339 Ormindale Way
Mississauga, Ontario
L5V 1J2
CANADA

Jones and Bartlett Publishers
International
Barb House, Barb Mews
London W6 7PA
UK

Jones and Bartlett's books and products are available through most bookstores and online booksellers. To contact Jones and Bartlett Publishers directly, call 800-832-0034, fax 978-443-8000, or visit our website, www.jbpub.com.

Substantial discounts on bulk quantities of Jones and Bartlett's publications are available to corporations, professional associations, and other qualified organizations. For details and specific discount information, contact the special sales department at Jones and Bartlett via the above contact information, or send an email to specialsales@jbpub.com.

The authors, editor, and publisher have made every effort to provide accurate information. However, they are not responsible for errors, omissions, or for any outcomes related to the use of the contents of this book and take no responsibility for the use of the products and procedures described. Treatments and side effects described in this book may not be applicable to all people; likewise, some people may require a dose or experience a side effect that is not described herein. Drugs and medical devices are discussed that may have limited availability controlled by the Food and Drug Administration (FDA) for use only in a research study or clinical trial. Research, clinical practice, and government regulations often change the accepted standard in this field. When consideration is being given to use of any drug in the clinical setting, the health care provider or reader is responsible for determining FDA status of the drug, reading the package insert, and reviewing prescribing information for the most up-to-date recommendations on dose, precautions, and contraindications, and determining the appropriate usage for the product. This is especially important in the case of drugs that are new or seldom used.

Additional credits appear on page xix, which constitutes a continuation of the copyright page.

Production Credits

Executive Editor: Kevin Sullivan
Acquisitions Editor: Emily Ekle
Associate Editor: Amy Sibley
Editorial Assistant: Patricia Donnelly
Production Director: Amy Rose
Production Editor: Carolyn F. Rogers
Senior Marketing Manager: Katrina Gosek
Associate Marketing Manager: Rebecca Wasley
Composition: Jason Miranda, Spoke & Wheel

Manufacturing and Inventory Coordinator:
  Amy Bacus
Photo Research Manager and Photographer:
  Kimberly Potvin
Cover Design: Anne Spencer
Cover Image: © Catherine Watson Genna, BS, IBCLC
Printing and Binding: Malloy, Inc.
Cover Printing: Malloy, Inc.

Library of Congress Cataloging-in-Publication Data
Supporting sucking skills in breastfeeding infants / [edited by] Catherine Watson Genna.
    p. ; cm.
  Includes bibliographical references and index.
  ISBN-13: 978-0-7637-4037-5 (pbk. : alk. paper)
  ISBN-10: 0-7637-4037-3 (pbk. : alk. paper)
  1. Breastfeeding. 2. Lactation. 3. Breastfeeding promotion. I. Genna, Catherine Watson.
  [DNLM: 1. Breast Feeding. 2. Infant, Newborn. 3. Lactation--physiology. WS 125 S959 2008]
  RJ216.S885 2008
  649'.33--dc22
                                2007026533
6048

Printed in the United States of America.
11 10 09 08 07   10 9 8 7 6 5 4 3 2 1

Contents

Chapter 3 | **Impact of Birth Practices on Infant Suck**   **57**

Linda J. Smith

Chapter 4 | **How Infants Learn to Feed: A Neurobehavioral Model**   **79**

Christina Smillie

Chapter 5 | **The Infant–Maternal Breastfeeding Conversation: Helping When They Lose the Thread**   **97**

Rebecca Glover and Diane Wiessinger

Chapter 6	The Goldilocks Problem: Milk Flow That Is Not Too Fast, Not Too Slow, but Just Right, or Why Milk Flow Matters and What to Do About It	131

Lynn Wolf and Robin Glass

Chapter 7	Breastfeeding Preterm Infants	153

Kerstin Hedberg-Nyqvist

Chapter 8   The Influence of Anatomical and Structural Issues on Sucking Skills 181

Catherine Watson Genna

Chapter 9   Minimally Invasive Treatment for Posterior Tongue-Tie (The Hidden Tongue-Tie)   227

Elizabeth V. Coryllos, Catherine Watson Genna, and Judy LeVan Fram

FOREWORD

Diane Wiessinger

If we were writing a handbook on bicycle riding for aliens, we would first study bicycling in all its complexity—how to mount, balance, turn, and stop. The first edition of our book would probably include considerable detail about what a bicycle is and how it works. That would be followed by precise instructions on, for instance, the exact placement of the ball of the left foot on the pedal as the right leg is swung over the bicycle. A few determined aliens would be able to put together a general picture from our mountain of minutiae (and our limited number of graphics and nonexistent film footage) and actually learn to ride; most would make clumsy attempts, feel defeated by our thoroughness, and quit.

Our second edition would emphasize certain aspects as being important, while leaving many of the details to the reader to work out with practice. This would be a much more useful book, but its continued emphasis on many steps would prevent most readers from gaining the grace and perspective of the average human 10-year-old bicyclist. Our third edition, I hope, would appear in two volumes: one for instructors, and one for would-be bicyclists. The instructors' volume would retain all the steps, but there would be no expectation that the bicyclists themselves would need to learn them all. For the bicyclists who needed extra help, a few brief and well-timed suggestions would allow them to be off and away without ever understanding exactly how they were doing it. The understanding part could be left to the instructors, whose modest but aptly chosen interventions were based on a thorough knowledge of all the small steps.

Breastfeeding is biology. Therefore, some mothers and babies have always needed help and will always need help, just as some of us need glasses or a math tutor. In our zeal to help those mothers and babies, we have spent decades dissecting breastfeeding and carefully detailing all of its parts: the anatomy and physiology of mother and baby, the angles of neck and mouth, the positions of arms and legs, the variations in breasts and nipples. Sometimes it seemed that the more we knew, the more trouble women had. Today, in addition to the familiar cry that

"I wanted to breastfeed but I didn't have enough milk," we too often hear "I wanted to breast-feed but my baby never latched." The reasons for this apparent shift are numerous, but we are beginning to recognize that our rigorous attending to every detail, and our eagerness for mothers to do the same, is sometimes part of the problem.

Time for a change. Mothers and babies, as you'll see in this book, already possess an advanced understanding of breastfeeding, provided we don't intervene unnecessarily. At the same time, mothers are perhaps more lacking in confidence than they have ever been—confidence in their bodies generally, confidence in their babies' abilities, and confidence in their inherent "mothering wisdom." Books for mothers are just beginning to portray the larger, right-brained picture of breastfeeding, with less emphasis on a rigid, left-brained list of steps and more emphasis on the innate abilities of mother and baby. But that leaves the instructors with perhaps a greater-than-ever need to know the supporting details for those mothers and babies who need them.

This book is for us, the instructors, to help us recognize when certain steps in the breast-feeding balance have gone awry, to provide detailed ideas on correcting them, and to give us deep enough knowledge over a broad enough area that we can choose the right level of inter-vention and leave the rest of the process alone.

It is not enough, of course. Only as we become a breastfeeding culture will the final pieces fall into place. Right now, our friend the alien comes to an earth on which only a few people ride bicycles. Most of the advertising, most of the language, most of the images are of easy-to-learn, readily available tricycles. But imagine the alien who comes to earth and sees everyone around him riding bicycles! He tries and falls, but he keeps trying. Eventually he sails off, steady and confident. Why did he succeed? Not only because he read a general guide that provided him with the big picture. Not only because his instructor had a nice, thick book of potentially helpful interventions. But because he saw around him, everywhere he went, people of all sizes and shapes and ages on bicycles. He learned to his very core that this is what people do, that this is what people enjoy, and that, if all of them can do it, then he can do it too. Maybe with just a little bit of help.

INTRODUCTION

Catherine Watson Genna

Breastfeeding is *normal* infant feeding. All that most infants need to breastfeed are a receptive state and the correct sequence of environmental signals. Infants placed on their mother's abdomen after unmedicated births are able to crawl up to the breast, attach deeply, and suck correctly. If those infants were either exposed to narcotic medications or separated from their mother for even a few minutes, they have greater difficulty finding the breast, and if they were both drugged and separated most fail even to attempt the normal seeking behavior.

The normal ability to self-attach, although strongest immediately after birth, does not become extinct for several months. It has been used successfully with older infants to overcome their learned resistance to attempting to latch. However, the older and more savvy an infant becomes, the more important cognitive processes become to feeding. Giving the right signals when an infant is in a receptive state can allow the neurobehavioral feeding program to overcome the infant's frustration with trying to get the breast to "work."

Inability to breastfeed is a red flag for further infant problems; breastfeeding is an essential component of normal infant life and its absence means something is fundamentally wrong with the infant's world. Minor anatomical variations such as ankyloglossia (tongue-tie) and recessed or small mandible can make breastfeeding more challenging. Breastfeeding management can often be modified to allow an infant with these conditions to feed successfully. Infants with respiratory issues such as laryngomalacia or tracheomalacia can usually be successful breastfeeders, with positional and temporal modifications. Infants who are unable to breastfeed with proper management need careful examination of their cardiac, respiratory, musculoskeletal, gastrointestinal, metabolic, and neurological functioning. Any medical illness that causes pain can interfere with an infant's state control and make feeding more difficult. Some ill infants can work toward breastfeeding, some infants will not be capable for some time or at all, and their mothers can be supported to provide their milk in whatever way the infant can feed.

This book is for any healthcare professional who works with infants. It is deliberately multidisciplinary because many different professionals work with infants and need to understand normal feeding, normal sucking, and how to help infants with problems. Specialization, although necessary, fragments knowledge, and teamwork is then required to assemble a whole picture. This book is intended to provide the information each team member needs about normal infant feeding to facilitate that teamwork, and to assemble in one volume many of the strategies that assist infants in sucking and feeding correctly.

Each profession has maxims that have been passed down through the generations without scrutiny. The authors of this work have endeavored to return to the research to try to share the most reliable information possible. Unfortunately, much of the research on infant feeding confuses cultural and biological norms. The text draws on both clinical experience and empirical evidence, and endeavors to differentiate clearly between the two.

I encourage you to read the book in order, and then return and re-read the assessment section at the end of Chapter 1 to help consolidate the information in a complete framework for breastfeeding evaluation.

ACKNOWLEDGMENTS

No project of this magnitude is a solo endeavor. I'd like to thank the contributors to this volume for their willingness to share their wisdom on paper, and on time, despite their international lecture schedules.

I'd like to thank Kathleen Bruce and Katherine Auerbach for starting Lactnet, and allowing a fertile cross-pollination that brought me into contact with many of the great minds in the field. I thank all the Lactnet and PPLC (private practice lactation consultant) participants who share their knowledge, speculations, research, and discoveries every day.

Thanks to the mothers who've trusted me with their precious infants. Babies have been my best teachers.

To my firstborn, Vincent, who made me a mother and set my feet on this path for my life, and my "baby," Alyssa, for confirming that breastfeeding is far more than nutrition.

To my husband, Dave, for your unwavering support, even when you had to learn to cook so we didn't starve as book deadlines approached.

Special thanks to Lisa Sandora for doing incredible amounts of research, and to Linda Kittrell and Jennifer Heffron in Bethesda North Medical Library at TriHealth Hospitals for their assistance locating many articles for us.

I am grateful to Linda Smith for acting as the midwife for this baby. For encouraging me that it was indeed time to birth a book on sucking issues, and not wait until we *know everything,* and for leading me through the publishing process.

Thank you Kathy Kendall Tackett for providing labor support! You were a great doula, sharing your experience gleaned through laboring on many books, while helping me find my own flow.

And finally, thanks to Tricia Donnelly, my editorial liaison at Jones and Bartlett, for patiently answering my millions of questions, and to Carolyn Rogers and her copyediting team, for their kind help in getting all the little details right!

Contributors

Nils Bergman, MB, ChB, MPH, DCH, MD
Health Systems Research Unit, Medical Research Council of South Africa (affiliate)
Professional Advisory Boards: LLL South Africa, Breastfeeding Associations of South
  Africa, International Lactation Consultant Association
Cape Town, South Africa

Elizabeth V. Coryllos, MS(s), MD, FAAP, FACS, FCCP, FAASP, FRCS(s), IBCLC
Associate Professor
Department of Surgery
Stony Brook University Medical Center of the State University of New York
Emeritus Director, Department of Pediatric Surgery
Winthrop University Hospital
Mineola, NY

Judy LeVan Fram, MEd, PT, IBCLC
Private Practice Lactation Consultant
Brooklyn, NY

Robin Glass, MS, OTR, IBCLC
Assistant Professor
Department of Rehabilitation Medicine
University of Washington
Children's Hospital and Regional Medical Center
Seattle, WA

Rebecca Glover, RN, RM, IBCLC
Private Practice
Perth, Western Australia

Kerstin Hedberg-Nyqvist, RN, PhD, IBCLC
Assistant Professor of Paediatric Nursing
Department of Women's and Children's Health, University Children's Hospital, Pediatrics
Uppsala, Sweden

Chele Marmet, MA, IBCLC*
Co-founder, Lactation Institute
Encino, CA

Lisa Sandora, MA, CCC-SLP, IBCLC
Speech-Language Pathologist and Lactation Consultant
TriHealth Bethesda North Hospital
Cincinnati, OH

Ellen Shell, MA, IBCLC*
Co-founder, Lactation Institute
Encino, CA

Christina Smillie, MD, FAAP, FABM, IBCLC
Medical Advisory Board, La Leche League International
Board of Directors, Academy of Breastfeeding Medicine
Medical Director, Breastfeeding Resources
Stratford, CT

Linda J. Smith, BSE, FACCE, IBCL
Steering Committee, Coalition to Improve Maternity Services (CIMS)
Bright Future Lactation Resource Centre
Dayton, OH

Diane Wiessinger, MS, IBCLC
Common Sense Breastfeeding
Ithaca, NY

---

* Retired, not recertified

Nancy Williams, MA, CCE, MFT, IBCLC
Pregnancy Support Centers of Lompoc and Santa Ynez Valley, Board of Directors LLL
  of Southern California/Nevada
Adjunct Faculty, Psychology Department
Chapman University College
Orange, CA

Lynn Wolf, MOT, OTR, IBCLC
Assistant Professor
Department of Rehabilitation Medicine
University of Washington
Children's Hospital and Regional Medical Center
Seattle, WA

Photo Credits

Figure 5-9: Reprinted with permission by Rebecca Glover, IBCLC.

Figure 5-10: © Catherine Watson Genna, BS, IBCLC

Figure 5-11: © Catherine Watson Genna, BS, IBCLC

Figure 5-12: Reprinted with permission by Barbara Wilson-Clay, BSEd, IBCLC.

Figure 5-13: © Catherine Watson Genna, BS, IBCLC

Chapter 6

Figure 6-1: Reprinted with permission from Wolf, L.S., & Glass, R.P. (1992). *Feeding and swallowing disorders in infancy: Assessment and management.* Austin, TX: Pro-Ed.

Figure 6-2: Reprinted with permission from Lau, C., Alagugurusamy, R., Schlanler, R.J., Smith, E.O., & Schulman, R.J. (2000). Characterization of the developmental stages of sucking in preterm infants during bottle feeding. *Acta Paediatrica,* 89(7), 846–852.

Figure 6-3: Reprinted with permission from Wolf, L.S., & Glass, R.P. (1992). *Feeding and swallowing disorders in infancy: Assessment and management.* Austin, TX: Pro-Ed.

Figure 6-4: Reprinted with permission from Wolf, L.S., & Glass, R.P. (1992). *Feeding and swallowing disorders in infancy: Assessment and management.* Austin, TX: Pro-Ed.

Figure 6-5: © Catherine Watson Genna, BS, IBCLC

Chapter 7

Figures 7-1 through 7-8: Reprinted with permission by Kerstin Hedberg-Nyqvist, RN, PhD, IBCLC.

Chapter 8

Figures 8-1 through 8-49: © Catherine Watson Genna, BS, IBCLC

Figure 8-50a and b: Reprinted with permission by Esther Grunis, IBCLC.

Figures 8-51 through 8-56: © Catherine Watson Genna, BS, IBCLC

Chapter 9

Figures 9-1 through 9-11: © Catherine Watson Genna, BS, IBCLC

Chapter 10

Figures 10-1 through 10-12: © Catherine Watson Genna, BS, IBCLC

Chapter 11

Figures 11-1 through 11-10: © Catherine Watson Genna, BS, IBCLC
Figure 11-11a, b, c: Reprinted with permission by Mellanie Sheppard, BS, IBCLC.
Figures 11-12 through 11-48: © Catherine Watson Genna, BS, IBCLC

Chapter 12

Figures 12-1 through 12-31: Used with permission of the Lactation Institute/Chele Marmet.

Chapter 13

Figure 13-1: Courtesy of Nancy Williams, MA, IBCLC.

Color Plates

Plates 1 through 7: © Catherine Watson Genna, BS, BS, IBCLC
Plate 8: Reprinted with permission from "Morphological analyses of the human tongue musculature for three-dimensional modeling," by Takemoto, H., *Journal of Speech, Language, and Hearing Research, 44,* p. 105. Copyright 2001 by American Speech-Language-Hearing Association. All rights reserved.

Breastfeeding: Normal Sucking and Swallowing

Catherine Watson Genna and Lisa Sandora

Normal Sucking

All mammals share a neurobehavioral program for sucking. They are competent to get to the teat—without maternal assistance—attach to it, and transfer milk. Humans are no exception. When born without labor medications and placed immediately on mom's abdomen, a human infant goes through the following behavioral sequence leading to breastfeeding (Ransjo-Arvidson et al., 2001):

1. Hand to mouth movements
2. Tongue movements
3. Mouth opening
4. Focusing on the nipple
5. Crawling to the nipple
6. Massaging the breast to evert the nipple
7. Licking
8. Attaching to the breast

Labor medications and separation from mother disrupt this sequence and can lead to incorrect sucking patterns (Righard & Alade, 1990). Later return to skin-to-skin contact can reestablish the original behavioral sequence and allow the infant to learn to attach (see Chapter 4).

Much of the difficulty with inducing infants to breastfeed is due to failure to understand their behavioral sequence and the environmental triggers for each behavior. Human infants expect positional stability—complete prone positioning against mom's abdomen or chest allows the infant better neck control and refined jaw and tongue movements. When infants self-attach, they extend their neck and lead with their chin. When the chin contacts the breast, the baby starts seeking the nipple. When the nipple contacts the philtrum (the ridge between nose and upper lip) the baby gapes widely and grasps the nipple and the surrounding tissue with the tongue, seals to the breast, and begins to suck. Infants use tactile (touch) and olfactory (smell) cues to help them identify the nipple.

One can use these expectations to assist babies who have difficulty latching on. The "infant helplessness" model leads moms to try to do too much for the baby, and many mothers handle their breast like a bottle, trying to center the nipple in the baby's mouth. Healthy, neurotypical infants simply need snug support against mom's ribcage and tactile proximity to the breast, preferably so that the nipple is at the philtrum and the chin is on the breast, and they are able to open well and grasp the breast with only minimal assistance (snuggling closer by mom as they come to breast). When infants are unable to self-attach, special techniques can be used to assist them. These are covered in Chapter 5.

Although a neurobehavioral program guides the initial attachment and sucking experiences, learning rapidly occurs. Human infants are able to experiment with different sucking pressures and different lip, tongue, and jaw movements to maximize the amount of milk they obtain, or to reduce an uncomfortably fast flow. Some of these compensations will be adaptive for the infant and comfortable for the mother; some will not, and will require intervention. This book focuses on interventions that have proven helpful in practice.

In order to intervene in any process, it is important that normal be well understood. Ideally, the infant orients to the nipple (rooting response), opens his or her mouth widely (gape response) and brings his or her tongue down to the floor of the mouth and extends it over the lower lip to grasp the breast. As the mouth closes, the anterior tongue cups the breast, and the body of the tongue grooves to conform to and hold the breast. The breast is enclosed between the grooved tongue, cheeks, and palate, forming a teat. The nipple is as far back in the mouth as possible, generally to the posterior hard palate.

Once attached, the infant lifts his or her tongue tip against the breast. A rapid elevation wave passes along the length of the tongue from front to back, perhaps moving milk toward the nipple. The anterior tongue remains grooved around the breast, and the soft palate contacts the posterior tongue. This makes a sealed chamber of the area around the nipple. The mid-tongue then drops as the jaw opens slightly (while the anterior tongue and lips remain sealed on the breast) to decrease the pressure in the mouth and pull milk from the breast. The tongue is still grooved from front to back, which allows the milk that sprays from the nipple to gather in a small pool, or bolus. The soft palate elevates and the pharyngeal walls contract to meet it in order to close off the nasopharynx, or nasal air space. Finally, the vocal folds snap shut, the epiglottis covers the vocal folds, the larynx elevates, and the tongue dumps the bolus of milk into the pharynx for transit to the esophagus during swallowing.

Anatomy

The newborn human mouth is particularly well designed for sucking (see **Figure 1-1**). The tongue is large in relation to the size of the oral cavity. When the mouth is open, the tongue and breast fill it completely, stabilizing tongue movements. The normal resting position of the tongue is with the tip over the lower lip, where it can easily contact the breast.

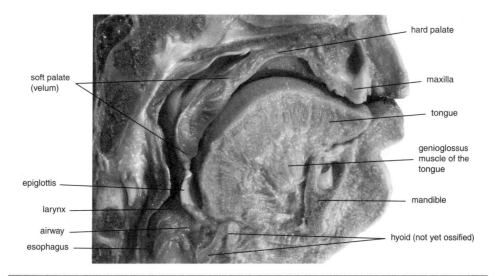

hard palate

soft palate
(velum)

maxilla

tongue

genioglossus
muscle of the
tongue

epiglottis

mandible

larynx

airway

hyoid (not yet ossified)

esophagus

Figure 1-1   Midsaggital section, oral anatomy of a 7-month fetus.

The cheeks contain fat pads that add to the thickness of the cheek wall and help guard against collapse of the cheeks when the oral cavity is enlarged by tongue depression (see **Figure 1-2**). If the cheeks collapse, the oral cavity becomes smaller, and the negative pressure less. Recent ultrasound studies have demonstrated that the negative pressure in the mouth is vital to milk transfer (Ramsay & Hartmann, 2005). The fat pads of the cheeks also provide lateral (side) borders for the tongue to keep the tongue in midline during sucking. Although newborns can perform lateral (side to side) tongue movements, these are generally not used during feeding until solids are begun after 6 months of age. The *buccinators* are the muscles of the cheek, which compress the cheeks when activated, to maintain contact between cheek and breast during breastfeeding and to keep food in contact with the teeth during chewing. The buccinators are innervated by the facial nerve.

Figure 1-2
Buccal fat pads provide
lateral stability to the
tongue in newborns.

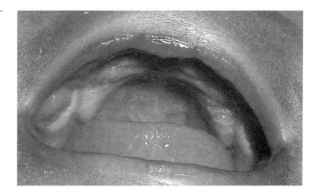

The lips are soft and flexible, and the lower lip is generally flanged outward on the breast, allowing contact with the soft mucous membrane. The upper lip is usually in a more neutral position when attachment is correct. (An overly turned out upper lip is a sign of a shallow latch, and can favor excessive use of the lips to press milk out of the breast.) Around the outside of the soft lips is a complex circular muscle made up of many fibers, named the *orbicularis oris*. Partial contraction of this muscle helps maintain the lips' seal on the breast. The mentalis muscle at the base of the lower lip elevates and protrudes the lip, and is very active during breastfeeding. These muscles are innervated by the facial nerve.

The mandible (lower jaw) is usually short in newborns, due to the position of the chin on the chest in utero, which may mechanically restrict jaw growth. This is compensated for by the infant's predominant flexor muscle tone pattern, which favors jaw opening over closing. Poor grading (fine control over the speed and amount) of movement also favors a large gape. The masseter muscle relaxes to depress the mandible, and contracts to elevate it during sucking. Both masseters working together allow symmetrical jaw movement during sucking; unilateral action causes the sideways jaw movements of chewing. The temporalis muscle closes the mandible during sucking. Both muscles are innervated by the trigeminal nerve's third (mandibular) branch.

Tongue and jaw motions are linked through mutual attachments to the hyoid bone to make it easier for the infant to use the tongue and jaw in concert during sucking. The mandible raises during the compression (positive pressure) phase of sucking, and drops during the suction (negative pressure) phase. The tongue is a complex muscular structure. In the past, a distinction was made between extrinsic and intrinsic tongue muscles, but careful dissections using advanced staining techniques have revealed that fibers from muscles that were thought to arise outside the tongue become incorporated into the body of the tongue (Hiiemae & Palmer, 2003; Takemoto, 2001).

Major muscles of the tongue include the genioglossus, which pulls the tongue down during the negative pressure phase of sucking; the superior longitudinal muscles, which lift the tongue tip; the inferior longitudinals, which lower the tongue tip and help move it from side to side; the vertical muscles, which help thin the tongue; and the transverse muscles, which along with the genioglossus and the extrinsic muscles help to groove the tongue (see **Figure 1-3**). Most of the fibers of the intrinsic tongue muscles are fast responding, allowing rapid changes in tongue configuration (Stal, Marklund, Thornell, De Paul, & Eriksson, 2003). An understanding of the arrangement and relationships of the major tongue muscles allows facilitation of correct sucking in infants with difficulties. See **Plate 8** for a three-dimensional representation of the arrangement of the muscles of the tongue, courtesy of Hironori Takemoto, PhD.

Newborns have unique airway protection. The epiglottis and soft palate touch at rest, and the upper airway is very short. This helps to direct milk to the esophagus and reduces the risk of aspiration. This airway configuration also encourages the infant to extend the neck, which reduces resistance to air flow in the airway and brings the small mandible forward to have as much contact with the breast as possible. Tongue and mandible contact with the breast needs to be as complete as possible for proper mechanical advantage during sucking.

Figure 1-3
Facial muscles involved in
feeding.

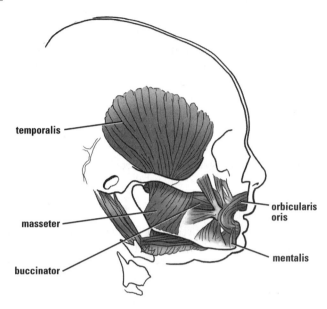

temporalis

orbicularis
oris

masseter

mentalis

buccinator

Suckling or Sucking: Differences Between Suckling at the Breast and Sucking at the Bottle

The speech and occupational therapy literature often repeats the idea that suckling (the front to back, wavelike movement of the tongue) changes to sucking (a straight up and down movement of the tongue and jaw) at around 3 months of age. A Japanese study (Iwayama & Eishima, 1997) of breastfed and bottle fed infants done on bottles showed transition to this pattern in infants over 3 months, but this might have been due to mechanical differences between breast and bottle, and increased size of the infants' oral cavity in relationship with the static artificial nipple. Electromyography (EMG) studies have confirmed that muscle activation is different between breastfeeding and bottle feeding, with less use of the mentalis and masseters and more use of the buccinators and oribicularis oris in bottle feeding (Gomes, 2006; Inoue, Sakashita, & Kamegai, 1995; Nyqvist, 2001). Lactation consultants have long been skeptical of the idea that there are two age-dependent forms of sucking at the breast. The author's (Genna's) ultrasound suck research has shown an up and down tongue and jaw pattern only in a subset of tongue-tied infants using excessive jaw excursions, which disappears in favor of the biphasic wavelike pattern after frenotomy. Breastfeeding children up to 4 years old have been studied so far with no evidence of a change in sucking pattern at breast. For this reason, *suckling* shall be used to mean the act of feeding at breast, and sucking as the oral motor activity that transfers milk, with the understanding that breastfeeding is the biological norm for human beings, and that normal sucking is the sucking that occurs at breast.

Deglutition (Swallowing)

For professionals working with children with feeding issues there are two terms that are useful to understand: feeding and swallowing. *Feeding* refers to what takes place during the *oral preparatory phase*, from sucking up to bolus formation, and the *oral phase*, propelling the bolus posteriorly in the mouth. In contrast, *swallowing* encompasses all four phases: the oral preparatory, oral, pharyngeal, and esophageal phases from when the milk enters the mouth until it enters the stomach (see **Figure 1-4**). The primary focus of the lactation consultant is to assess the feeding aspects (the oral preparatory and oral phases); however, it is useful to have an understanding of the entire process. Generally, evaluation of the pharyngeal and esophageal phases are carried out through instrumental tests such as the videofluoroscopic swallow study (VFSS), discussed later in this chapter. Tests are typically ordered by a physician and performed and interpreted by speech-language pathologists or occupational therapists.

The anatomical structures used for feeding are also used for breathing and speech production. An infant is faced with the challenge of using these structures in a highly orchestrated way in order to maintain oxygenation as well as acquire adequate intake to grow. Sucking is the initial stage of a four-part swallowing process (Corbin-Lewis, Liss, & Sciortino, 2005; Logemann, 1998). Swallowing has four phases that must take place in a synchronous, organized fashion for safe feeding to occur. The focus of this discussion is to explore infant anatomy and physiology as it relates to the sucking and swallowing process.

Although both sucking and swallowing occur prenatally, they are not necessarily occurring together. In utero, both sucking and swallowing have been observed in fetuses as early as 12.5 weeks of age. A full-term fetus swallows 450 ml of amniotic fluid in a day (Bosma, 1986). This volume is greater than early postnatal daily intake. This discrepancy is most likely due to the need for the neonate to coordinate sucking, swallowing, and breathing.

Morris (1998) gave an excellent description of the anatomy and physiology of swallowing. She described the swallowing system as a single tube with two cavities at the upper end (nose and mouth) that divides two tubes at the lower end, the esophagus for eating and the trachea for breathing. There are valves throughout the tube for closing off areas so that safe breathing can occur when it's time to breathe and safe eating when it's time to move food to the esophagus. These valves also allow for pressure build-up in the various cavities along the tube so that the bolus can be moved to the esophagus safely and bypass the airway. For example, the lips, cheeks, palate, and tongue form a seal to create negative pressure to remove milk from the breast and then the pressure changes help to propel the bolus into the pharynx (throat). Breakdown of any of these systems of valves along the way will disrupt sucking, swallowing, and/or breathing.

Although there is limited human research, animal studies show that the neurological control of the swallow may not be fully developed for 30–60 days postnatally (Newman, 1996). Newman reports various studies where the nerves innervating the pharynx (throat) were stimulated or when fluid was introduced into the throats of newborn animals. The newborns responded with apnea (stopping of breathing), in contrast with 1–2-month-old

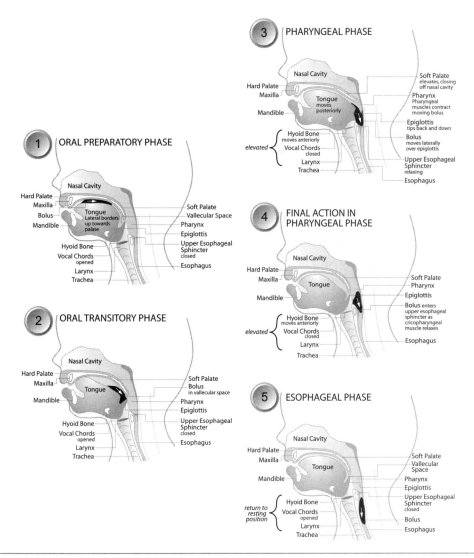

Figure 1-4   The four phases of swallowing.

animals who responded by swallowing. Newman also cited a study that looked at the myelination of the vagus nerve fibers, a relay center for breathing and swallowing (Becker, Zhang, & Pereyra, 1993), in infants who died of sudden infant death syndrome (SIDS) in the first 9 months. When the autopsies of the SIDS victims were compared with age-matched controls, they found incomplete myelination of the nerve fibers of the vagus nerve, which may indicate incomplete maturation. Becker speculated that this incomplete maturation could be an explanation for problems related to incoordination of breathing, sucking, and swallowing in the first month or so of life that appear to resolve in typically developing infants. This has been observed and reported in clinical practice.

Neural Control of Sucking and Swallowing

Cranial nerves in the brainstem provide the sensory and motor fibers that innervate and provide feedback to the face, mouth, pharynx, larynx, and stomach. Two sets of specialized nerved tracts in the brain stem, referred to as the "swallowing centers," direct movements for swallowing. Sensory fibers from the cerebral cortex, cerebellum, and brainstem influence coordination of swallowing (Morris & Klein, 2000, p. 47).

Reflexive Control of Sucking and Swallowing

The newborn infant depends primarily on reflexes for feeding. Reflexes are prewired templates for life-sustaining movements in the infant that gradually become integrated into voluntary movement patterns (**Table 1-1**).

The *rooting* reflex is stimulated by touch to the face and mouth, and causes the infant to turn toward the breast, open the mouth, depress and extend the tongue, and grasp the breast.

The *transverse tongue* reflex occurs when the lateral edge of the tongue is stroked. The infant's tongue should move toward the source of stimulation. *Tongue protrusion* occurs when the anterior tongue is touched. The *phasic bite* reflex is not elicited during sucking unless the infant retracts the tongue and exposes the gum ridge to stimulation. These reflexes diminish by around 6 months in preparation for introduction of solid foods.

Like sucking, *swallowing* is not a simple reflex, but encompasses complex, highly orchestrated sensory and motor events that are under both voluntary and involuntary control (Arvedson & Brodsky, 2002).

The *cough* reflex is of great importance to feeding because it allows the infant to expel material that has entered the airway and/or been aspirated. This protective reflex is triggered by sensory receptors (chemoreceptors) in the larynx, causing the vocal folds to snap shut and a cough to propel the foreign material out of the airway (Arvedson & Lefton-Greif, 1998).

The *gag* reflex is the other protective reflex that prevents the infant from swallowing an object or bolus larger than the pharynx can handle.

The Four Phases of Swallowing

In order to develop an understanding of the four phases of the swallow, a listing of the phases and the structures involved in each phase are presented below (Stevenson & Allaire, 1991):

Oral Preparatory Phase:
- Lips
- Tongue/mandible

TABLE 1-1 Oral-Motor, Cranial Nerve, and Reflex Evaluation

Reflex	Stimulus	Behavior	Cranial Nerves Involved	Present At
Protective Reflexes				
Cough	Fluid in larynx or bronchii	Upward movement of air to clear the airway	X Vagus	35–40 weeks gestation
Gag	Touch back of tongue	Mouth opening, head extension, floor of mouth depresses	IX Glosso-pharyngeal X Vagus Cortex	26–27 weeks gestation
Adaptive Reflexes				
Phasic bite	Stimulate gums	Rhythmic up and down jaw movement	V Trigeminal	28 weeks gestation
Transverse tongue	Stroke sides of tongue	Tongue moves toward side of stimulus (lateralizes)	XII Hypoglossal	28 weeks gestation
Tongue protrusion	Touch tongue tip	Tongue protrudes from mouth	XII Hypoglossal	38–40 weeks gestation
Rooting	Stroke cheek or near mouth	Infant senses stimuli and localizes toward source, opens mouth (gapes), extends and depresses tongue to grasp breast, creates seal against breast	V Trigeminal VII Facial XI Accessory XII Hypoglossal	32–37 weeks gestation (MMP)
Suckling	Touch to junction of hard/soft palate	Wavelike tongue movement, coordinated with up/down jaw movement	V Trigeminal VII Facial IX Glosso-pharyngeal XII Hypoglossal	18 weeks gestation

Source: Adapted from Hall, 2001.
Note: MMP, Majorie Meyer Palmer, NOMAS Certification Course 2006.

- Cheeks
- Hard palate

Oral Transitory Phase:

- Tongue/mandible

Pharyngeal Phase:

- Soft palate (velum)
- Pharyngeal muscles surrounding the throat
- Epiglottis
- Laryngeal muscles
- Arytenoid mass (made up of the false vocal folds, true vocal folds, and arytenoid cartilages; the arytenoid cartilages sit on top of the true vocal folds posteriorly, and open the airway during breathing and close the airway during swallowing)
- Upper esophageal sphincter

Esophageal Phase:

- Esophagus

How the Four Stages of Deglutition Work

Oral preparatory phase. Rooting, attachment, and sucking comprise the beginning of the oral preparatory phase. During sucking, the medial portion of the tongue forms a trough or groove for channeling the milk posteriorly. Milk is delivered onto the tongue as the midtongue drops to create negative pressure in the mouth.

Is It Tongue Stripping (Positive Pressure) or Suction (Negative Pressure) That Removes Milk?

Studies have described infants as using a stripping, wavelike tongue motion (Bosma, Hepburn, Josell, & Baker, 1990; Hayashi, Hoashi, & Nara, 1997; Newman, 1996; Weber, Woolridge, & Baum, 1986) during feeding. Ramsay (Ramsay & Hartmann, 2005) indicates that milk is not removed by the stripping motion of the tongue. Their ultrasound studies indicated that milk flows due to the creation of suction (negative pressure) when the tongue and jaw drop during sucking.

The movements that appear to be tongue stripping may in reality be the tongue modulating pressure changes that create suction. As research continues, the mechanisms for milk removal from the breast will be further elucidated.

What Is Peristalsis?

Peristalsis is defined as "progressive contraction down a muscular tube." This is the activity seen in the esophagus as the bolus is progressively moved toward the stomach. Logemann (1998) points out that it is inaccurate to use this term in reference to the movement of the bolus in the oral and pharyngeal phases of the swallow, because anatomically they are not muscular tubes. Rather, there are pressure changes propelling the bolus. This can be seen by the rolling wave of the tongue in the oral cavity creating the negative pressure described in the previous box, which move the bolus over the base of the tongue (Logemann). Therefore, the term *peristalsis* will only be used in this text to describe what occurs in the esophageal phase, and tongue movements will be described as wavelike.

Oral transitory phase. Wavelike mechanical movements and pressure changes created by the tongue propel the bolus to the back of the oral cavity.

Pharyngeal phase. In newborns, the presence of the bolus at the valeculae at the base of the tongue triggers the swallow. The following mechanisms for protection of the airway are engaged (Arvedson & Brodsky, 2002):

1. Breathing stops.
2. The soft palate (velum) elevates to close off the nasal cavity and prevent the bolus from going into the nose (nasopharyngeal reflux).
3. The true and false vocal folds (cords) come together to close over the trachea.
4. The hyoid bone moves up and anteriorly.
5. The larynx (suspended from the hyoid bone by muscles and cartilage) is elevated by this same upward movement.
6. As the tongue moves posteriorly, the epiglottis also moves back and downward over the larynx to divert the bolus laterally and back toward the esophagus.
7. The pressure of contractions of the pharyngeal wall moves the bolus to the esophagus.
8. The upper esophageal sphincter opens, and the bolus enters the esophagus.

It is important that the pharyngeal phase of the swallow be well coordinated, because this is the phase during which there is the greatest risk of aspiration. The infant's ability to propel the bolus to the tongue base (valeculae) is important for setting the pharyngeal phase in motion and signaling the onset of the cascade of movements that protect the airway and direct the bolus to the esophagus (Arvedson & Brodsky, 2002).

Esophageal phase. The bolus moves through the esophagus (food tube) toward the stomach, consisting of the following stages:

1. Peristaltic movement of the bolus through the esophagus
2. Opening of the lower esophageal sphincter to allow the bolus to enter the stomach

Dysphagia

Dysphagia, or swallowing disorder, can range from mild to severe. The feeding specialist, a speech-language pathologist or occupational therapist, sometimes in cooperation with a specialist physician, assesses the swallowing mechanism during the oral and pharyngeal phases. The clinical examination involves observing oral movements in isolation and while the infant is feeding. If a swallowing problem is suspected, instrumental procedures are carried out to identify the source of the swallowing disorder and which phase or phases are disrupted. **Table 1-2** shows the evaluation procedures that are used to identify dysphagia. For a more extensive discussion of these instrumental procedures, refer to *Pediatric Videofluoroscopic Swallow Studies: A Professional Manual with Caregiver Guidelines* (Arvedson & Lefton-Greif, 1998).

Cervical Auscultation

Listening over the neck with a stethoscope is a useful method for scrutinizing swallowing sounds that can easily be used by lactation consultants. Normal swallowing sounds like a rapid biphasic click. Wet, bubbling sounds can indicate air passing through an incompletely cleared pharynx (Bosma, 1986), and short, discreet bouts of stridor during the swallow can indicate that fluid has leaked into the larynx (laryngeal penetration). In addition, delayed initiation of the swallow, inefficient swallowing (multiple swallows needed to clear the pharynx), and slower than normal swallowing can be identified. Integration of swallowing and breathing can be clearly heard. Infants with clinical symptoms due to dysphagia (repeated respiratory infections, feeding refusal) that do not resolve with management changes (prone feeding to assist bolus handling, applying pressure on the breast near the areola to obstruct some ducts during rapid milk flow, treatment of tongue-tie if indicated, calibration of milk supply to meet infant need if hyperlactation is responsible) should be referred for VFSS to determine whether oral feeding is safe. Exclusively breastfed infants rarely have repeated respiratory infections even if they are aspirating, because human milk is less irritating to the human respiratory epithelium than other foods. In this case, breastfeeding can continue, but caution is warranted when weaning (feeding any liquid or food other than human milk) begins.

TABLE 1-2   **Instrumental Procedures for Identifying Dysphagia**

Instrumental Procedure	Parts of Swallow Studied
Upper gastrointestinal study (Upper GI)	Esophagus, stomach, duodenum
Videofluoroscopic swallow study	Oral preparatory, oral, pharyngeal, upper esophageal phases of swallowing
	Identifies cause of dysphagia and aspiration
Ultrasound	Oral preparatory and oral phases of swallowing
Cervical auscultation (CA)	Sounds of breathing and swallowing in pharyngeal phase
Fiber-optic endoscopic evaluation of swallowing (FEES)	Looks at pharyngeal and laryngeal structure before and after the swallow

Feeding Assessment

Feeding assessment is a complex process that involves observation of oral structure and oral motor functioning, as well as global body condition including muscle tone, energy level, appropriate arousal, and aerobic capacity. All body systems participate in feeding, not just the gastrointestinal and renal systems whose involvement is obvious. Feeding is aerobic exercise for the human infant, so the heart, lungs, and circulatory system are vital for providing the oxygen necessary for the work of feeding. The musculoskeletal system participates both in providing stability for the infant and in performing specific movements that allow milk to be transferred from the breast to the infant's mouth and into the GI tract while excluding it from the respiratory passages. Cellular respiration (mitochondrial enzymes) provide the energy for each cell from their metabolism of blood-borne glucose, which is maintained by the liver and pancreas and the hormonal systems of the body. The nervous system must work properly to direct the activities of all the other systems.

A healthy infant, given a normal environment, can perform the necessary functions to maintain life and health, one of which is feeding. As mammals, human infants have the ability to move to, attach to, and remove milk from the mammae, or breasts. Conversely, if a newborn given a normal environment cannot breastfeed, the index of suspicion is increased that all is not well. Healthy infants indicate hunger by feeding behaviors, which include lip smacking, tongue movements, hands to mouth, squirming, and throwing themselves from an adult's shoulder down to the breast. These behaviors were once seen as hunger "cues," but now it is understood that they are functional behaviors that are part of the competent infant's feeding sequence. When mothers are educated to work with these normal behaviors, attachment to the breast becomes far easier.

This section will provide a framework for evaluating the infant's feeding behaviors at the breast. The purpose is to provide the reader with a system for evaluating the dynamics of feeding and swallowing from a breastfeeding perspective, so an intervention plan can be developed.

Most infants seen by lactation consultants have minimal or mild disorders. These may be transient problems such as incoordination of suck-swallow-breathe due to inexperience or poor feeding secondary to labor medications, or they may be persistent, such as the abnormal tongue movements from a tight lingual frenulum. These infants may have difficulty transferring milk at the breast but may be able to functionally bottle feed, offering false reassurance. Abnormal tongue movements may persist without intervention. In contrast, infants with moderate to severe problems are likely to have difficulty with both breast and bottle feeding and are more easily identified. Tracheomalacia or laryngomalacia may first become apparent as feeding volumes increase over the first few days of life. Lactation consultants (LCs) may therefore be the first to identify the short sucking bursts and stressed respiration typical of a respiratory anomaly. It is important for all members of the healthcare team to work together in the baby's best interest. Breastfeeding is usually an achievable goal, given practice, milk expression to support milk production, and supplementation in a manner supportive of normal feeding skills.

Breastfeeding promotes normal physiological development and optimal growth and function of the orofacial structures. Each step in normal development depends on the step before, and though the child may be able to function using compensatory strategies, these compensations do not promote optimal development. Therefore, early intervention is likely to avoid the need for more extensive therapy later.

Ideally, a *feeding team* addresses significant feeding and/or swallowing issues. A feeding team is a group of specialists who work together to develop an individualized feeding program for the infant or child. A pediatrician or neonatologist may serve as the medical coordinator. A speech-language pathologist, occupational therapist, nurse, and dietitian are included in the basic team. Other team members may include a social worker, psychologist, physical therapist, gastroenterologist, neurologist, otolaryngologist, pulmonologist, allergist, endocrinologist, and dentist. Team members evaluate the infant's skills from their professional perspective and report the results to the team. For example, the otolaryngologist may assess the integrity of the infant's oral, pharyngeal, and laryngeal structures through endoscopy and report to the team any abnormalities in anatomy and physiology as well as suggestions for treatment. The feeding team devises a plan of action that will address the infant's needs (Arvedson & Lefton-Greif, 1998; Morris & Klein, 2000). In order to participate as a feeding team member, the LC should have an understanding of normal feeding, techniques for assessing problems, and interventions for facilitating development of feeding skills.

Factors Affecting Feeding

Gestational Age

In order to assess the infant's feeding behavior, the clinician should have an understanding of how the infant develops and what to expect in terms of reflexive oral behaviors, state, endurance, and coordination of sucking, swallowing, and respiration. The younger the gestational age of the infant, the more his or her feeding skills are likely to be disrupted by lower aerobic capacity, lower muscle tone, lower energy, and decreased neurological maturity.

Pre-existing Medical Diagnosis

Information about medical conditions that affect feeding competence will shed light on the infant's capabilities, challenges, and behaviors. It is useful to keep the diagnosis in mind but approach the infant as an individual with his or her own set of feeding skills. It is helpful to know if and how the medical condition typically affects feeding and swallowing, while realizing that there is always a continuum of effects and the individual may be mildly, moderately, or severely affected in each area.

Screening Tools versus Assessment Tools

A *screening tool* identifies individuals at risk for feeding and swallowing problems by a rapid observation of signs and symptoms. An *assessment tool* provides more in-depth information as to the nature of the problem so that a plan of corrective or facilitative action can be taken (Logemann, 1998).

Current breastfeeding assessments are technically screening tools that have been devised primarily to identify when breastfeeding behaviors are present in mother and infant and if the potential for breastfeeding to occur is present. These are predominantly observational scales where the lactation consultant or nurse indicates the presence or absence of behaviors associated with breastfeeding. These screening tools have primarily been designed for use in the early postpartum period and may be viewed as a signal that breastfeeding is not "getting off to a good start." Dyads identified as at risk can then be referred for further assessment and intervention to protect mother's milk production in the sensitive calibration phase and ensure the infant's nutrition.

Examples of breastfeeding screening tools that can be used with term infants are as follows:

- Infant Breastfeeding Assessment Tool
- Latch Assessment Documentation Tool
- Via Christi Breastfeeding Assessment Tool
- Mother-Baby Assessment Tool

The Preterm Infant Breastfeeding Behavior Scale (Nyqvist, Rubertsson, Ewald, & Sjöden, 1996) is an observational tool for use with preterm infants to identify prebreastfeeding and early breastfeeding behaviors.

For a complete in-depth description of these and other breastfeeding scales, consult *Breastfeeding Management for the Clinician: Using the Evidence* by Marsha Walker (2006, pp. 116–126).

Other Oral Motor Assessment Tools

Speech pathologists and occupational therapists have used observational feeding tools to observe infant bottle feeding behaviors in the preterm and term population. The Neonatal Oral-Motor Assessment Scale (NOMAS) was developed to assess bottle feeding, though the author states that it can be used with breastfeeding infants as well (Palmer, 2006). The NOMAS is used to rate tongue and jaw movements during both non-nutritive and nutritive sucking. Infants with problems are diagnosed with disorganized sucking if they have deficiencies of rate and rhythm or dysfunctional sucking if they display abnormal tongue or jaw movements that interrupt the feeding (Palmer, 1998).

Another observational tool, the Early Feeding Skills (EFS) Assessment (Thoyre, Shaker, & Pridham, 2005) is a cue-based approach to feeding assessment and intervention in preterm hospitalized infants. The EFS is a checklist for determining infant readiness and tolerance for feeding based on infant physiologic, motor, and state regulation; oral-motor abilities; and coordination of suck-swallow-breathe.

Facilitation versus Compensation

Techniques for assisting with feeding issues fall under two categories:

- *Facilitative strategies:* Techniques that encourage normal development
- *Compensatory strategies:* Techniques that allow for more optimal feeding but do not change the underlying problem

Examples of facilitative strategies used with breastfeeding babies include:

- Skin-to-skin contact with the mother to increase arousal and interest in the breast
- Regulation of suck-swallow-breathe bursts (also called external pacing) with clinician-imposed pauses prior to coughing, drooling, or color changes in the infant
- Oral motor exercises to increase the range of oral movements
- Oral stimulation to increase strength and tone
- Decreasing oral sensory difficulties to allow deeper attachment to the breast (Adapted from treatment strategies in Hall, 2001)

Examples of compensatory strategies used with breastfeeding babies include:

- Approaching the infant when he or she is alert and ready to breastfeed
- Maintaining a quiet environment conducive to attending to feeding
- Attempting alternative positioning to compensate for infant or maternal anatomical variations
- Swaddling and flexing the infant when stress cues are exhibited
- Using a nipple shield when the infant has difficulty grasping the breast due to tongue-tie
- Using a nipple shield when the infant is preterm
- Providing cheek support when the baby has low tone, carefully observing for the ability to handle flow rate
- Providing jaw support for wide jaw excursions to prevent loss of attachment

These strategies are examples of what can be done to improve feeding skills. The determination of what strategies are appropriate for an individual infant can be made when a complete assessment is carried out.

Clinical Breastfeeding Assessment

An in-depth breastfeeding assessment will give the clinician more specific information about the infant's feeding ability at the breast. Detailed assessment facilitates the formulation of a plan of action for alleviating the problem. According to Arvedson and Lefton-Greif in their book *Pediatric Videofluoroscopic Swallow Studies* (1998), there are two basic questions asked during a feeding and swallowing evaluation: "What is the cause of the problem?" and "How can it be fixed?" This approach can also be adapted to the clinical breastfeeding assessment.

The steps of a clinical breastfeeding assessment follow:

1. Determine whether the breastfeeding problem is the result of:

    *   Basic positioning or attachment issues
    *   An underlying anatomical problem in the infant (or a problematic interaction with the mother's anatomy)
    *   An underlying neurological problem in the infant

2. Analyze the steps needed to alleviate the problem:

    a. Correct basic attachment, positioning, and management.
    b. Identify and implement compensatory techniques for anatomical problems and/or refer to another professional for further evaluation and treatment (e.g., frenotomy).
    c. Identify and implement facilitative techniques to improve neurological development and/or refer to another professional with specific expertise in this area.

3. Collaborate with parents on an individualized plan for them to follow at home to meet their breastfeeding goals with both short-term and long-term objectives.

4. Provide education, anticipatory guidance, and demonstration/return demonstration of techniques to be followed.

5. Arrange for follow-up.

In their book *Prefeeding Skills,* 2nd edition, Morris and Klein (2000) stated, "Assessment and treatment are sides of the same coin. Each assessment contains treatment probes to discover the most effective approaches to remediating the difficulties that have brought the child and family for the evaluation" (p. 174). This perspective can also apply to the clinical breastfeeding evaluation, where compensatory and facilitative techniques can be incorporated by the clinician. Both compensatory and facilitative techniques should be practiced during the assessment in order to determine their effectiveness in enhancing feeding skills. If successful, they can be incorporated into the feeding plan.

The clinical assessment consists of several areas of evaluation. Some clinicians carry out all of the following areas, whereas some focus only on specific areas:

- Oral-motor observation of infant and digital suck examination
- Breast examination of mother
- Breastfeeding assessment of infant and mother, including assessment of milk transfer
- Assessment of feeding using compensatory techniques, facilitative techniques, and alternate feeding devices (when appropriate)
- Milk expression (when appropriate)

Global Observations of the Infant

As part of the initial portion of the assessment, it is useful to globally observe the infant's:

- Tone
- Grading of movement
- Symmetry
- State and level of arousal/alertness
- Respiratory pattern
- Color

This information will be used as a baseline for comparison when the infant is engaged in feeding. A global assessment is useful because it can yield information that will contribute to the clinician's understanding of what may be happening during a feeding. The following information provides some guidelines to look for.

Tone

An infant with low muscle tone may let the extremities hang, recruit accessory muscles to help maintain stability, or use fixing to help compensate (see Chapter 11). There may be hypotonia in the facial area where the infant appears expressionless. At the breast, the hypotonic infant may lose suction as well as milk from the mouth. A hypertonic infant may exhibit arching when put to the breast and have a retracting jaw when sucking. Hypertonic infants may seem stiff, and may have difficulty opening the mouth wide (gaping) and initiating sucking bursts. These effects and compensations are usually easily visible, as are excessive excursions (downward movement) of the mandible that cause the lip seal to be disrupted. See **Figures 1-5** through **1-7** for examples of infants with hypotonia and normal muscle tone.

Figure 1-5
Infant with benign neonatal hypotonia.
Note that the mouth hangs open and arms fall to
the side of the body.

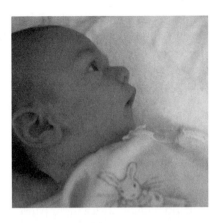

Figure 1-6
Infant with normal muscle tone. Note the crisp
creases from normal contraction of the muscles of
facial expression.

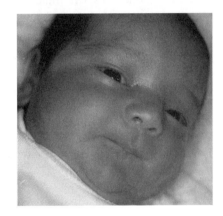

Figure 1-7
Infant with hypotonia due to Down syndrome.
Note the expressionless look due to low tone of
facial muscles.

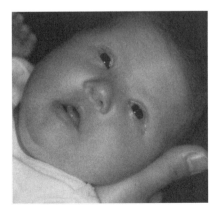

Infants may increase their tone in response to stress. Facial expression (wide or narrowed eyes, furrowed forehead) will usually help differentiate a stressed infant from a hypertonic one.

Grading of Movement

Infant grading (smoothness) of motion generally depends on stability. Neurologist Amiel-Tison noted that head and neck support improved fine motor control in neonates (Gosselin, 2005). When prone on the mother's trunk or abdomen, infants are capable of remarkably accurate movement. Head lift can't generally be maintained more than a second or two, but that is long enough for the baby to bob his or her way to the breast. The quality of grading will also be apparent in jaw movement. Movements should be smooth and equal, in midline, with a slight pause or bounce or accentuation of the downward jaw excursion as the mouth fills with milk.

Symmetry

Symmetry across midline is an indication of equal nerve and muscle activity on each side of the body. Nerve palsies, birth injuries, and adverse effects of restricted in utero positioning such as torticollis may all cause asymmetry and feeding difficulties (See **Figures 1-8, 1-9**).

Figure 1-8
Facial and neck asymmetry from torticollis.

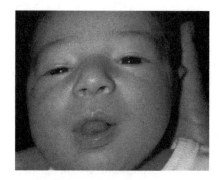

Figure 1-9
Normal symmetry.

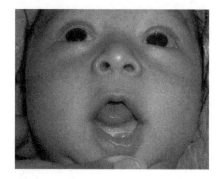

State and Level of Arousal

Infants who are transferring milk usually are alert, with open eyes and an intent facial expression. As the feeding progresses and the baby becomes sated, the fingers generally relax open, the eyes close, and the muscle tone softens. Infants who are hyperaroused may cry or be unable to inhibit rooting and move on to the next step of attachment. Most LCs have seen infants who shake their heads furiously trying to identify the nipple when it is already in the mouth. Sliding the baby's body toward mom's contralateral breast, and bringing the lower lip closer to the areolar margin (and farther from the nipple) will often allow the tongue to contact the breast and the baby to attach. Infants who are underaroused may fall asleep before attaching. Infants who find feeding threatening or stressful will show motoric, behavioral, and autonomic signs, including color changes, increased respiratory rate, tone changes, yawning, tuning out, and crying (see Chapter 10).

Respiratory Pattern

An infant's respiratory rate (RR) must be slow enough to coordinate with sucking and swallowing (see **Table 1-3**). Though most infants are not able to feed with an RR over 80, if the infant is willing to breastfeed, he or she is probably capable of doing so.

Color

Changes in skin color can reflect reduced oxygenation or stress. These are most apparent around the mouth, eyes, and nipples, and in the hands and feet. Mottling usually reflects a chilled infant. Pallor, duskiness, and cyanosis (blueness) are signs of reduced tissue oxygenation. Flushed and ruddy colorations are usually a sign of autonomic instability. A gray infant may have a cardiac problem. (See **Plates 1** and **3** for photos of cyanosis.)

Neurological Screen of the Infant

Probing the infant's reflexes reveals valuable information about the infant's neurological status. Table 1-1 on page 8 summarizes the information necessary to assess the cranial

TABLE 1-3 Respiratory Pattern	
Resting Respiratory Rates for Infants	**Breaths per Minute**
Term infant	30–40
Preterm infant	40–60
Ill infant	60–80

Source: Adapted from Hough, 1991, in Arvedson & Lefton-Greif, 1998.

nerves and reflexes the infant uses in feeding (adaptive reflexes) and airway protection (protective reflexes). An alert infant who does not exhibit adaptive behaviors may have a neurological deficit.

Oral Assessment of the Infant

A visual examination of the infant's oral structures will provide useful information regarding the structures at rest and in isolated movements. The clinician may want to also do a digital examination of the infant sucking non-nutritively to assess tongue range of motion. Sucking behavior is better assessed when fluid (from a dropper or syringe) is used during a digital suck exam. This allows evaluation of sequential tongue movements, adaptability to different flow conditions, and coordination of sucking, swallowing, and breathing. It is normal for infants to modulate sucking pressure in response to milk flow. During non-nutritive sucking, the neurotypical infant keeps increasing sucking pressure in an attempt to get milk, and will decrease sucking pressure when milk is delivered.

Tongue

A well-coordinated tongue that has full range of motion is of great importance in feeding and the oral preparatory and oral stages of swallowing. Note the tongue's appearance, any anatomical variations, and symmetry or asymmetry of movements. The clinician can observe the tongue while interacting with the infant, or may need to elicit them with a gloved finger. The following movements can be observed/elicited and any inabilities or limited abilities to perform them can be recorded as well as possible causes:

- Ability to protrude or extend tongue (during quiet alert state interactions or when the lower gum ridge is stimulated with the clinician's fingertip; see **Figure 1-10**)
- Ability to lateralize tongue (when the outer gum ridge is stroked from center to side by the clinician's digit; see **Figure 1-11**)
- Ability to elevate tongue (observe for elevation of the tongue tip to the palate if the infant cries or attempt to stimulate this action by touching the upper gum ridge with a gloved finger; see **Figure 1-12**)

Anatomical variations of the tongue. Relative tongue length may impact feeding skills. A short tongue may restrict ability to attach to the breast, and a long tongue may be held on the palate and may not develop normal coordination. Asymmetry of the tongue can be structural or can result from an underlying neurological problem, in which case the tongue deviates to the stronger side (**Figure 1-13**). A flat tongue may indicate low tone or a severe tongue-tie (**Figure 1-14**). Infants with decreased muscle tone may also protrude their tongue at rest. Preterm infants may adopt an open mouth posture with the tongue protruded in an effort to open the airway when there are respiratory issues. Tongue tip elevation in a preterm infant indicates stressed respiratory status and unreadiness to feed. (See **Plate 7** for a photo of an infant fixing the tongue to the palate.)

Figure 1-10
Normal tongue extension.

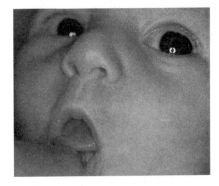

Figure 1-11
Normal lateralization.

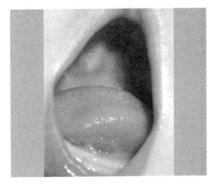

Figure 1-12
Normal elevation.

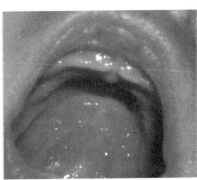

An infant with posterior tongue elevation (humping) at rest will block the oral cavity and make attachment difficult (**Figure 1-15**). A tongue with a thick, bunched configuration that distributes its muscle mass posteriorly when retracting is usually restricted by a tight lingual frenulum. Tongue retraction also prevents the tongue from grasping the breast and is a common cause of latch failure. It is often postulated that infants who have had unpleasant oral experiences will use the tongue to block access to the mouth. Although this is not proven, infants are sentient beings and deserve to be treated with respect.

Figure 1-13
Asymmetrical tongue movement due to
tongue-tie.

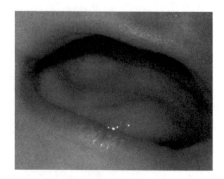

Figure 1-14
Flat tongue due to both tongue-tie and hypotonia.

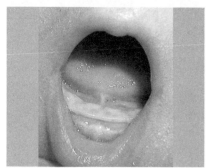

Figure 1-15
Tongue retraction and posterior elevation
(humping) due to tongue-tie.

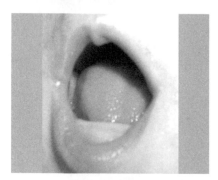

Figure 1-16
Bunched tongue due to tongue-tie. Note how the
entire length of the tongue is pulled down in
midline by the frenulum.

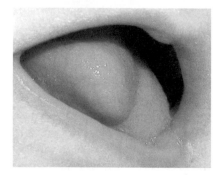

Range of motion is perhaps the most important factor in infant ability to breastfeed with tongue-tie. A thin elastic frenulum will generally impact tongue movement less than a thick, fibrous one. Elasticity of the floor of the mouth may partially compensate for a restrictive lingual frenulum. If the floor of the mouth is tight and the frenulum is short and inelastic, the infant is at risk for very poor tongue function. The extent of the lingual frenulum along the underside of the tongue is another important determinant of function, with a longer attachment generally restricting tongue elevation and extension more than a shorter one of equal thickness and elasticity.

A severely restrictive lingual frenulum will usually keep the tongue behind the gum line, especially as the mouth opens. The tongue will appear flat, or bunched into an unusual configuration (**Figure 1-16**). Touching the future tooth bearing surface of the exposed lower gum ridge triggers reflexive biting, which is normally inhibited by the presence of the tongue tip. The combination of inability to elevate the tongue for wavelike movements and the triggering of the normal phasic bite reflex causes these infants to chew at the breast.

Tremors of the tongue and/or mandible. Neurologically immature or impaired infants can exhibit tremors during activity or at rest, due to insufficient muscle activation by the brain (see Chapter 11). Tremors can also occur due to fatigue in tongue-tied infants who recruit accessory muscles and use less ergonomic compensatory sucking strategies. Tremor is a reliable sign the infant is working too hard to feed. Oral anatomy and oral motor function should be thoroughly assessed when tremors occur, and growth should be followed closely.

Lips

Lips are gently applied to the breast with the lower lip flanged completely outward and the upper neutral. A tight superior labial frenulum can produce sucking blisters on the mucosal surface of the upper lip (**Figure 1-17**). Infants with restrictive tongue attachments may use sweeping motions of the upper lip during sucking, causing a sucking blister on the vermillion border of the upper lip. Observe the lips and note any anatomical variations. Make note of any asymmetry, which is often due to nerve damage and muscle weakness that causes the lip to deviate (pull) toward the stronger side. Increased or decreased tone can occur with neurological deficits.

An indentation of the upper lip vermillion (gull wing sign), especially when paired with a paranasal bulge, can indicate the presence of an occult submucosal cleft (Stal, 1998) (**Figure 1-18**). A cleft of the lip may or may not influence the infant's ability to breastfeed, depending on the existence of a concomitant submucous cleft of the palate, and how well the mother's breast tissue fills the defect.

Nose

The nose should be symmetrical and the infant should be able to breathe at rest without flaring of the nares (nostrils). Flared nares (**Figure 1-19**) indicate increased effort of breathing. Note any congestion, discharge, sounds of effortful nasal respiration, and the presence of nasal regurgitation (**Figure 1-20**), which can indicate soft palate dysfunction.

Figure 1-17
Tight labial frenulum. Note the large blister on
the center of the upper lip.

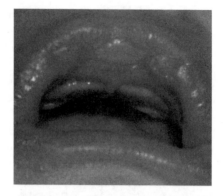

Figure 1-18
Gull wing sign and paranasal bulge in a toddler
with soft palate dysfunction.

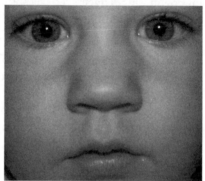

Cheeks

Full-term infants have fat pads within the buccal muscles that give them their full, rounded
appearance. Their purpose is to provide lateral stability during the first few months. Preterm
infants, depending on gestational age, may not have fully developed fat pads, and may suffer
cheek collapse during sucking that reduces their ability to create intraoral negative pressure.
Record any anatomical variations, asymmetries, or tonal differences between the cheeks.

Jaw

Tongue and jaw movements are linked and synchronized during sucking. Infants typically
have a receded jaw, but one that is unusually receded can reduce the mechanical advantage
of the jaw during sucking. Reduced alignment of the maxilla and mandible can reduce milk
transfer. It is unusual for an infant to have a protruded jaw. Asymmetry of jaw opening may
indicate congenital torticollis (Wall & Glass, 2006) (**Figure 1-21**). Other signs of torticollis include the infant's head turning to one side with a flattened occiput on that side (plagiocephaly) and the head tilting toward the opposite side with neck shortening/limited range
of movement. Additional signs include asymmetrical placement of eyes and ears, with one
eye appearing larger than the other (**Figure 1-22**). The unilateral upward tilt of the lower

Figure 1-19
Flared nostrils.

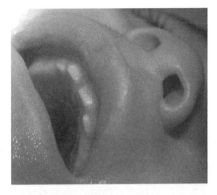

Figure 1-20
Simultaneous regurgitation from mouth and nose.

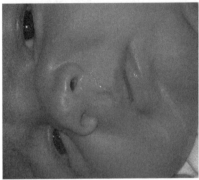

jaw and alveolar ridge in infants with torticollis contributes to feeding difficulty. These infants require referral for occupational or physical therapy.

Wide jaw excursions that disrupt the attachment or clenching where the jaw moves minimally are problematic. The disorganized infant with immature sucking abilities may have inconsistent jaw movements, arrhythmical movements, or difficulty initiating movements (**Figure 1-23**).

Hard and Soft Palates

The hard palate is continuous with the alveolar (gum) ridge in the front and the soft palate (the movable portion) posteriorly. The movement of the soft palate may be noted if a gag reflex is elicited or when the infant cries. Clefts are the most obvious deviation affecting the palates (**Figure 1-24**). Even a submucosal cleft may affect the infant's ability to produce suction and effectively breastfeed (see Chapter 8). Two strategies for better visualizing the posterior palates include digital photography and stimulation of the gag reflex at the soft palate with a cotton swab. Asymmetries in soft palate movements (just as in the tongue) can indicate a neurological deficit.

Figure 1-21
Mandibular asymmetry due to congenital muscular torticollis.

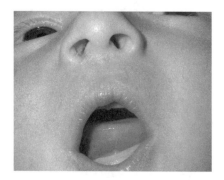

Figure 1-22
Subtle asymmetry in infant with feeding difficulties.

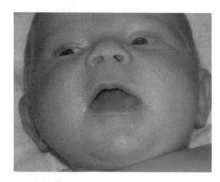

Figure 1-23
Excessive jaw excursion causes the infant to lose contact with the breast with his tongue and upper lip.

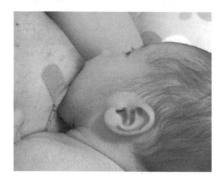

A highly arched or narrow hard palate is an indication of abnormal or restricted tongue movement (**Figures 1-25** and **1-26**). The tongue normally shapes the palate, widening it into a broad U shape. It is unclear if there is any contribution of a high palate to breastfeeding difficulty in and of itself, and in the author's (Genna's) research, narrow infant palates due to tongue-tie have spontaneously broadened in the month after frenotomy. A high narrow palate may be hypersensitive to stimulation due to lack of tongue contact in utero. The

Figure 1-24
Cleft of the soft palate.

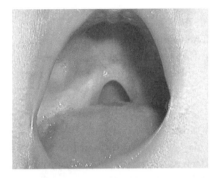

Figure 1-25
High arched, narrow palate due to tongue-tie.

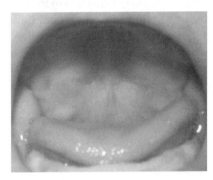

Figure 1-26
High arched, unusually shaped palate caused by a genetic deletion syndrome (Phelan-McDermid syndrome).

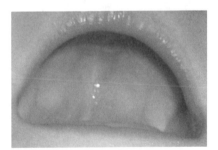

resultant hyperactive gag reflex may make the infant reluctant to accept the breast deeply into the mouth, and may interfere even more with the acceptance of firmer objects.

A preterm or ill infant whose history includes intubation or orogastric tube feedings may have a channel palate from pressure from the narrow tube. Infants who have experienced repeated invasive oral procedures may develop hypersensitivity and aversion that may influence their willingness to accept anything into their mouths.

Breast Assessment of the Mother

The focus of this text is the infant; however, breastfeeding requires a dyad. Anatomical mismatches between the mother and the infant influence the infant's feeding abilities. Look at the mother's breasts to see how well the infant's limitations may be accommodated.

Breast Characteristics

Mild breast hypoplasia may be less problematic with a vigorous infant than a challenged one. Increased intramammary spacing (over 1.5 inches) increases the index of suspicion for decreased glandular development in the breasts, as does breast asymmetry (see **Figures 1-27, 1-28, 1-29**). Persistent maternal Tanner stage 4 breasts (bulbous areolas) may improve feeding ability for some infants, and disadvantage others. Flat or inverted nipples (see **Figures 1-30, 1-31**) will be more challenging for a tongue-tied or hypotonic infant to grasp, whereas long nipples may be difficult for a child with a hyperactive gag. Wide, inelastic nipple tissue may make feeding ineffective for infants with small mouths until they grow into them. Placement of the nipple on the breast will determine what positions will be most effective for the individual dyad. Maternal motor skills and previous breastfeeding exposure and experience all contribute to the support she can offer her infant.

Compensatory Strategies

Based on the above assessments, the following techniques could be employed to enhance breastfeeding given the anatomical limitations of mother and/or baby:

- Positioning to enhance support and maximize attachment
- Nipple shield to make nipple/areola more graspable
- Reverse pressure softening (RPS) (Cotterman, 2004) or brief prepumping to soften nipple/areola area to make it more elastic
- At-breast supplementation to improve milk transfer

Breastfeeding Assessment

Tools

When sucking problems exist, pre- and postfeeding weights need to be measured in the same clothing on a sensitive digital scale designed for test-weighing. A penlight or otoscope is helpful in visualizing oral structures. A neonatal head stethoscope is helpful for cervical auscultation (listening at the neck) to assess swallowing sounds and coordination of swallowing and breathing. A digital camera or camcorder helps to preserve information for future re-evaluation, and photos or videos may be provided to the mother as teaching tools or the infant's physician as documentation. Even experienced clinicians may notice important details that were initially missed when reviewing such documentation.

Figure 1-27
Mild hypoplasia with wide intramammary space.

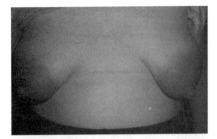

Figure 1-28
Breast asymmetry, with use of a Lact-Aid nursing trainer due to lower milk production in the smaller breast.

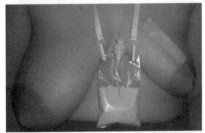

Figure 1-29
Severe breast hypoplasia.

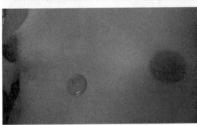

Figure 1-30
Inverted nipple.

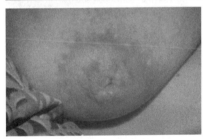

Figure 1-31
Breast engorgement flattens the nipple and makes attachment difficult.

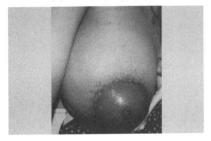

Observation

Attachment and positioning are essential to infant performance at breast. Look at infant support and alignment; complete contact between mother's body and infant's chin, chest, trunk, and abdomen; hip flexion around the mother's side; and maternal ergonomics and comfort (**Figures 1-32** and **1-33**). Note how much assistance the mother requires to provide optimal support for her infant.

Stimuli that best trigger the inborn neurobehavioral feeding program in human infants include skin-to-skin contact with the mother, chin contact with the breast, and nipple contact with the philtrum (ridge between upper lip and nose). When given these cues, a hungry infant will gape widely, extend and depress the tongue, grasp the breast and seal to it with the tongue and lips, and begin sucking.

Tongue

The infant's tongue position during approach to the breast is one of the most important factors in successful attachment: The tongue is down in the mouth over the lower gum or lip. At the point of latch the anterior portion of the tongue lifts upward to contact the breast as the tissue is drawn into the mouth. Optimal attachment is vital to filling the mouth and stabilizing the tongue so it can function as well as possible.

If the Infant Initiates Sucking Before Attaching, and Is Unable to Latch

Facilitative strategy: Ask the mother to wait until the infant stops sucking, and then begin again. Because sucking is reflexive in the first few months, the infant may persist in the pattern without assistance from the mother.

If the Tongue Tip Elevation Obstructs Attachment

When the infant is not lowering the tongue tip, try the following strategies to encourage the infant to lower it:

Facilitative strategy:
- Allow the infant more time to organize oral movements and drop the tongue to begin nuzzling and licking the breast.
- Tickling down the tongue tip with an adult finger immediately before attachment might help if the infant does not spontaneously drop the tongue.
- Fingerfeeding can be useful for habitual tongue tip elevation, by teaching the baby that food belongs on top of the tongue.
- Observe respirations to determine if the infant's rate of breathing is rapid and he or she is not inclined to feed.

Compensatory strategy:
- A silicone nipple shield may provide stronger tactile input and allow the infant to slide the tongue under the teat during the learning period.

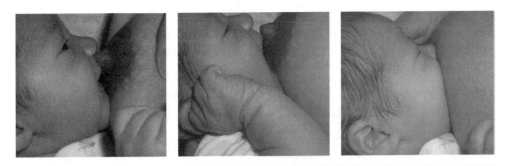

Figure 1-32 Good alignment allows the infant to self-attach to the breast.

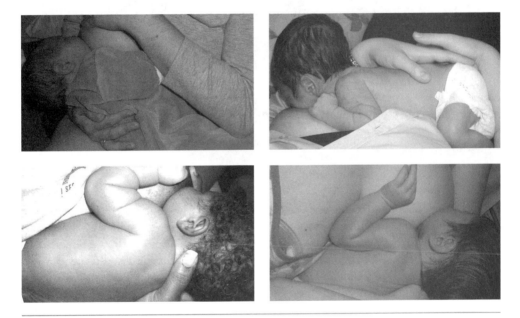

Figure 1-33 Placement of the infant where the breast naturally falls, and supporting him against the mother's body, is usually more ergonomic for the mother and gives the infant optimal stability.

Ankyloglossia (tongue-tie) usually has a negative effect on feeding; although some tongue-tied infants are able to latch and transfer milk, most are less efficient than their peers with unrestricted tongue motion (Ramsay, 2004). Others are unable to attach to breast at all (**Figure 1-34**). Some attach but fail to transfer enough milk to sustain growth and stimulate maternal supply, or cause maternal nipple or breast damage due to repetitive stress from abnormal movements of the tongue. Ask the mother about her sensations during feeding. Pinching or biting sensations may be due to excessive positive pressure from the tongue or jaws; friction (often described as feeling like sandpaper or a cat's tongue on the nipple) may be due to compensatory in-out movements of the tongue; and feeling percussive movement against the nipple may be due to excessive posterior tongue elevation (humping; see Chapter 8).

If the Tongue Is Retracted/Unable to Grasp the Breast

Facilitative strategy: Massage the anterior tongue with a fingertip until it extends over the lower gum. Finger-feed for one or more feedings.

If the Tongue Tip Is Humped/Blocking the Infant's Oral Cavity

Facilitative strategy: Massage the posterior tongue. finger-feed with counter-pressure to humped area of the tongue.

If the Tongue Tip Is Elevated, Blocking the Infant's Oral Cavity

Facilitative strategy: Tickle the tongue tip down, and calm the infant.

Lips

Hoover found that breastfeeding was pain-free if the infant's lip angle was 130 to 160 degrees (Hoover, 1996). In young infants, the angle of the lips will often be hidden by the cheeks, which contact the breast and remain rounded. The nasolabial crease should remain soft, and the upper lip should be neutral to slightly everted on the breast and should be relatively immobile during sucking. Older infants and toddlers generally do not touch the breast with their cheeks during breastfeeding. Their lip angle should be at least 130 degrees to ensure maternal comfort. See **Figure 1-35** for an example of ineffective latch and **Figure 1-36** for an example of optimal latch.

Overuse of the upper lip is associated with large sucking blisters, and is easily visible as a sweeping motion of the lip during feeding, and may be associated with in and out movement of the breast.

Facilitative strategy: Increase the depth of attachment, check for tongue-tie, and work on strengthening tongue movements.

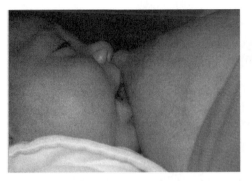
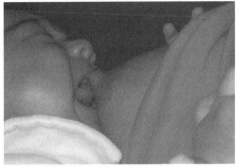

Figure 1-34 This infant with tongue-tie cries in frustration from the absence of his expected cue (tongue tip on breast), which causes his tongue to elevate and block the mouth.

Figure 1-35
An overly flanged upper lip is a sign of shallow attachment or overuse of the lip to compensate for tongue immobility. This infant's head is flexed, bringing his nose into the breast and the chin away, reducing mechanical advantage.

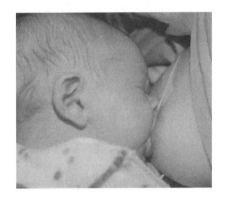

Figure 1-36
Optimal latch for a young infant. The upper lip is neutral, cheeks are rounded, head is slightly extended, chin is on the breast, and nose is free.

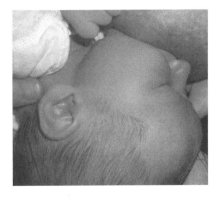

Jaw

Latching infants need to open widely in order to grasp enough breast tissue to efficiently transfer milk. Jaw movements should be smooth, with a slight pulse on the downward component and a slight pause with the jaw open as the mouth fills with milk. Grading of jaw opening and closing should be smooth. Infants displaying jerky movements, snapping at the temporomandibular joint, or sideways or circular jaw movements should be referred for speech therapy.

Cheeks

In newborns, the cheeks should press against the breast, hiding the lower lip, which is completely everted. Cheeks should remain smooth during sucking. Shallow attachment will cause a tight everted upper lip, excessive movement of the upper lip, tight nasolabial creases, and dimpling of the cheek during sucking (**Figures 1-37** and **1-38**). Dimpling of the cheek could also indicate buccinator (cheek muscle) weakness and instability, or failure of the anterior tongue to cup the breast.

Feeding at the Breast

Sucking speed is inversely proportional to milk flow. Before the milk ejection reflex (MER), the infant may suck rapidly, with two sucks per second and infrequent swallows. The sucks are shallower, with less jaw excursion than sucking after the MER. During rapid milk flow, the infant generally sucks about once per second, with a 1:1:1 suck:swallow:breathe ratio. During slower but still significant milk flow, it can be 2:1:1. A ratio of 3:1:1 is considered the break-even point, where energy expended in feeding equals calories taken in. Larger numbers of sucks between swallows generally indicate little milk transfer. However, at the end of a

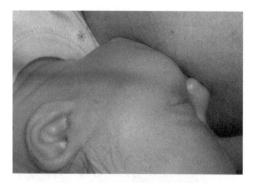

Figure 1-37 Dimpled cheek from shallow attachment. Note that the shoulders are rotated away from the mother.

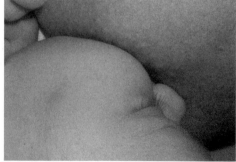

Figure 1-38 Same infant, better alignment and attachment.

normal feeding, the infant may "linger over dessert," ingesting very high fat milk, and ideally should *not* be taken off the breast. A sated infant will release the breast voluntarily. Normal sucking bursts consist of 10–20 suck:swallow:breathe triads, followed by a 3–5-second respiratory pause. Swallowing sounds are normally subtle, with a quiet "cuh" sound representing the soft palate closing off the nasopharynx to prevent milk from entering the nose. As the baby adjusts to a new milk ejection, swallowing may become slightly louder.

Observation of the infant's burst pause pattern can reveal cardiorespiratory instability—sucking bursts will be short, 3–5 sucks, and respiratory pauses prolonged. Immature infants may use a transitional sucking pattern consisting of 5–8 sucks and swallows with breathing mostly between sucking bursts (Palmer, 1993). Difficulty coordinating sucking, swallowing, and breathing can manifest as gulping, coughing, color changes, aerophagia (air swallowing), and short bursts of stridor (high-pitched breathing, in this case occurring as the vocal folds snap shut to keep milk out of the airway during a poorly timed swallow). The difficulty can stem from maternal hyperlactation and rapid milk flow, or more frequently, from infant inability to handle a normal flow. Infants with mild difficulties will usually respond to being removed from the breast or feeding in a prone or sidelying position. Infants with severe difficulties with flow may refuse to feed or become fussy during feeding.

Ineffective Sucking or Low Maternal Milk Flow?

Ask the mother to express milk for a few minutes. If several ounces are obtained, the problem is likely with the infant. If several milliliters are obtained, the problem may be with the mother or the supply may have responded to the infant's inability to drive it.

A periodontal syringe or syringe and feeding tube can be used diagnostically at the breast in such cases to see how baby suckles with a better milk flow. If the baby does well with the additional flow, supplementing at the breast preserves breastfeeding while the supply is rebuilt.

If the infant is still not capable of transferring milk, milk production will falter if expression does not occur frequently—approximately eight times per day (Hill, Aldag, Chatterton, 2001). Alternating feeding with expressed milk and brief breastfeeding for practice may be a better use of the dyad's energy.

Respiratory Pattern

Infants take breathing breaks whenever they need to in order to maintain normal blood oxygen levels, as long as the flow of milk is under their control. It was once thought that infants could swallow and breathe simultaneously, due to the anatomical proximity of the soft palate and epiglottis. Although this arrangement does help protect them from aspiration, intricate coordination is still required between swallowing and breathing, as the paths for food and air cross in the pharyngeal region. Therefore, swallowing requires a brief interruption of breathing. Breastfed infants frequently swallow after inspiration or expiration is completed, limiting the potential for aspiration.

Colostrum is viscous and present in relatively low volumes, probably allowing a training period for safer practice of this coordination. Weber et al. (1986) identified improvements in coordination of breathing and feeding in breastfed infants over the first 5 days of life.

Respiration during sucking pauses should be quiet, unlabored, and perhaps slightly more rapid than the breathing during the sucking bursts. Infants with high baseline respiratory rates or increased work of breathing might not be able to afford the respiratory pauses of frequent swallowing. They will generally use short sucking bursts and longer respiratory pauses to meet their conflicting needs for nutrition and oxygen, respectively. No attempts should be made to prod the infant. When the respiratory rate returns to baseline, the infant will begin to suckle again. This ability to self-regulate is one of the reasons that physiologic stability is greater during breastfeeding than during bottle feeding. Infants with reduced aerobic capacity generally need to be fed more frequently to make up for their longer pauses and reduced work capacity.

Signs of respiratory difficulties include:

- Rapid respiration during pauses
- Stridor or other respiratory noises (may be due to airway instability)
- Harsh and wet respiratory sounds (may be due to velopharygneal insufficiency or aspiration)
- Increased effort of breathing (retractions of the chest or in the suprasternal notch)
- Mouth breathing (nasal blockage or deviated septum) (**Figure 1-39**)
- Short sucking bursts
- Loss of milk through the lips or nose
- Apnea, bradycardia, and desaturation
- Color changes
- Panting or purring (cardiac issue causing pulmonary hypertension)

If the infant does not have the aerobic capacity to breastfeed, prompt medical assessment is warranted. Evolving cardiac issues (aortic stenosis, transposition of the great vessels) become life threatening as the ductus arteriosus closes.

Indications of Satiety

In addition to pre- and postfeeding weight, observation of infant body language will provide clues that the infant has taken sufficient milk. When sated, a young infant will release the breast, rest his or her face on mom's breast, and go to sleep (**Figure 1-40**). In addition, the hands generally relax from a fisted posture to gentle flexion of the fingers as the baby is satisfied. Older infants will let go of the breast and woo mom into interaction. During the more distractible stages of development (4–6 months) the baby may come on and off the breast, alternating eating with engaging mom's attention or paying attention to other interesting environmental happenings.

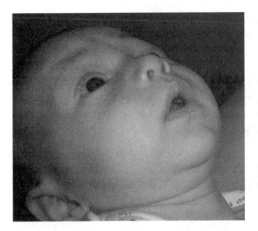

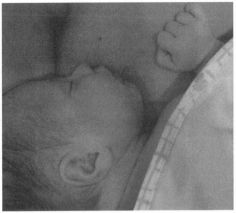

Figure 1-39 Infant with upper respiratory obstruction displays mouth breathing and worried facial expression.

Figure 1-40 Infants remove themselves from the breast when satiated.

Infants who regularly fall asleep at breast without removing themselves might not be getting sufficient milk, particularly if they protest or begin to suckle again when attempts are made to remove them or put them down.

Developing a Feeding Plan with the Mother

Careful assessment with attention to the infant's structure and functioning, the feeding skills that are present, and those that are yet to develop provides a framework for choosing interventions. The feeding plan provides compensations and facilitations to ensure the infant's present nutrition while building future feeding skills.

Basic management issues are easily solved with maternal education and practice with improved positioning and attachment. More complex feeding problems require a multi-step plan. Some possible components of the plan include:

- Referral to physicians if anatomical or neurological issues are suspected.
- Alternative feeding methods used while working toward transition to exclusive breastfeeding.
- Maintenance of milk production by pumping with a hospital-grade, metal piston-driven breast pump, at least eight times each day.
- Encouraging skin-to-skin contact and comfort sucking at the breast when the infant is not hungry to maintain interest in breastfeeding.

- Positioning and attachment techniques based on the results of evaluation.
- Determine whether oral exercises are appropriate. Specific oral exercises are selected to reduce maladaptive movements and encourage correct ones.

New procedures should be demonstrated and the parent(s) should return-demonstrate them to assure that the techniques are understood. Written instructions should be provided. Provisions for follow-up should be made. Progress can be followed by telephone with return visits when the plan needs revising or updating.

A firm background in both the individual components as well as the gestalt of normal feeding is required for lactation consultants working with infants with sucking difficulties. Providing normal cueing in the form of ideal positioning and skin-to-skin contact with the mother is the first step to promoting normal feeding. Next, compensatory and facilitative strategies are applied as probes and added to the feeding plan if effective and well tolerated by both mother and infant. If normal feeding is not restored by these interventions, the infant should be referred to a feeding team for further evaluation.

References

Arvedson, J. C., & Brodsky, L. (2002). *Pediatric swallowing and feeding: Assessment and management* (2nd ed.). Albany, NY: Singular Thomson Learning.

Arvedson, J. C., & Lefton-Greif, M. A. (1998). *Pediatric videofluoroscopic swallow studies: A professional manual with caregiver guidelines.* San Antonio, TX: Therapy Skill Builders (Harcourt).

Becker, L. E., Zhang, W., & Pereyra, P. M. (1993). Delayed maturation of the vagus nerve in sudden infant death syndrome. *Acta Neuropathologica (Berlin), 86*(6), 617–622.

Bosma, J. F. (1986). Development of feeding. *Clinical Nutrition, 5,* 210–218.

Bosma, J. F., Hepburn, L. G., Josell, S. D., & Baker, K. (1990). Ultrasound demonstration of tongue motions during suckle feeding. *Developmental Medicine and Child Neurology, 32*(3), 223–229.

Corbin-Lewis, K., Liss, J. M., & Sciortino, K. L. (2005). *Clinical anatomy and physiology of the swallowing mechanism.* Clifton Park, NY: Thompson.

Cotterman, K. J. (2004). Reverse pressure softening: A simple tool to prepare areola for easier latching during engorgement. *Journal of Human Lactation, 20*(2), 227–237.

Gomes, C. F. (2006). Surface electromyography of facial muscles during natural and artificial feeding of infants. *Journal of Pediatrics (Rio J), 82*(2), 103–109.

Gosselin, J. (2005). The Amiel-Tison neurological assessment at term: Conceptual and methodological continuity in the course of follow-up. *Mental Retardation and Developmental Disabilities Research Review, 11*(1), 34–51.

Hall, K. D. (2001). *Pediatric dysphagia resource guide.* San Diego: Singular.

Hayashi, Y., Hoashi, E., & Nara, T. (1997). Ultrasonographic analysis of sucking behavior of newborn infants: The driving force of sucking pressure. *Early Human Development, 49*(1), 33–38.

Hiiemae, K. M., & Palmer, J. B. (2003). Tongue movements in feeding and speech. *Critical Reviews in Oral Biology and Medicine, 14*(6), 413–429.

Hill, P. D., Aldag, J. C., & Chatterton, R. T. (2001). Initiation and frequency of pumping and milk production in mothers of non-nursing preterm infants. *Journal of Human Lactation, 17*(1), 9–13.

Hoover, K. (1996). Visual assessment of the baby's wide open mouth. *Journal of Human Lactation, 12*(1), 9.

Inoue, N., Sakashita, R., & Kamegai, T. (1995). Reduction of masseter muscle activity in bottle-fed babies. *Early Human Development, 42*(3), 185–193.

Iwayama, K., & Eishima, M. (1997). Neonatal sucking behaviour and its development until 14 months. *Early Human Development, 47*(1), 1–9.

Logemann, J. A. (1998). *Evaluation and treatment of swallowing disorders* (2nd ed.). Austin, TX: Pro-Ed.

Morris, S. E. (1998). *Issues in the anatomy and physiology of swallowing: Impact on the assessment and treatment of children with dysphagia.* Retrieved February 8, 2007, from: www.new-vis.com/fym/papers /p-feed10.htm

Morris, S. E., & Klein, M. D. (2000). *Prefeeding skills* (2nd ed.). San Antonio, TX: Therapy Skill Builders.

Newman, L. A. (1996). Infant swallowing and dysphagia. *Current Opinion in Otolaryngology & Head and Neck Surgery, 4,* 182–186.

Nyqvist, K. H., Rubertsson, C., Ewald, U., & Sjöden, P.-O. (1996). Development of the Preterm Infant Breastfeeding Behavior Scale (PIBBS): A study of nurse-mother agreement. *Journal of Human Lactation, 12*(3), 207–219.

Nyqvist, K. H. (2001). Early oral behaviour in preterm infants during breastfeeding: An electromyographic study. *Acta Paediatrica, 90*(6), 658–663.

Palmer, M. M. (1993). Identification and management of the transitional suck pattern in premature infants. *Journal of Perinatal and Neonatal Nursing, 7*(1), 66–75.

Palmer, M. M. (1998). A closer look at neonatal sucking. *Neonatal Network, 17*(2), 77–79.

Palmer, M. M. (January 2006). NOMAS® certification course. Raleigh, NC.

Ramsay, D. T., & Hartmann, P. E. (2005). Milk removal from the breast. *Breastfeeding Review, 13*(1), 5–7.

Ramsay, D.T., Langton, D., Jacobs, L., Gollow, I., & Simmer, K. (2004). Ultrasound imaging of the effect of frenulotomy on breastfeeding infants with ankyloglossia. In *Abstracts of the Proceedings of the 2004 ISRHML Conference.*

Ransjo-Arvidson, A. B., Matthiesen, A.-S., Lilja, G., Nissen, E., Windström, A.-M., & Uvnas-Moberg, K. (2001). Maternal analgesia during labor disturbs newborn behavior: Effects on breastfeeding, temperature, and crying. *Birth, 28*(1), 5–12.

Righard, L., & Alade, M. O. (1990). Effect of delivery room routines on success of first breast-feed. *Lancet, 336*(8723), 1105–1107.

Stal, P., Marklund, S., Thornell, L. E., De Paul, R., & Eriksson, P. O. (2003). Fibre composition of human intrinsic tongue muscles. *Cells, Tissues and Organs, 173*(3), 147–161.

Stal, S. (1998). Classic and occult submucous cleft palates: A histopathologic analysis. *The Cleft Palate—Craniofacial Journal, 35*(4), 351–358.

Stevenson, R. D., & Allaire, J. H. (1991). The development of normal feeding and swallowing. *Pediatric Clinics of North America, 38*(6), 1439–1453.

Takemoto, H. (2001). Morphological analyses of the human tongue musculature for three-dimensional modeling. *Journal of Speech Language and Hearing Research, 44*(1), 95–107.

Thoyre, S. M., Shaker, C. S., & Pridham, K. F. (2005). The early feeding skills assessment for preterm infants. *Neonatal Network, 24*(3), 7–16.

Walker, M. (2006). *Breastfeeding management for the clinician: Using the evidence.* Sudbury, MA: Jones & Bartlett.

Wall, V., & Glass, R. (2006). Mandibular asymmetry and breastfeeding problems: Experience from 11 cases. *Journal of Human Lactation, 22*(3), 328–334.

Weber, F., Woolridge, M. W., & Baum, J. D. (1986). An ultrasonographic study of the organisation of sucking and swallowing by newborn infants. *Developmental Medicine and Child Neurology, 28*(1), 19–24.

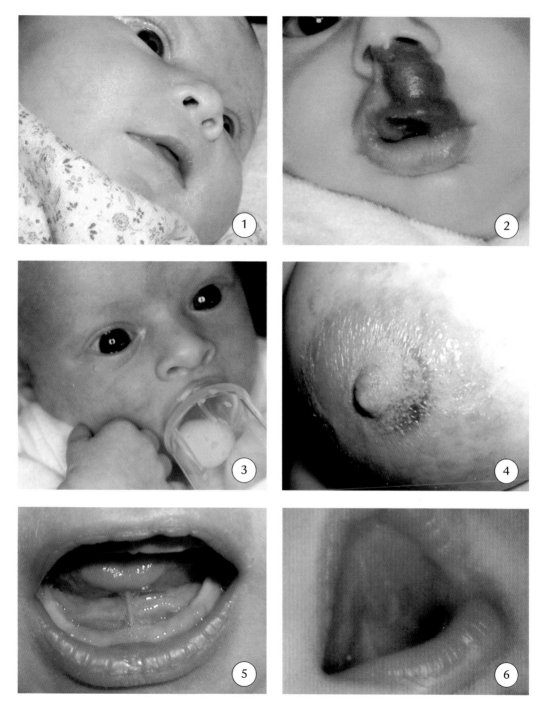

Plate 1: Circumoral and periorbital cyanosis. **Plate 2:** Ulcerated hemangioma.
Plate 3: Fixation of the orbicularis oris causes mild cyanosis around the mouth.
Plate 4: Breast injury from sliding of the tongue and jaw in a micrognathic infant.
Increased head extension changed sucking mechanics and allowed spontaneous healing.
Plate 5: Blanching of the tongue tip on attempted elevation in a severely tongue-tied infant.
Plate 6: Tongue tip elevation in an infant with a shorter than average mandible.

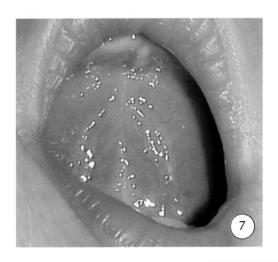

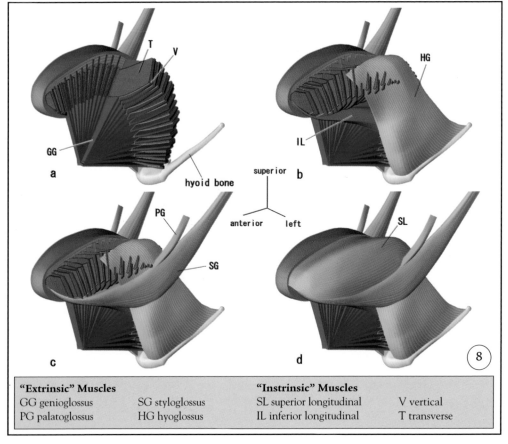

"Extrinsic" Muscles		**"Instrinsic" Muscles**	
GG genioglossus	SG styloglossus	SL superior longitudinal	V vertical
PG palatoglossus	HG hyoglossus	IL inferior longitudinal	T transverse

Plate 7: Tongue tip fixing to stabilize the airway in a micrognathic infant. Note the muscular tension in the tongue. **Plate 8:** Spatial arrangement of muscle fibers in human tongue. *Source:* Reprinted with permission from "Morphological analyses of the human tongue musculature for three-dimensional modeling," by Takemoto, H., *Journal of Speech, Language, and Hearing Research, 44,* p. 105. Copyright © 2001 by American Speech-Language Hearing Association. All rights reserved.

Chapter 2

Breastfeeding and Perinatal Neuroscience

Nils Bergman

Introduction

Breastfeeding is a brain-based behavior of the newborn, an inborn ability that is regulated by the limbic system of the brain. Newborns are born with the behavioral capability to breastfeed. However, this capability is fragile, and requires the uninterrupted presence of the mother, with specific stimuli at early critical periods working to reinforce the inborn ability. The behavior can easily be modified, modulated, or abolished. The normal innate behavior that the newborn exhibits at the breast, which develops and matures in the first day, is "breastfeeding." One of its components is "suckling" but this breastfeeding is far more; it is the total occupation of the newborn. It is the restoration of this behavior that is the objective of the authors of this book.

I will use the term *suckle* or *suckling* to refer to the somatic behavior of the infant on the breast. Accepting the word *sucking* as an activity for breastfeeding may cause confusion, and reinforces the cultural myth that bottle feeding and breastfeeding are equivalent. There is no science or research supporting the safety of bottle feeding; it simply is assumed to be normal.

Likewise, many maternity ward routines and hospital practices are not supported by scientific research or evidence-based medicine (Kroeger & Smith, 2003). Numerous assumptions concerning fetal and newborn brain development have been derived to justify our practices, rather than the other way around. Recent neuroscience has very dramatically shifted, leaving most of our practices without justification. These practices cause a host of behavioral problems in babies, not least evidenced by breastfeeding problems, and failure of newborns and infants to suckle normally.

I will summarize the main points of this new neuroscience in this chapter.

Early Developmental Mechanisms

Genes and DNA

After conception, there is a very rapid differentiation and development of the fetal brain. For the first 10–14 weeks, development is determined by heredity, by genes expressed from the DNA of the fetus. Genetic influences continue to operate beyond this time, but are modified by experience-based connection, stabilization, and myelination.

Neural Cells

The functional cell of the brain, for our purposes, is the neuron. Neurons form in the brain until 28 weeks of gestational age, and not beyond (with few exceptions). Once formed they migrate to other parts of the brain, and in the process connect to sensory organs. They are "sensitive cells," and when sensitized they trigger an action potential, or "fire." Various sensations will make various cells fire. That firing causes first "budding" and then axon formation on one end and dendrification on the other. Ongoing firing makes more branches and at the ends of branches synapses form, which when fired repeatedly result in stabilization of the synapse, or "wiring." Ultimately almost all the neurons of the brain will be connected to each other in a network. The neuroscientists term this with unusual brevity: "Cells that fire together, wire together" (Schatz, 1992).

Neuronal Plasticity

Genetic determination does continue after 14 weeks, but its importance in the development process is overtaken by two more important processes, the first of which is described in the previous section; the second can be described as "use it or lose it."

From very early in gestation, there is a parallel process of programmed cell death and elimination of redundancy, or pruning. By 40 weeks of gestational age, half the precious neurons that were formed have been lost! Some neurons undergo programmed cell death, and are dismantled and removed. A suboptimal level of stimulation results in fewer branches and poorer connections in the remaining neurons. A certain critical repetition of firing is needed to stabilize the synapse, which is then immune from elimination or removal. This process continues throughout development (McCain & Mustard, 1999).

Neuronal plasticity therefore relates to the interplay between firing and wiring of neurons, and removing those that are not used (Teicher, 2002). From 28 weeks the number of neurons is maximal, from 40 weeks the number of synapses peaks, and from then on neuronal plasticity refers to pruning and removing neurons and their synapses. (This is also called "sculpting," in that the end result comes from removing unwanted parts.) The parts of the brain that now capture the stimuli become pathways, and they may or may not myelinate, which makes them faster and more complex pathways. The end result of this process is a "hard-wired" brain. It used to be thought that the brain can regenerate and repair, as amazing recovery in function is observed in many cases. However, this is a misconception: Although a very young brain can wire new pathways with residual neural cells, this ability is rapidly lost. The brain stem (controlling breathing and heart rate, etc.) is hard wired at the time of birth. The limbic system of the brain, which controls basic autonomic functions and moods and emotions and self-control, is hard wired by the age of 3 years. The cerebral cortex (and the cerebellum) retain a small degree of neuronal plasticity into adult life, and cortical synapses continue to form as needed (McCain & Mustard, 1999).

Essentially, the genes set a process in motion that sets the scaffolding of the brain, but the final result as to what cells remain and how cells are connected has become experience determined, the result of neuronal plasticity (Teicher, 2002). This is in sharp contrast to the belief that most medical professionals have derived from their training that if brain development is genetic, then it does not matter too much if some experience along the way is poor. Although the growth in absolute brain size after birth is clearly seen, the assumption that there is addition of new neurons is false.

Developmental Competence

Throughout the developmental sequence, whether embryo, fetus, newborn, or infant, the organism is regarded from a biological perspective as "complete" for that stage (Alberts, 1994; Als et al., 1994). A fetus succeeds very well in the uterus, where its behaviors ensure well-being and development. These behaviors are actually neurobehaviors, because they are governed by the developing midbrain and limbic system. The organism is not designed to succeed outside the uterus while it is a fetus. It may seem a bit obvious, but the key principle is that each stage of development is completely dependent on being in the right place.

Developmental competence requires the successful accomplishment of the requirements of each stage, in order to be able to work toward competence at the next level. In many school systems you have to pass the current grade if you are to have the background skills to pass the next grade. Similarly, suboptimal development at any stage of the organism will impact the development trajectory in a negative way.

Throughout this development, it is the experience of the organism that drives the development. This experience translates to sensory stimuli sent to the brain, which is first and foremost a sensory organ. The fetus has extraordinary sensory discrimination. Various sensory systems come on line during the second trimester; by the beginning of the third the fetus's discrimination in terms of kinesthesia, smell, and sound are greater than at any other time in life, present and future (Graven, 2004; Philbin, 2004; Schaal, Hummel, & Soussignan, 2004). In effect, the brain "makes sense of sensations." However, the brain is secondly a social organ; the sense the brain makes of its experiences is about relationships.

Neurobehavior

The newborn's behavior arises from the limbic system, and expresses itself through three main systems: the autonomic nervous system, the hormonal system, and the somatic (or muscular) system. Although these can be studied separately, and parts of each in detail, what is essential to appreciate is that there is a program that integrates autonomic, hormonal, and somatic expression, and it is the program as a whole that achieves the required homeostasis, well-being, and development.

There are three such programs and they are mutually exclusive, meaning that the body cannot operate more than one at a time. Each will have its own set of hormones, its own autonomic wiring, and its own muscular or somatic functions (Despopoulos & Silbernagl, 1986). The analogy to computer software is apt: A computer works on a single task at a time, be it word processing, spreadsheet, or a database, though it switches back and forth so rapidly it can seem otherwise.

The *nutrition* program is the default setting. This is governed by a parasympathetic or vagal nervous system, and ensures that the body keeps balance and homeostasis, that food is digested, and that temperature is controlled. There are many hormones active in this program, including insulin and growth hormone.

The *defense* program actively and immediately switches off other programs. It is governed mainly by the sympathetic nervous system; its hormones include adrenaline and cortisol, and its somatic expression is summarized in the well-known phrase "fight or flight."

The *reproduction* program is sensitive, uses both parts of the autonomic nervous system, and has a host of hormones depending on the circumstances, including estrogen and oxytocin.

It is critically important to understand that the place or habitat determines which of these three programs will operate. Biologists use the term *habitat* for place, and habitat determines the neurobehavior of the organism. This behavior is focused on ensuring well-being through the fulfillment of basic biological needs. It is the habitat the organism occupies that provides these needs; *niche* then refers to the behaviors appropriate to the habitat (Alberts, 1994). Thus, the fetus acts successfully in the uterus to ensure balance and homeostasis, and to achieve oxygenation, warmth, nutrition, and protection. These are termed *basic biological needs*.

At birth, mammals experience a habitat transition. What is evident from biological studies is that the newborn is in control of its destiny, and that control depends entirely on being in the right habitat. Newborn rats will, without maternal assistance, move towards their mother's belly to find warmth, to suckle, and to ensure protection (Alberts, 1994). In the process, they will evoke or elicit care-giving behaviors from the mother.

Timetables

Another important factor determining brain development is time and timing. The ongoing presence of the mother is part of the essential experience for the developing organism. The sound of the mother's heartbeat gives an ongoing awareness of time (Rivkees, 2004). The mother's daily rhythms and routines imprint themselves on the developing brain. Maternal biorhythms influence the developing fetus (Browne, 2004). The infant's brain develops sleep cycling during the last trimester, with cycles lasting between 60 and 90 minutes. These become more differentiated and developed after birth, and are important for the wiring of the brain (Rivkees). Lastly, DNA and genes initiate development, and experience continues it, but there is also an underlying timetable. Timing is embedded in innate or genetic timetables, a kind of biological clock that creates a developmental agenda (McCain & Mustard, 1999). These have also been described as "brain expectations" (Schaal et al., 2004).

Critical Periods

This development agenda or timetable has "critical periods," which are defined as "windows of opportunity in early life when a child's brain is exquisitely primed to receive sensory input in order to develop more advanced neural systems" (McCain & Mustard, 1999, p. 29). The timetable primes particular parts of the brain in the specific sequence required to achieve higher levels of function and therefore structure. During such times the brain is "exquisitely susceptible to adverse factors," and these can both "positively and negatively impact the structural organization of the brain" (Schore, 2001a, p. 12). The neuroscientists have in fact identified this by studying adult brain pathology and tracing back in time; they conclude that "alterations in the functional organization of the human brain ... [is] ... correlated with the absence of early learning experiences. Social stressors are far more detrimental than nonsocial aversive stimuli" (Schore, 2001b, p. 204). The "infant's immature brain is exquisitely vulnerable to early adverse experiences, including adverse social experiences" (Schore, 2001b, p. 208).

In the study of such early experiences and critical periods, there is generally a "salient stimulus," a particular stimulation required along a specific pathway to fire and wire over a particular period (McCain & Mustard, 1999). However, "the wiring of the brain's pathways is best supported when it can integrate quality sensory input through several pathways at once, particularly during critical periods of development" (McCain & Mustard, p. 31).

Many physicians and researchers do not accept the concept of a critical period as described in animals as applying to humans. In lower order animals such periods may be extremely short and transient, and it is felt that humans develop far more slowly and therefore this does not apply. This assumption is, however, an assumption; it has not been proven. The term *sensitive period* is often more accepted.

The Critical Period of Birth

For any mammal, the transition from uterine to extra-uterine life is a critical period in more ways than one. The fetus is suddenly transposed from placental nutrition in a liquid environment to new means of nutrition in an air environment. There are critical adaptations the organism must achieve, and for many species there is a significant mortality in the process. However, from a neurological use of the term, birth is the "ultimate critical period." The events of the innate timetable have been converging to prepare for birth. From an evolutionary perspective, this was an extremely dangerous event, and there is an extremely precise series of steps and events that must be accomplished for survival. At birth, all the senses of the newborn are exquisitely primed to receive new stimuli, and the infant feels everything maximally, without filters. (Filters develop quickly, an early form of learning, as synapses are pruned.) Each of the senses will have a key role to ensure that pathways are fired, which in turn will enable subsequent higher levels of functioning.

Skin-to-Skin Contact and Smell

The salient stimuli that the newborn timetable requires at birth are mother's smell (perhaps reassuring of continuity) and skin-to-skin contact, which will provide touch, warmth, stability, and movement. The nerve fibers of smell and touch lead directly to the amygdala, the seat of emotional memory and fear conditioning (Schore, 2001a), which fires a pathway to the prefrontal-orbital tract: the first part of an efficiently wired right brain. This takes 8 weeks to hardwire optimally; the mother's continuous presence is needed to achieve the optimal pathway. However, all the senses make a package of "quality sensory input through several pathways at once" (McCain & Mustard, 1999, p. 31) that reinforce the pathway and connect the pathway to others. These stimulations will fire and wire the brain and create the first beginnings of vital pathways, which need ongoing stimulation to establish and hardwire. Clearly, there is only one place where this package exists: mother. And at birth, the baby needs the full exposure to these stimuli without filters.

Self-Attachment

All mammals at birth behave in very specific stereotyped ways, unique to their species, involving movements towards the mother and the nipple, with subsequent suckling. In many mammals this is immediately evident at birth. The human being is a mammal, and as such is no different from other mammals. Due to relative biological immaturity, the human newborn requires approximately an hour of undisturbed time (Widstrom et al., 1987) for the infant to begin suckling; it can require more time in other mammals.

The reproductive program is operative at this critical time in both mother and newborn. The salient stimuli required of the particular pathways in the critical period stimulate specific areas of the limbic system. This makes the autonomic nervous system adjust or regulate to achieve homeostasis, the required hormones are produced, and the appropriate somatic or body movements take place. It is only the latter that we can observe as "behavior," but that behavior is dependent on the autonomic and hormonal events.

Given the maternity ward routines developed in the last 100 years, this was unknown until the work of Winberg, Widstrom, Righard, and others in the late 1970s (Righard & Alade, 1990). The observed behavior is generally termed *self-attachment*. The suckling observed at the end of self-attachment can be regarded as evidence of achievement of the requirements of the particular critical period, of having "passed the grade."

It is, however, not the complete picture, which is greatly more complex. The next grade follows immediately: Neurons need repetitive firing in order to stabilize and wire into pathways. The salient stimuli should continue. After successful self-attachment, the newborn will go into a sleep cycle. The important part of the sleep cycle is "quiet sleep," and it is in this phase of the cycle that synapse connections are observed. Healthy sleep cycles occur only when the salient stimuli remain in place. Newborns will wake spontaneously after 4 to 6 hours on average. In separated newborns the postnatal sleep may be 12 hours or more. Separated infants experience chaotic sleep patterns, and may not achieve the wiring that came from the firing.

We noted earlier that the place determines behavior, stimuli activate the autonomic nervous system and the hormones, and make muscles do the right thing. The purpose of these behaviors is to ensure the basic biological needs of the organism (Alberts, 1994):

- Oxygenation
- Warmth
- Nutrition
- Protection

When these needs are met, the infant will continue to function (breastfeed), which will ensure that these needs continue to be met, which further ensures that the brain structure continues to develop, which provides for both better breastfeeding and for the ability to function at subsequently more complex levels.

It is more than this, however. For example, other critical pathways have been stimulated, which may not have been evident in observable muscular behaviors. The metabolic (autonomic and hormonal) adjustment of achieving cardiorespiratory balance and thermal regulation and other homeostasis in general requires approximately 6 hours of continued maternal-infant skin-to-skin contact after birth (Bergman, Linley, & Fawcus, 2004). Other evidence of critical period sensitivity: A single dose of glucose given to newborns at 3 hours of age had a negative impact on the breastfeeding rate at 3 months of age (Martin-Calama et al., 1997). The psycho-immune axis is activated at this early stage; skin-to-skin contact in the first day improved immunity during the first year of life (Sloan, Camacho, Rojas, & Stern, 1994; Syfrett & Anderson, 1993).

Bonding

Klaus and Kennell (1976) described major differences in maternal behavior following early continuous contact. Anderson (1975) at an early stage of this research described the mother-infant dyad as "mutual caregivers." Mammalian research shows clearly that the newborn has as great an effect on the mother as vice versa. The pair should be regarded a "single psychobiological organism" (Teicher, 2002). Mammalian research also elucidates the purpose of this critical period: It is to establish the "breastfeeding program." Mammals that are disturbed during such critical periods fail to establish breastfeeding and die. Mammalian young (and primates in particular) generally wean of their own volition. Our Western culture weans early and does not recognize the need to breastfeed for 2 years or more; our researchers would not imagine looking for such an outcome.

I personally feel, based on comparative mammalian biology and neuroscience, that the self-attachment described above results in a neurological synergistic process that equates to the mammalian term *bonding*. The brain processes involved here are at the level of the "old mammalian brain" embedded in the limbic system and the midbrain. Further, I regard this as quite distinct from attachment, which in neurological terms is related to cerebral cortical pathways, and may be uniquely human. Bonding greatly enhances the quality of attachment, but also results in long-term behavioral differences, such as increased duration of breastfeeding. These effects are determined at the level of the limbic system.

Where early contact is missing, critical period bonding will not occur, but attachment can make compensations for this. Attachment will become the key factor in sculpting the brain, and is a cerebral cortical process, rather than a limbic system process. Without the optimal limbic wiring, the attachment may not be optimal for the maternal-infant dyad. The attachment may be wholly good and optimal, but the neural pathways for breastfeeding are not cortical, they are limbic: Attachment cannot achieve prolonged breastfeeding, bonding can. Obviously cortical choices and external circumstances have major influences, which makes teasing out the relative contributions difficult!

Human beings are generally not regarded as behaving by "instinct," as in the meaning of an animal behavior over which there is no control. We are uniquely human in that we are able to make a cerebral cortical conscious choice. However, the old mammalian brain is in accord and synchrony with our biology and our well-being, and has an impeccable evolutionary track record. When cerebral choice goes against the old mammalian brain, we may be "straining mother-infant dyads beyond their limits of adaptability" (Lozoff, Brittenham, Trause, Kennell, & Klaus, 1977, p. 1), and we are likely to be doing harm.

There is ongoing debate as to how long mother and newborn should stay together after birth. The World Health Organization (WHO) and the United Nations Children's Fund (UNICEF) in the Baby-Friendly Hospital Initiative (BFHI) initially recommended 30 minutes, subsequently extended to 60 minutes. The question should in fact be the opposite: The debate should be about when separation between mother and infant should take place, if at all and ever. From a neurological point of view separation should not take place at all in the newborn period. It is purely our Western culture and entrenched hospital practices, unsupported by any kind of science or research, which assumes that separation is required or normal.

Later Developmental Mechanisms

In the first weeks of life a number of new neurological processes are important in understanding the newborn and in supporting its development and breastfeeding.

State Organization

State organization refers to the infant's ability to appropriately control the levels of sleep and arousal (Ludington-Hoe & Swinth, 1996). This is related also to sleep cycling. The organism will cycle through various states, and each state has a specific purpose, as well as specific risks. During the first 90 minutes of life the healthy undrugged newborn will be in the active awake state, and this corresponds with the critical period: a conscious and aware absorption of sensory stimuli. Thereafter regular cycling enhances development (Lehtonen & Martin, 2004); extremes of deep sleep and hard crying should be avoided (Schore, 2001b).

Attention

Als et al. (1994) identify the ability to achieve attentive control as the key agenda or achievement in the first weeks of life. The human being is above all a social being, and the ability to relate starts with this capability. This is an important achievement towards attachment.

Attachment

Mothers (and other family members) behave in very specific ways to newborns; for example, they speak in a particular kind of voice and seek out eye contact. The response from the infant creates a kind of reverberation, or a two-way game. The result is attachment. It starts on the first day, and continues in ever more complex and variable forms through the first few years of life.

> In the first months of life, attachment is the primary driving force in sculpting the brain of the infant into its final configuration (Teicher, 2002).

Through the processes in neuronal plasticity the pathways for optimal right brain development will be laid down (Schore, 2001a). Breastfeeding is the basic and fundamental activity or behavior that ensures continuity and a sense of well-being that will optimize the result of the brain sculpting. It also provides (almost by the way!) species-specific and unique nutritional requirements, designed for brain growth.

Touch and contact facilitate "the flow of affective information from the infant . . . to the mother. The language of mother and infant consists of signals produced by the autonomic nervous system of both parties" (Schore, 2001a, p. 32). A feature of human development is that the autonomic nervous system (which regulates heart rate and breathing and all homeostasis) is wired to the cranial nerves. Thus the mother's face and movements and emotional "face play" registers through the infant's cranial nerves to the autonomic and hormonal homeostasis of the baby, and vice versa (Porges, 2001).

Hence, Myron Hofer concludes from years of study:

> The mere presence of the mother not only ensures the infant's well-being, but also creates a kind of invisible hothouse in which the infant's development can unfold. This is a private realm of sensory stimulation constructed by the mother and infant from numberless exchanges of subtle clues. For a baby the environment is the mother. What seems to be a single physical function, such as grooming or nursing, is actually a kind of umbrella that covers stimuli of touch, balance, smell, hearing and vision, each with a specific effect on the infant. Through "hidden maternal regulators" a mother precisely controls every element of her infant's physiology, from its heart rate to its release of hormones, from its appetite to the intensity of its activity (Gallagher, 1992, p. 15).

The key developmental mechanism that sustains the "invisible hothouse" is the neurobehavior called suckling. This behavior is place dependent, and for the first weeks of life requires maternal-infant skin-to-skin contact.

Conclusion: The mammalian brain is designed to be sculpted into its final configuration by the effects of early experiences. These experiences are embedded in the attachment relationship.

Protest-Despair Response

In the first section of this chapter, three limbic system programs were described. Further, it is the habitat that determines which of those programs controls the body. The reproduction and nutrition programs have been described earlier in this chapter, and the habitat that elicits them is the mother's chest, or maternal-infant skin-to-skin contact. At birth and in the weeks beyond, the human organism only recognizes two habitats: mother, or other.

Separation from mother to any other habitat will immediately elicit the defense program. This has been extensively studied in animals since the 1950s (Bowlby, 1969; Harlow, 1958), and is described as "protest-despair." The organism knows its life and survival depend on the right habitat, and the first response is protest, by crying and by extensor activity. The crying is intended to alert the primary caregiver of the crisis and threat to life and health. Protest as such is not necessarily harmful, and may even be necessary for optimal development of resilience, unless it is repetitive and prolonged (Schore, 2001b). When protest does not give the desired result, despair follows. The sequence is regarded as a single neurological behavior, or program. In despair, the organism shuts down all metabolic systems for prolonged survival, conserving calories by lowering temperature and heart rate, with inhibition of crying and immobilization, feigning death.

At birth, the protest-despair behavior is easily demonstrated. In my own research, separation in the first hour of life results in a very brief protest response followed by a profound parasympathetic despair response, evidenced by slower heart rate and a drop in core temperature of 1 or 2 degrees Celsius within 5 minutes (faster than possible by evaporative and radiative cooling).

The reason for this may lie in the development stages of the autonomic nervous system (Porges, 1998). At birth, the human has only developed the first part, the unmyelinated or "primitive" vagus nerve, which provides the parasympathetic nervous system pathway to the body. In nutrition mode it governs the body's metabolism; in defense mode it shuts down metabolism completely, and causes "dissociation" or immobilization. Only at 8 weeks of age does the second part become active: the sympathetic nervous system. When activated, this is the system that produces a muscular response: the well known "fight or flight." At 6 months of age a third stage appears, the myelinated vagus. This is the part that connects to the cranial nerves and higher cerebral centers, and allows the organism to choose between immobilization or fight or flight, or complex alternatives determined by interpretation of the social relationships in the stress situation.

Therefore, any separation of the baby will invoke the defense program.

Hyperarousal Dissociation

For many years, the medical establishment regarded the human being as "exalted and unique" in nature, and no parallels on protest-despair were drawn or researched from mammal studies to the human being. This is ironic, because Harlow started his research on monkeys after observing human orphans in Germany after the Second World War.

However in the 1990s, major research on the human brain took place, in a variety of disciplines, including psychiatry and psychopathology (Schore, 2001a, 2001b). Without reference to mammalian studies, the exact parallels are reported, only using different words. Protest is called *hyperarousal,* and despair is called *dissociation.* The research shows that in hyperarousal the brain is hypermetabolic, with massive activation of the sympathetic nervous system. In dissociation, the sympathetic system remains maximal, but the parasympathetic is equally massively activated, trying to make the brain hypometabolic. This creates "chaotic biochemical alterations in the developing brain; a toxic neurochemistry..." (Schore, 2001b, p. 212). The massive firing of the stress pathways reinforces them to the point where they rapidly become exempt from elimination and so are hardwired. The result is that more adaptive and alternative pathways do not get the opportunity to develop, and the organism is left with primitive, monotonous, and simplistic responses to stress and an inefficiently regulating right brain, which impact both future psychiatric and future somatic health across the life span. Potential pathways that would have been conducive to health, waiting for stimuli in critical periods, will now atrophy, and may be removed altogether. The exact biochemical mechanisms for how this happens have been described. Schore (2001b) defines "infant mental health" as the ability to vary response to stress, and this depends on an efficiently regulated right brain. Hyperarousal-dissociation prevents the development of this ability.

Modern neuroscience also emphasizes the importance of the critical period. Absence of positive stimulation at such a time may be as harmful as the presence of a negative stimulus. In so far as negative experiences result in hardwired pathways persisting into adult life, neuroscientists conclude that adverse social experiences have worse effects than "non-social aversive stimuli" (Schore, 2001b, p. 206) such as hypoxia, intracranial bleeds, or chemicals. In the early developing brain, there are neural precursor cells able to replace damaged cells to some extent, and the long-term outcome is potentially better than that of an equivalent injury later in life. When "bad" pathways are hardwired, the good pathways are dismantled and removed, and long-term permanent problems result. Schore writes: "Neuroscience is currently exploring early beginnings of adult brain pathology ... (and showing) ... alterations in the functional organization of the human brain ... correlated with the absence of early learning experiences" (2001b, p. 204).

The fetal metabolic programming or "Barker hypothesis" (Barker, Eriksson, Forsen, & Osmond, 2002) comes from epidemiological studies of birth records followed through to adult life, and provides further support. If the uterine environment has been suboptimal in any way, this can hardwire the brainstem and limbic system in ways that will adversely impact health across the lifespan. The WHO has recognized a new pandemic dubbed

"Syndrome X" or metabolic syndrome—a combination of hypertension, obesity, and diabetes. It is possible that the early pathways for autonomic control of blood pressure and hormonal control of fat cells and glucose metabolism were laid down under stress conditions in the perinatal period. These persist, and set the future adult on a trajectory of a "thrifty" limbic regulation of metabolism that in an environment of plenty results in Syndrome X.

Practice Recommendations

What are the implications of this new knowledge? One of the primary axioms of the medical profession is *primum non nocere,* first do no harm. What we really want to do is to prevent things from going wrong in the first place. Mothers and infants should never be harmed by being separated; their bonding and attachment should be supported. The behaviors described in this chapter will then emerge, and they can be supported and encouraged according to circumstances.

When some serious circumstances should arise, and for overriding reason separation is necessary, then our knowledge of neuroscience should guide the rehabilitation of the neurobehavior of suckling, and restoration to mother or another primary caregiver should be achieved as soon as possible.

Once things have gone wrong, very specific management and skills will be needed, as described in this book. But these do require some basic fundamentals to be in place; if we want to elicit the limbic neurobehavior of breastfeeding, we must restore its habitat.

Space does not permit detailed discussion on this, but a book by Kroeger and Smith (2003) summarizes research that has been done on current maternity ward routines and makes suggestions consistent with a better understanding of modern neuroscience. Separation causes stress in mother and infant. Maternal anxiety has adverse effects, including potentially decreased milk production. But her stress is evident also to the baby, and reinforces the baby's hyperarousal-dissociation. Chapter 3 contains more information on the effect of birth interventions on infant neurobehavior.

The present reality is that most newborns experience prolonged separation. The kind of questions that need to be answered are:

- How much separation can the newborn tolerate?
- How long does it take for the newborn organism to recover from separation?

When the newborn infant is separated from the mother, autonomic and hormonal systems rapidly achieve dissociation. One hormone in particular is worthy of mention: somatostatin (Uvnas-Moberg, 1989). This hormone acts directly on the gut, and has a powerful inhibitory action on the 20 or more hormones that regulate every aspect of gut function. It also inhibits production of growth hormone. Its own direct effects are to inhibit gastrointestinal secretion, inhibit gut motility, reduce blood flow to the gut, and reduce absorption from the gut. The result of this is gastric retention, vomiting, and constipation.

Somatostatin is relatively easy to measure. It has been found that after restoration of the right habitat, it takes at least 20 and probably 30 minutes to eliminate somatostatin from the system. It is probable that other dissociation hormones will behave in the same way, but they have yet to be measured. Autonomic effects are likely to recover more quickly. The advice, therefore, would be that for any intervention or therapy, the first 30 minutes should start with doing absolutely nothing, apart from placing the baby on the mother's chest and making them both comfortable. If after 30 minutes both are sleeping, therapy should await their spontaneous awakening.

There are reports of warm baths having a positive effect on restoration. This may well enhance the quality of the restored maternal-infant environment, evoking memories in the child. This may perhaps be more effective if the infant is some weeks old and has mastered state and attentional behaviors, and therefore can engage more directly. There may be other measures that are supportive in restoring the maternal-infant connection, and foster attachment.

> "Society reaps what it sows in the way that infants and children are treated. Efforts to reduce exposure to stress and abuse in early life may have far-reaching impacts on medical and psychiatric health and may reduce aggression, suspicion and untoward stress in future generations" (Teicher, 2002).

References

Alberts, J. R. (1994). Learning as adaptation of the infant. *Acta Paediatrica,* (Suppl. 397), 77–85.

Als, H., Lawhon, G., Duffy, F. H., McAnulty, G. B., Gibes-Grossman, R., & Blickman, J. G. (1994). Individualized developmental care for the very low-birth-weight preterm infant. Medical and neurofunctional effects. *Journal of the American Medical Association, 272*(11), 853–858.

Anderson, G. C. (1975). A preliminary report: Severe respiratory distress in transitional newborn lambs with recovery following nonnutritive sucking. *Journal of Nurse Midwifery, 20*(2), 20–28.

Barker, D. J., Eriksson, J. G., Forsen, T., & Osmond, C. (2002). Fetal origins of adult disease: Strength of effects and biological basis. *International Journal of Epidemiology, 31*(6), 1235–1239.

Bergman, N. J., Linley, L. L., & Fawcus, S. R. (2004). Randomized controlled trial of skin-to-skin contact from birth versus conventional incubator for physiological stabilization in 1200- to 2199-gram newborns. *Acta Paediatrica, 93*(6), 779–785.

Bowlby, J. (1969). *Attachment and loss* (Vol. 1: Attachment). New York: Basic Books.

Browne, J. V. (2004). Early relationship environments: Physiology of skin-to-skin contact for parents and their preterm infants. *Clinics in Perinatology, 31*(2), 287–298, vii.

Despopoulos, A., & Silbernagl, S. (1986). *Color atlas of physiology* (3rd rev. enl. ed.). Stuttgart, Germany: Georg Thieme Verlag.

Gallagher, W. (1992). The motherless child. *The Sciences, 32*(July/August), 12–15.

Graven, S. N. (2004). Early neurosensory visual development of the fetus and newborn. *Clinics in Perinatology, 31*(2), 199–216, v.

Harlow, H. F. (1958). The nature of love. *American Psychologist, 13,* 673–685.

Klaus, M. H., & Kennell, J. H. (1976). *Maternal-infant bonding.* St. Louis, MO: C.V. Mosby.

Kroeger, M., & Smith, L. J. (2003). *Impact of birthing practices on breastfeeding.* Sudbury, MA: Jones & Bartlett.

Lehtonen, L., & Martin, R. J. (2004). Ontogeny of sleep and awake states in relation to breathing in preterm infants. *Seminars in Neonatology, 9*(3), 229–238.

Lozoff, B., Brittenham, G. M., Trause, M. A., Kennell, J. H., & Klaus, M. H. (1977). The mother-newborn relationship: Limits of adaptability. *Journal of Pediatrics, 91*(1), 1–12.

Ludington-Hoe, S. M., & Swinth, J. Y. (1996). Developmental aspects of kangaroo care. *Journal of Obstetric, Gynecologic, and Neonatal Nursing, 25*(8), 691–703.

Martin-Calama, J., Bunuel, J., Valero, M., et al. (1997). The effect of feeding glucose water to breast-feeding newborns on weight, body temperature, blood glucose and breastfeeding duration. *Journal of Human Lactation, 13*(3), 209–213.

McCain, M. N., & Mustard, J. F. (1999). *Reversing the real brain drain: Early years study final report.* Ontario: Ontario Children's Secretariat.

Philbin, M. K. (2004). Planning the acoustic environment of a neonatal intensive care unit. *Clinics in Perinatology, 31*(2), 331–352, viii.

Porges, S. W. (1998). Love: An emergent property of the mammalian autonomic nervous system. *Psychoneuroendocrinology, 23*(8), 837–861.

Porges, S. W. (2001). The polyvagal theory: Phylogenetic substrates of a social nervous system. *International Journal of Psychophysiology, 42*(2), 123–146.

Righard, L., & Alade, M. O. (1990). Effect of delivery room routines on success of first breast-feed. *Lancet, 336*(8723), 1105–1107.

Rivkees, S. A. (2004). Emergence and influences of circadian rhythmicity in infants. *Clinics in Perinatology, 31*(2), 217–228, v–vi.

Schaal, B., Hummel, T., & Soussignan, R. (2004). Olfaction in the fetal and premature infant: Functional status and clinical implications. *Clinics in Perinatology, 31*(2), 261–286, vii.

Schatz, C. (1992). The developing brain. *Scientific American, 267*(3), 60–67.

Schore, A. N. (2001a). Effects of a secure attachment relationship on right brain development, affect regulation, and infant mental health. *Infant Mental Health Journal, 22*(1–2), 7–66.

Schore, A. N. (2001b). The effects of early relational trauma on right brain development, affect regulation, and infant mental health. *Infant Mental Health Journal, 22*(1–2), 201–269.

Sloan, N. L., Camacho, L. W., Rojas, E. P., & Stern, C. (1994). Kangaroo mother method: Randomised controlled trial of an alternative method of care for stabilised low-birthweight infants. Maternidad Isidro Ayora Study Team. *Lancet, 344*(8925), 782–785.

Syfrett, E. B., & Anderson, G. C. (November 1993). Early and virtually continuous kangaroo care for lower-risk preterm infants: Effect on temperature, breastfeeding, supplementation and weight. American Nurses Association, paper presented at the biennial conference of the Council of Nurse Researchers, Washington, DC.

Teicher, M. (2002). Developmental neurobiology of childhood stress and trauma. *Psychiatric Clinics of North America, 25,* 397–426.

Uvnas-Moberg, K. (1989). Gastrointestinal hormones in mother and infant. *Acta Paediatrica Scandinavica, 351*(Suppl.), 88–93.

Widstrom, A. M., Ransjo-Arvidson, A. B., Christensson, K., Matthiesen, A. S., Winberg, J., & Uvnas-Moberg, K. (1987). Gastric suction in healthy newborn infants. Effects on circulation and developing feeding behaviour. *Acta Paediatrica Scandinavica, 76*(4), 566–572.

Chapter 3

Why Johnny Can't Suck: Impact of Birth Practices on Infant Suck

Linda J. Smith

Introduction

The impact of birthing practices on the breastfeeding mother-baby dyad can be clustered into several categories: infant maturity, chemical effects of drugs on the central nervous system, injuries and physical (mechanical) forces affecting oral-motor function, indirect factors such as maternal hydration affecting breast pliability, and consequences of separation that often occurs when the birth is traumatic.

The effects of medications and mechanical interventions are cumulative and synergistic. There is a paucity of research that addresses any direct relationship of birth practices to breastfeeding outcomes. Jordan et al. (2005) describe the dilemma of establishing cause and effect:

> Because "failure to breastfeed" is not recognized as a possible harmful effect of medication, there are few methodological precedents in this area. The complex, but under researched, physiological process of establishing lactation is not generally considered vulnerable to pharmacological influences. The transitory nature and "ordinariness" of "switching to bottle feeding" render the usual algorithms for identifying adverse drug reactions inadequate, inapplicable or even irrelevant. Susceptibility to bottle feeding is often regarded as determined exclusively by socio-cultural factors. The possibility of an additional dose-related impact of medication has not previously been explored in this context. (p. 931)

Professional segmentation is a major barrier to accurately evaluating breastfeeding-related outcomes of birth practices, despite the fact that "mothers and babies form an inseparable biological and social unit" (World Health Organization [WHO], 2003, p. 3). During pregnancy and breastfeeding, professional specialties tend to focus on either the mother or the baby, rarely both (Kroeger & Smith, 2004). Obstetricians and anesthesiologists rarely are involved in establishing successful breastfeeding in the early hours and days postbirth. Pediatricians are rarely involved in decisions regarding labor management. Anesthesiologists are even further removed from postbirth and pediatric outcomes than obstetricians.

Midwives in many countries provide continuity of care, but may lack in-depth education about infant suck issues. In many places, little overlap exists between prebirth and post-birth care providers, leaving the establishment of breastfeeding to fall through the cracks. Mechanisms and tools for identifying sucking problems are rare and inconsistently applied.

Induction of Labor and Infant Maturity

Induction of labor often results in an unready mother and immature baby. An immature baby is likely to exhibit an immature and disorganized suck-swallow-breathe pattern. Induction is more traumatic for the baby, is more likely to cause cranial and cerebral injuries, is likely to expose the baby to narcotic drugs, and results in poor feeding ability. The induced baby is more likely to be separated from the mother. If there is inadequate lactation support, the baby's nutrition is compromised and risks of jaundice and even kernicterus increase.

Medical reasons for induction include prolonged rupture of membranes without labor; postdates, meaning greater than 42 completed weeks of gestation; maternal hypertension; maternal health problems such as diabetes; chorioamnionitis (intrauterine infection); and intrauterine growth restriction. Elective inductions for primigravidas increase the risk of cesarean surgery by 2–4 times (American College of Obstetricians and Gynecologists [ACOG], 2002a, 2002b; Coalition for Improving Maternity Services [CIMS], 2003).

Induction of labor may be performed with drugs (e.g., oxytocin), hormones (e.g., prostaglandin in several forms), mechanical stimulation (e.g., stripping or artificial rupture of membranes), or ingested substances (e.g., castor oil). When labor is induced or augmented by drugs, uterine contractions are stronger, longer, closer together, and more painful. This results in more mechanical and chemical stress on the baby, less time for the baby to recover between contractions, more desire for chemical pain relief by the mother, and increased risk of mechanical (instrument) delivery if the labor does not start or continue on its own.

Infant maturity is one indicator or trigger of spontaneous onset of labor. Simply put, when the baby is ready for extrauterine life, labor begins on its own. If compelling medical reasons indicate a significant advantage to inducing labor artificially, then by definition the baby is unlikely to be fully mature. Elective induction of labor before 41 weeks of gestation has *not* been shown to improve outcomes for the mother or baby (Fraser et al., 1999). Immaturity itself, alone and in combination with other consequences of induction, affects the infant's ability to feed.

Artificial rupture of membranes to induce or augment labor increases the risk of intrauterine infection, which is a risk factor for cerebral palsy and a host of other consequences, and only slightly shortens labor. Induction with oxytocin increases the risk of infant jaundice and is implicated in a rising number of babies with kernicterus, or staining of the brain, causing severe neurological impairment and even death. Vinod Bhutani, MD, and colleagues studied a cluster of babies with kernicterus and found five common risk factors (American Academy of Pediatrics, 2004; Keren et al., 2005):

1. Oxytocin use to induce labor
2. Vacuum extractor use at delivery
3. Less than 38 weeks gestation
4. Large for gestational age (LGA)
5. Maternal desire to exclusively breastfeed

Exclusive breastfeeding did not cause the infants' injuries; rather, immature, injured infants were unable to effectively breastfeed and inadequate lactation support resulted in severe underfeeding of vulnerable infants. Induction of labor is sometimes done for less than compelling medical reasons, resulting in a near-term or "borderline" baby with immature or disorganized feeding abilities and a higher risk of readmission to the hospital (Boies, Chantry, Howard, & Vaucher, 2004). Some lactation professionals have reported an impression of a weaker milk ejection after a long induction. Whether that observation is valid has not been determined through research. The U.S. Food and Drug Administration (FDA) ruled that prostaglandin E1 (PgE1, misoprostol, Cytotec), commonly used to soften the cervix during induction of labor, is "contraindicated for use in pregnancy because of serious adverse effects" including torn uterus, hysterectomy, and death of mother or baby (U.S. FDA, 2005).

When a decision is made to induce labor, regardless of the reason, a cascade of interventions is triggered, which usually includes:

- Unnaturally strong, closely spaced uterine contractions that cause increased pressure on the baby's head (presenting part) and leaves less time for the infant to recover between contractions.

- Increased maternal pain, which triggers a desire/need for more chemical pain relief.

- Early and continuous epidural, resulting in maternal immobility, intravenous hydration and even overhydration, a longer and slower labor, increased maternal and infant fever because of the epidural, and reduced maternal and infant endorphins.

- High likelihood of assisted delivery by forceps or vacuum extraction devices. These devices cause infant pain, bruising, injury, and possibly disruption of CNS structures.

- Increased risk of cesarean surgery (Kaul et al., 2004).

Thus, when labor is induced, the infant is more likely to be immature, probably drugged, possibly injured, and likely to be separated from the mother at birth. Each of those factors, individually and collectively, impairs the mother-baby dyad, compromises the initiation of breastfeeding, and makes the transition into external gestation (Montagu, 1986), more challenging.

Chemicals/Drugs: Direct Effects on Sucking, Swallowing, and/or Breathing

All drugs administered to a pregnant or laboring woman reach the fetus/baby. This is not a new issue. Five decades ago, Virginia Apgar introduced a scoring system for newborn conditions to evaluate anesthetic treatment of laboring women, and urged caution on the use of labor anesthetics (Apgar, 1953). The APGAR score measures Activity (muscle tone), Pulse (heart rate), Grimace (reflex irritability), Appearance (skin color), and Respiration (breathing). However, APGAR scores do not measure the infant's feeding ability.

Drugs administered during labor appear in umbilical cord blood within a few seconds to a few minutes (Loftus, Hill, & Cohen, 1995). Labor anesthetics and narcotics are chosen for their effect on sensory nerves, with an effort to find drugs that do not affect motor nerves and with the least likely effect on the child:

> An ideal anesthetic for childbirth blocks only those nerves subserving pain, leaving all other functions intact. No current drug or technique has that degree of selectivity. Among available methods, however, a properly managed epidural anesthetic comes closest. (Caton, Frolich, & Euliano, 2002, p. S27)

Although various combinations of drugs have been studied, there appears to be no one single protocol or combination that is consistently used.

Narcotics and anesthetic drugs given by intravenous injection have long been known to depress respiratory function, thereby compromising the infant's ability to coordinate sucking, swallowing, and breathing (Nissen et al., 1995). Regardless of the route of administration, the effects on the infant are dose-related. Drugs given by epidural vs. IV require a larger absolute dose for effect. The pediatric half-life of some narcotics is far longer than the maternal half-life; therefore, the drugs continue to affect the baby long after the mother has metabolized them. For example, the pediatric half-life of bupivacaine and mepivacaine is 8.1 hours and 9 hours, respectively. Fentanyl's half-life is dose-related and can be up to 18 hours or more. Drugs are cleared via infant metabolism, taking about five half-lives for approximately 97% of the drug to clear. Sepkoski and colleagues (1992) documented the effects of bupivacaine using the Neonatal Behavioral Assessment Scale, and found that deficits in motor and orientation clusters were dose-related and persisted for 30 days. They stopped measuring the effects at 30 days, so the duration of any potential negative effects remains unclear.

There is mounting evidence that narcotics, especially those administered into the epidural space, affect the infant's neurobehavior including ability to suck, swallow, and breathe in a coordinated manner. Ransjo-Arvidson et al. (2001) documented that "several types of analgesia given to the mother during labor may interfere with the newborn's spontaneous breast-seeking and breastfeeding behaviors and increase the newborn's temperature and crying" (p. 5). Radzyminski (2005) correlated low neurobehavioral scores with poorer breastfeeding behaviors. Baumgarder, Muehl, Fischer, and Pribbenow (2003) reported that "Labor epidural anesthesia had a negative impact on breastfeeding in the first 24 hours of life even though it did not inhibit the percentage of breastfeeding attempts in the first hour" (p. 7). In other words, the babies had the *opportunity* to breastfeed but were *unable* to latch and suck.

Direct evidence that narcotics compromise breastfeeding is accumulating. Jordan et al. (2005) reported that "intrapartum fentanyl may impede establishment of breastfeeding, particularly at higher doses" (p. 927). Beilin et al. (2005) published in *Anesthesiology* that among experienced breastfeeding mothers, higher does of fentanyl were associated with stopping breastfeeding before 6 weeks.

When narcotic pain relief is administered, especially via epidural injection, other drugs are commonly used as well. Oxytocin is often administered to augment contractions and speed up labor, and has been associated with hyperbilirubinemia in the infant. Whether this is a direct effect of oxytocin or a result of an immature baby is still unclear (Davies, Gomersall, Robertson, Gray, & Turnbull, 1973). Intravenous fluids are administered to prevent supine hypotension. Overhydrated mothers may experience more breast edema, causing difficulty in breastfeeding (Cotterman, 2004). Although there is no research exploring the direct effect of IV fluids on breastfeeding, indirect adverse consequences have been documented:

- Excessive water loads in IV treated women (Cotterman, 2004; Cotton, Gonik, Spillman, & Dorman, 1984; Gonik, Cotton, Spillman, Abouleish, & Zavisca, 1985)

- Increased risk of overload with IV fluids leading to infant hypoglycemia, hyponatremia , and jaundice (Jawalekar & Marx, 1980; Lucas, Adrain, & Aynsley-Green, 1980; Ludka & Roberts, 1993; Singhi, 1988; Singhi et al., 1982, 1985)

When the mother has an epidural catheter in place her mobility is restricted, causing her to remain supine, which further retards the progress of labor and is associated with increased fetal malpresentation with resultant abnormal pressures on the infant skeleton (Lieberman, Davidson, Lee-Parritz, & Shearer, 2005). The risk of instrument use and cesarean surgery is increased (Cheng, Shaffer, & Caughey, 2006; Lieberman, 2004), and the infant is further subject to abnormal mechanical pressures and possible injury from these procedures.

Epidural drugs reduce the infant's ability to cope with pain. Epidural drugs inhibit the mother's own naturally produced beta-endorphins during labor (Goland, Wardlaw, Stark, & Frantz, 1981) and the levels of beta-endorphins in colostrum and milk (Zanardo, Nicolussi, Carlo et al., 2001; Zanardo, Nicolussi, Giacomin et al., 2001). Research shows that breastfeeding is comforting (Gray, Watt, & Blass, 2000) and breastmilk itself is analgesic (Gray, Miller, Philipp, & Blass, 2002). Therefore, the infant's ability to suck is compromised by epidural drugs; the pain-relieving components in milk are reduced; and the baby is more likely to be separated from the mother. The likely result is an infant who suffers more pain and is unable to relieve that pain through normal breastfeeding.

Physics and Forces: Mechanical Effects of Birth Practices and Procedures

Normal birth requires molding of the fetal skull with associated shifting of the four segments of the occiput, both parietal bones, and three segments of each temporal bone (Netter, 1989). The parietal bones override the basilar portion of the occiput and the two halves of the frontal bone, allowing the fetal head to "corkscrew" through the maternal pelvis (**Figure 3-1**).

The hypoglossal nerve (XII) controls tongue movement, including the patterns necessary for latch and sucking. In the infant, cranial nerve XII lies in the space between segments of the occipital bone that later fuse to form the hypoglossal canal in adults. Disruption of the occipital segments could lead to nerve entrapment of the hypoglossal nerve(s), which in turn could cause or contribute to ineffective, mispatterned, and/or disorganized contraction patterns in the tongue muscle group. During cesarean surgery, the surgeon's hands lift on the condylar segments, possibly disrupting the cranial base and altering alignment and function of the hypoglossal nerve, which could affect milk transfer (Evans, Evans, Royal, Esterman, & James, 2003).

Three cranial nerves and the jugular vein pass through the jugular foramen, which lies between the occipital segments and the temporal bones:

- Glossopharyngeal nerve (IX), with sensory fibers in the posterior palate and tongue, which, among other functions, trigger the gag response

Figure 3-1
External view of occiput at birth.

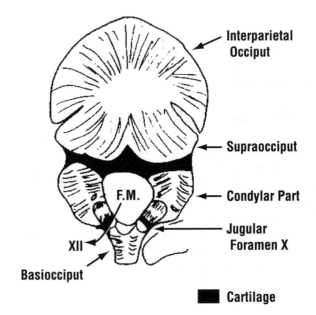

- Vagus nerve (X), with sensory fibers to the heart, lungs, trachea, bronchi, larynx, pharynx, gastrointestinal tract, and external ear and motor fibers to the larynx, heart, lungs, trachea, liver, and gastrointestinal tract

- Spinal accessory nerve (XI) innervates the trapezius and sternocleidomastoid (SCM) muscles, which stabilize the infant's head and maintain airway patency

- Jugular vein, affecting venous return and fluid balance in the cranium

Recent mechanical analysis of the forces of labor on the fetal skull confirm clinicians' observations of the effects of molding (Lapeer & Prager, 2001). After birth, sucking and crying help expand the cranial vault and allow the bones to gradually move back into alignment over the first 1–2 weeks postbirth (Ward, 2003).

Cranial asymmetry of the occipital, temporal, and/or parietal bones is often accompanied by disrupted alignment of the cranial base (Fryman, 1966). In the first 1–3 days of life, cranial asymmetry is associated with primiparity, assisted delivery, and long labor. Early posterior cranial flattening or other unusual head shapes can progress to deformational plagiocephaly (asymmetry without suture fusing). Cranial asymmetry is more common in males, twins, and on the right side, and may be associated with torticollis (shortening of the sternocleidomastoid muscle). Cephalohematoma is a well-known risk factor for posterior deformational plagiocephaly. Multiple births and uterine constraints have been reported as risk factors for plagiocephaly but not for true synostosis (premature fusion of the sutures; Peitsch, Keefer, LaBrie, & Mulliken, 2002).

Excessive pressures to the fetal head, which can be caused by uterine tetany, forceps delivery, or excessive external fundal pressure, can increase fetal intracranial pressure (Amiel-Tison, Sureau, & Shnider, 1988). Use of a vacuum extractor substantially increases the amount of force applied to the occipital segments, and entails a documented risk of complications. Hall et al. (2002) reported that "Data strongly suggests that success of breastfeeding is associated with events in the first two weeks of life, if not the first 3 to 5 days" (p. 659). Vacuum vaginal delivery was a strong predictor of early cessation of breastfeeding (Hall et al., 2002). The U.S. Food and Drug Administration published a Public Health Advisory about vacuum delivery devices in 1998, specifically warning that use of these devices increases risk for two major life-threatening complications: subgaleal hematoma (subaponeurotic hematoma) and intracranial hemorrhage (brain bleeds) (FDA, 1998).

Instrument delivery with forceps causes lateral compression of the parietal and three segments of each temporal bone. Forceps use can cause bruising and nerve damage to the sides of the infant cranium, causing the jaw to deviate to the paralyzed side when the mouth is open (Tappero & Honeyfield, 1993).

Lactation consultants have observed that babies with poor suck may have cranial, postural, or jaw asymmetry. Wall and Glass (2006) reported that of 11 babies with mandibular asymmetry and torticollis seen in a Seattle lactation clinic, "10 of the 11 mothers had complications of labor and birth, including prolonged labor in 6 cases, resulting in 1 forceps-assisted birth and 4 cesarean births" (p. 329).

More definitive research on the effect of mechanical (physical) forces of labor on the infant's ability to suck, swallow, and breathe needs to be conducted. In the meantime, our observations suggest that asymmetry in any part of the infant's body, especially the head and neck, may be one indication of nontrivial mechanical issues that contribute to poor suck.

Consequences of Separation

In utero, the baby (fetus) is literally bathed—internally and externally—in his or her mother's body, receiving food, oxygen, flavors from family foods, allergens, food preferences, oxygen, immunities unique to the family, comforting touch, random passive movement, sound, and even visual stimulation. The mother is the baby's entire environment. The baby swallows *and* breathes amniotic fluid, which matures the lungs and provides protein and tactile experiences in the gut. Some babies suck their fingers, which may be practice for coordinating suck, swallow, and breathe patterns later.

At birth, the baby's internal and external environment drastically and permanently changes. Suddenly sound and light are unmediated; the baby must coordinate sucking, swallowing, and breathing to obtain food and air, and his or her entire skin surface is bombarded by new, often harsh sensations. The skin elements with the largest representation in the sensory cortex of the brain are the hands and especially thumbs, lips, tongue, pharynx, and feet—precisely those body parts that are involved when a baby crawls to the breast and latches on after childbirth (Montagu, 1986). Now the baby is in a condition of exterogestation—maturing outside the womb (Montagu). The closer the external environment to the internal environment, the more the baby stabilizes and can turn his or her attention to growth and development. A normal baby placed in skin contact with his or her mother immediately after birth can crawl to the breast and begin breastfeeding in as little as 5 minutes or at least within the first hour or so (Bullough, Msuku, & Karonde, 1989; Righard & Alade, 1990). Immediate and sustained skin-to-skin contact is so central to establishing breastfeeding that the Baby-Friendly Hospital Initiative includes close physical contact in Step 4 and Step 7 (WHO, 2006). A 2003 Cochrane review found

> statistically significant and positive effects of early skin-to-skin contact on breastfeeding at one to three months post-birth (odds ratio 2.15); breastfeeding duration (mean weighted difference 41.99); maintenance of infant temperature in the neutral thermal range (odds ratio 12.18); infant blood glucose (mean weighted difference 11.07); (less) infant crying (odds ratio 21.89); and summary scores of maternal affectionate love touch during an observed breastfeeding within the first few days post-birth (standardized mean difference 0.73). (Anderson, Moore, Hepworth, & Bergman, 2003, p. 5)

There is no research justifying the separation of a healthy mother and baby, yet this is a very common practice. Separating babies, even for procedures as allegedly benign as weighing and measuring, disrupts the infant's sucking response (Righard & Alade, 1990, 1992). Separating the mother and baby postbirth is harmful to the mother and baby (Anderson, 1989) and painful for the infant (Jacobson & Bygdeman, 1998). Separation instantly and permanently raises stress hormones, including salivary cortisol. The separated baby experiences the trauma of hyperarousal and dissociation (protest-despair) simultaneously (Bergman, Linley, & Fawcus, 2004). Thus, separated babies are more stressed and separated mothers are more stressed. Breastfeeding is comforting for both mother and baby (Gray et al., 2000; Heinrichs, Neumann, & Ehlert, 2002).

In addition to alterations in oral motor functioning when separation occurs, separated babies cry more (Christensson et al., 1992). Crying increases risks of postbirth intracranial bleeds (Anderson, 1989). Symptoms of intracranial bleeds in term newborns include hypotonia or hypertonia, disturbed swallowing, disturbed sucking, transient apnea, and tremor or jerks (Avrahami, Amzel, Katz, Frishman, & Osviatzov, 1996).

As harmful as separation is to mother and baby individually, separation obviously impedes breastfeeding. Babies need to be physically close to their mother to breastfeed. Physical proximity, especially skin-to-skin contact, results in more episodes of breastfeeding, faster maternal response to baby's feeding cues, normal sucking patterns, thermal coregulation, immune protection for the infant, and more. Dr. Helen Ball conducted a randomized trial of infant sleep locations on a postnatal ward and concluded, "Suckling frequency in the early post-partum period is a well known predictor of successful breastfeeding initiation. Sleeping newborn babies in close proximity to their mothers (bedding-in) facilitates frequent feeding in comparison with rooming-in" (Ball, Ward Platt, Heslop, Leech, & Brown, 2006, p. 4). Safe bed-sharing facilitates maternal rest (Quillin & Glenn, 2004), infant rest and recovery (Christensson et al., 1992), and breastfeeding (McKenna & McDade, 2005). Conversely, separation stresses mothers and infants, and compromises breastfeeding.

Consequences of Other Birth-Related Practices

Suctioning an otherwise vigorous baby is associated with oral aversion, injury to the posterior oropharynx, removing normal immunologically important mucus, and failing to prevent meconium-aspiration pneumonia, even in babies born through meconium-stained amniotic fluid (Vain et al., 2004). Babies who have been suctioned and/or intubated may exhibit oral aversions, making breastfeeding difficult.

Circumcision, especially if performed without analgesia and before breastfeeding is well established, causes significant infant pain and interferes with breastfeeding and other behaviors (Anand et al., 2004; Howard, Howard, & Weitzman, 1994; Kroeger & Smith, 2004).

Radiant electronic warmers separate the infant from the mother, have inconsistent temperature regulation, expose the infant to hospital-borne pathogens, destabilize the infant (Bergman et al., 2004), and are less effective in keeping the infant warm than direct skin-to-skin contact on the mother's body. Furthermore, when a baby is in an electronic warmer, he or she is not breastfeeding.

Recovery from and Resolution of Birth-Related Infant Problems

The three most important and effective strategies to help an infant recover from birth-related insults are (1) skin-to-skin contact, (2) skin-to-skin contact, and (3) more skin-to-skin contact. Skin-to-skin contact between baby and mother does not preclude or replace treatment of any injuries. "Healthy infants should be placed and remain in direct skin-to-skin contact with their mothers immediately after delivery until the first feeding is accomplished....Delay weighing, measuring, bathing, needle-sticks, and eye prophylaxis until after the first feeding is completed" (Gartner et al., 2005, p. 5). Virtually all nonemergency procedures can be done with the baby resting on the mother's body or lying supine next to her, in her bed. Let the mother and baby get to know one another without interruption (Morrison, Ludington-Hoe, & Anderson, 2006). Staff and family should fully support the mother's cues and requests for privacy or companionship, food and drink, warmth, and so on. Nursing staff should specifically discourage anyone other than the mother (including other hospital staff) from handling, holding, feeding, or otherwise removing the baby from the mother's arms or bed. Safety should be assured for mother and baby, of course, by unobtrusive and careful observation from a short distance. Nothing should be introduced into the baby's mouth other than the mother's breast until some time after the baby's first effective breastfeed. The Baby-Friendly Hospital Initiative Steps 4, 6, 7, 8, and 9 address these strategies in detail.

The Ten Steps to Successful Breastfeeding (WHO/UNICEF, 2006)

1. Have a written breastfeeding policy that is routinely communicated to all health care staff.
2. Train all health care staff in skills necessary to implement this policy.
3. Inform all pregnant women about the benefits and management of breastfeeding.
4. Help mothers initiate breastfeeding within half an hour of birth.
5. Show mothers how to breastfeed and how to maintain lactation even if they should be separated from their infants.
6. Give newborn infants no food or drink other than breastmilk, unless medically indicated.
7. Practice rooming-in, allow mothers and infants to remain together—24 hours a day.
8. Encourage breastfeeding on demand.
9. Give no artificial teats or dummies to breastfeeding infants.
10. Foster the establishment of breastfeeding support groups and refer mother to them on discharge from hospital.

Mother and baby should remain together throughout the recovery period, even after cesarean surgery or other operative procedures. Breastfeeding should be on cue 24 hours a day. An undrugged baby kept with his or her mother may sleep deeply up to 3–4 hours after the first feed (Emde, Swedberg, & Suzuki, 1975), and then transition into and out of sleep for the next day or two with very frequent breastfeeding sessions. This is to be expected:

Up until the moment of birth, the baby received nourishment continually through the umbilical cord and intermittently by sucking and swallowing amniotic fluid. Colostrum is thick, almost gel-like, and is released in relatively small quantities that are easier to manage during the first days of coordinating sucking, swallowing, and breathing. As the mother and baby adapt to external gestation with frequent unrestricted breastfeeding, the dyad's mutual breastfeeding dance continues to improve and mature.

However, some babies are too immature, injured, drugged, and/or otherwise compromised to feed effectively. In that case, follow three rules:

1. Feed the baby.

2. Support the mother's milk supply.

3. Keep the dyad together while the baby's problems are identified and resolved.

Smith's ABC protocol may be useful (see **Figure 3-2**). The #1 rule is always "feed the baby." The #2 rule is "Try the easy solutions that do not involve equipment first." The following is a sequential, three-step strategy. Stop when the mother and baby decide that successful breastfeeding has been achieved. The goal is staying at or returning to Step 1—effective feeding directly at breast.

Step 1: Feed the Baby at the Breast (1–3 Days)

Goal: Rule out behavioral issues and minor mechanical issues. The first step is working with mother and baby together.

First, assure enough time at breast. If the baby isn't near the food, she or he can't eat! To obtain enough calories, the baby should be at breast about 140 minutes per 24 hours, or an average of about 11 minutes per hour (DeCarvalho et al., 1983). Many babies cluster feedings into 10–30-minute sessions, using one or both breasts, every 1 to 3 hours. After 6 weeks, babies may have one 4–6-hour sleep stretch per 24-hour day. Other patterns are common.

Warning signs:
- There are consistently fewer than 8 feedings per 24 hours.
- Feedings are consistently less than 5–10 minutes per breast.
- Mother removes baby from breast at a predetermined time.
- Any pacifier use.
- Mother is worried that baby "isn't getting enough milk."

What to do: Get the baby to the breast!
- Keep mother and baby in nearly constant skin-to-skin contact for 24–48 hours.
- Maximize the amount of time the baby is at breast: as continuous as possible.
- Stop all pacifier and bottle (artificial nipple) use. Pacifiers keep the baby away from the breast. All sucking should be at breast.

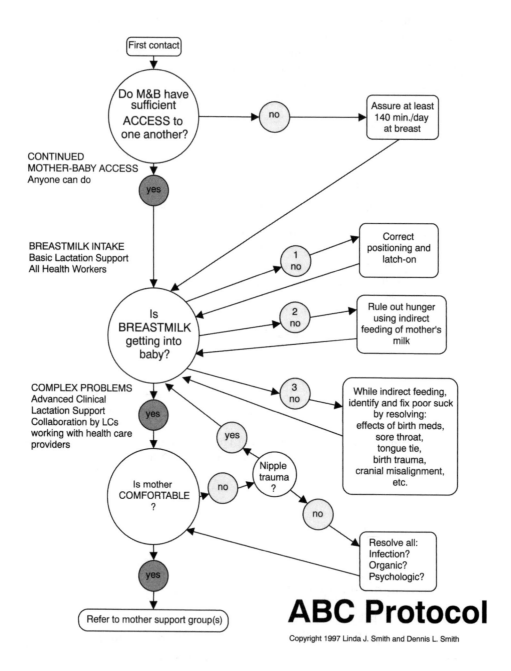

Figure 3-2   Smith's ABC protocol.

Warning: If the mother will not or cannot bring the baby to breast frequently for any reason, the baby is at immediate risk of inadequate caloric intake. Follow Rule #1: Feed the baby—with any reasonable source of nutrition, by any method—while addressing this issue. Breastfeeding is impossible without frequent breast contact. That's why it's called *breast*feeding.

Second, assure adequate milk transfer: The baby can be near food, but not actually eating. Audible swallowing should be heard for most of the feed at a rate of about one swallow per second, with pauses between bursts of swallows (Riordan, Gill-Hopple, & Angeron, 2005).

Warning signs:

- There are consistently fewer than 8 or more than 16 feedings per 24 hours.
- Feedings are *consistently* shorter than 5 minutes or longer than 30 minutes (Kent et al., 2006).
- Rapid sucking with little or no swallowing occurs most of the time.
- Baby sucks 3–4 times, falls asleep, *stays at breast,* and repeats this pattern.
- Mother's nipple is creased, cracked, flattened, or painful after feeding.
- Breast fullness does not change (soften) as a result of feeding.

What to do: Make sure milk is getting from the mother to the baby!

- Assure deep attachment (grasp) to the breast.
- Assure good alignment of the baby's body.
- Assure baby is sucking and swallowing properly.

When to go to Step #2:

- Corrected positioning *does not* result in gulping or swallowing.
- Corrected positioning *does not* eliminate nipple compression or pain.
- Baby pulls away from breast, screams, or cannot stay at breast.
- Baby does not come off breast spontaneously with obvious satiety.

Step 2: Feed the Baby Expressed Milk Indirectly (Not at the Breast; 1–3 days)

Goal: Continue to feed the baby while correcting short-term suck problems.

Because feeding at breast is not effective, working with the mother and baby separately is necessary. Poor sucking results in inadequate milk intake for the baby, and causes milk retention, engorgement, and a subsequently lowered milk supply in the mother. Hunger may cause a poor or disorganized sucking response, resulting in a self-fulfilling vicious circle. Step 2 breaks this cycle by assuring adequate calories for the baby while maintaining or increasing the mother's milk supply. The feeding method used in Step 2 should correct early interferences and/or avoid compromising future direct breastfeeding. A disorganized suck caused by hunger may resolve in 2–5 days if artificial nipples are completely avoided and sufficient calories are consumed; feeding at the breast can then begin again.

First, get milk. To increase milk supply, *remove milk from the breast more frequently and thoroughly.* Use a hospital-grade electric breast pump, preferably with a double collection kit. Hand-expression is an excellent method if the total collection time remains the same. Collect milk in a pattern similar to how a normal baby would feed: at least 140 minutes per 24 hours, or about every 2 hours during waking hours and once or twice at night. When the breasts begin to feel full, express again. At each session, collect until the milk flow ceases, or at least past one let-down response (Kent et al., 2006). If you feel milk dripping or leaking at any time, *collect immediately.*

Warning signs:

- Milk volume does not increase in 2–5 days of determined pumping/expressing.
- Nipple or breast pain occurs or continues.
- The mother is taking hormonal contraceptives.
- The mother ever had surgery on her breasts.

What does not matter:

- Mother's fluid intake, food quality, or food quantity
- Telling mother to "rest" and "relax"

Second, feed the baby with anything other than an artificial teat (nipple): The goal is to provide calories while permitting or encouraging normal wavelike tongue movements. Feed the baby with a small cup, dropper, or spoon. A nipple shield may also be effective.

In this author's professional opinion, use of a feeding tube device placed at breast is not effective in Step 2 because feeding tube devices do not remove milk from the breast. If a baby cannot get milk out of a breast filled with milk, it is unlikely she or he can get milk out of a tube placed at breast either. Research is lacking in this area.

Third, keep attempting to breastfeed the baby for comfort and practice. After giving 1–2 ounces by an alternate method, try breastfeeding. Assure meticulous latch and positioning. Breastfeeding should be comforting and is desirable even if few calories are obtained. Monitor baby's weight, stools, and urine with accurate equipment.

When to go to Step #3:

- Breastfeeding causes nipple pain, compression, soreness, or damage.
- Baby continues to be unable to attach and feed from the breast.
- Baby's suck does not improve after 2–5 days of increased calories.
- Baby has a difficult time feeding from alternate devices.

Step 3: Find Out Why the Baby Cannot Obtain Milk at the Breast

Goal: To identify and fix the cause of the underlying suck problem.

Continue to feed the baby with mother's milk, using any feeding device that accomplishes effective, nonstressful feeding. Follow the #1 rule—feed the baby. Consider *volume* of milk first, then *type* of milk, then feeding *method*. Denying a baby food to "improve the suck" is unjustified. Babies must receive adequate and appropriate caloric support while oral motor problems are solved. Help the mother maintain her milk supply in the most efficient manner. Because the baby's feeding problem has persisted despite previous strategies, further investigation is needed to identify whether this baby has a disorganized or dysfunctional suck. Disorganized and dysfunctional suck patterns are not corrected by using artificial nipples. An artificial nipple (teat) should be used only as a last resort for feeding. Many parents are at the "last resort" stage if Step 3 becomes necessary.

Step 3 includes complete and careful medical evaluation and close follow-up by the baby's primary care provider. Breastfeeding does not cause sucking problems. However, sucking problems jeopardize the baby's nutritional status. Virtually all infant problems, including poor oral motor responses, are exacerbated by inadequate nutrition. Ineffective or inappropriate feeding practices may further compromise undernourished babies with feeding problems. In nearly all situations, human milk is best even if direct feeding at the breast is not possible or must be modified. Maintaining mother's milk supply is usually the easiest part of managing Step 3 problems. The lactation consultant can continue to help the mother maintain a good milk supply and preserve and enhance whatever at-breast feeding is possible.

The reasons and remedies for suboptimal sucking responses in otherwise healthy babies are poorly studied. The underlying causes of poor sucking patterns may have long-term consequences to the baby that are unrelated to feeding. The following possibilities are areas to be explored in cooperation and collaboration with the entire healthcare team:

1. *Effects of birth medication:* Narcotic analgesia, epidural anesthesia, and general anesthesia can affect the baby's sucking and alertness for several hours to several weeks after birth.

   - *To identify:* History of birth medication.
   - *Remedy:* Time. If the baby cannot suck well, use an effective breast pump or hand-express to maintain milk supply. Feed that milk to the baby by an alternate nonteat method until the effects of the medication have worn off. There should be noticeable improvement within one week, even if total resolution takes longer. If there is no improvement, seek further evaluation.
   - *Cost:* Pump rental and patience.

2. *Sore throat from suctioning or intubation:* Vigorous suctioning or intubation may cause swelling or result in soreness in the mouth and/or throat. Some babies will react by biting, clenching their gums, and/or guarding their airway with strong tongue-tip elevation.

   - *To identify:* History of suctioning or intubation.

   - *Remedy:* Time and gentle, respectful oral experiences. A suctioned baby may not want anything in his or her mouth for a while, not even a breast. Cup feeding is usually the preferred strategy. Do not use pacifiers or artificial nipples in this situation!

   - *Cost:* Pump rental and patience.

3. *Head insult or injury during birth:* The use of forceps or vacuum extraction, prolonged pushing, excessive or persistent molding, or cephalohematoma may cause head pain and motor inhibition.

   - *To identify:* History of events during delivery and immediately postpartum.

   - *Remedy:* Time, gentle patience, and posture changes. Treat the baby as if she or he has a severe headache. Reduce sensory input by reducing noise and music, light, touch, and excessive motion. Try keeping the baby upright against a parent's bare chest, kangaroo-style, in a quiet, darkened place. These babies seem to feel and feed better when the sore side of the head or body is higher than the unaffected side. If the baby can nurse effectively in one position, use it frequently without trying for variety! Cool cloths on the baby's head may help. Some clinicians would suggest judicious use of infant pain relief medications. Cup feeding of pumped milk may be more comfortable for the baby than feeding directly at the breast.

   - *Cost:* Pump rental and patience.

4. *Oral structural problems, especially tongue-tie (ankyloglossia):* See Chapter 8 for more information about ankyloglossia.

   - *To identify:* Use a validated assessment tool. Visual clues: heart-shaped or square-tipped tongue, or tongue that cannot extend past lower lip without curling or denting. Functional clues: tongue peristalsis absent or reverse, tip cannot rise to palate, mother's nipples are creased and cracked across the tip or have unhealed wounds on the tip, or the baby cannot obtain milk at breast.

   - *Remedy:* Evaluation and treatment by a qualified healthcare professional. The professional will release the frenulum (perform a frenotomy, see Chapter 9) with sterile scissors and immediately have the baby put to breast. Frenotomy can be done within hours of the baby's birth. Maternal comfort and infant sucking effectiveness are often improved immediately, and continue to evolve over several days.

   - *Cost:* Medical/dental outpatient surgical treatment; may be covered by insurance.

5. *Misalignment of cranial bones during birth that does not spontaneously resolve in 1–2 weeks (Fryman, 1966):* This may cause pressure on cranial sensory and motor nerves as they pass through the foramina between the infant's skull bones and sutures, which in turn can affect sucking, swallowing, and digestion. The vagus nerve can also be affected.

   - *To identify:* Gagging, weak suck, abnormal tongue movements, facial asymmetry (Wall & Glass, 2006), postural asymmetry; head molding persisting past 1 week, arching, plugged tear ducts, baby cannot turn head both ways easily, palpable ridges along cranial suture lines.

   - *Remedy:* Evaluation and treatment by a doctor of osteopathy, physical therapist, cranial-sacral therapist, or other qualified provider trained in manipulative techniques on infants. These therapeutic modalities are subtle, gentle, and have produced remarkable results (Fraval, 1998; Wall & Glass, 2006). More research is needed.

   - *Cost:* Varies; may be covered by insurance.

6. *Other medical or health problems in baby:* These may include cardiac abnormalities, neurological problems, severe allergies, fungal or other mouth infections, or metabolic abnormalities. Some providers suggest that "feeding behavior is the first thing to go wrong" when a severe problem is developing in a baby. Always stay in close collaboration with the baby's primary care provider whenever Step 3 becomes necessary.

To summarize the protocol:

Step 1: Direct breastfeeding. Keep mother and baby together.

- Assure sufficient time at breast (quantity issue).
- Assure effective feeding at breast (quality issue).

Step 2: Indirect feeding of mother's own milk. Keep mother and baby together.

- Maintain or increase mother's milk supply.
- Feed the baby in a way that encourages proper tongue movements.
- Continue attempts to breastfeed directly.

Step 3: Find out why the baby cannot feed at breast. Keep mother and baby together.

- Continue indirect feeding with mother's milk while causes and remedies are investigated.
- Support the mother's milk supply, her efforts, and her motivation.
- Collaborate with other providers.

Summary

Obviously babies have to be born somehow. The best way to prevent complications arising from birth practices is to minimize the use of interventions in the first place. A normal birth usually leads to normal breastfeeding. However, complications during pregnancy, labor, and birth do occur, and properly used interventions can be life-saving for the mother and/or baby. Interventions, even appropriately used, can have a profound effect on the infant, the mother, and the course of breastfeeding. The rate at which interventions are used is the chief concern, not the interventions themselves. The World Health Organization and other health-policy bodies have published research-based data on the recommended rates of medically necessary interventions. In many places, local rates of induction, cesarean surgery, and epidural use far exceed "medically necessary" rates (CIMS, 2003).

In 2006, the WHO/UNICEF Baby-Friendly Hospital Initiative released updated, expanded, and integrated program guidelines, including an optional module on Mother-Friendly Care (WHO/UNICEF, 2006). The Mother-Friendly Module was developed with input and collaboration from the Coalition for Improving Maternity Services (CIMS). The Global Criteria for the BFHI Mother-Friendly Care Module contains these five principles:

- Encouraging women to have companions of their choice to provide continuous physical and/or emotional support during labour and birth, if desired

- Allowing women to drink and eat light foods during labour, if desired

- Encouraging women to consider the use of non-drug methods of pain relief unless analgesic or anaesthetic drugs are necessary because of complications, respecting the personal preferences of the women

- Encouraging women to walk and move about during labour, if desired, and assume positions of their choice while giving birth, unless a restriction is specifically required for a complication and the reason is explained to the mother

- Care that does not involve invasive procedures such as rupture of the membranes, episiotomies, acceleration or induction of labour, instrumental deliveries, or caesarean sections unless specifically required for a complication and the reason is explained to the mother (WHO/UNICEF, p. 36)

Lamaze International developed *Six Care Practices for Normal Birth*, each of which is fully supported by abundant research. "Lamaze International believes that the following care practices, adapted from the World Health Organization (WHO), promote, support, and protect nature's plan for birth:

1. Labor begins on its own

2. Freedom of movement throughout labor

3. Continuous labor support

4. No routine interventions

5. Non-supine (e.g., upright or side-lying) positions for birth

6. No separation of mother and baby after birth with unlimited opportunity for breastfeeding" (Lamaze International, 2006)

Regardless of what happens during childbirth, lactation consultants (LCs) have a key role in helping mothers and babies establish breastfeeding. LCs are trained and skilled in observing, assisting, and monitoring the mother-baby dyad as they move along the continuum from internal gestation to exterogestation. Lactation consultants play an important role in documenting and bearing witness to the mother and baby outcomes that may be affected by birth interventions, and in aiding the mother-baby dyad to overcome early and/or negative consequences of birth practices.

References

American Academy of Pediatrics, Subcommittee on Hyperbilirubin. (2004). Management of hyperbilirubinemia in the newborn infant 35 or more weeks of gestation (Clinical Practice Guideline). *Pediatrics, 114*(1), 297–316.

American College of Obstetricians and Gynecologists (ACOG). (2002a). *ACOG news release: Cesarean delivery more likely with labor induction of a large baby.* Washington, DC: Author.

American College of Obstetricians and Gynecologists (ACOG). (2002b). *ACOG news release: Commentary—Nonmedical indications help fuel rise in induction rate.* Washington, DC: Author.

Amiel-Tison, C., Sureau, C., & Shnider, S. M. (1988). Cerebral handicap in full-term neonates related to the mechanical forces of labor. *Bailliere's Clinical Obstetrics and Gynaecology, 2*(1), 145–165.

Anand, K. J., Runeson, B., & Jacobson, B. (2004). Gastric suction at birth associated with long-term risk for functional intestinal disorders in later life. *Journal of Pediatrics, 144*(4), 449–454.

Anderson, G. C. (1989). Risk in mother-infant separation postbirth. *Image: Journal of Nursing Scholarship, 21*(4), 196–199.

Anderson, G. C., Moore, E., Hepworth, J., & Bergman, N. (2003). Early skin-to-skin contact for mothers and their healthy newborn infants. *Cochrane Database of Systematic Reviews, 2,* CD003519.

Apgar, V. (1953). A proposal for a new method of evaluation of the newborn infant. *Current Researches in Anesthesia & Analgesia, 32*(4), 260–267.

Avrahami, E., Amzel, S., Katz, R., Frishman, E., & Osviatzov, J. (1996). CT demonstration of intracranial bleeding in term newborns with mild clinical symptoms. *Clinical Radiology, 51,* 31–34.

Ball, H. L., Ward Platt, M. P., Heslop, E., Leech, S. J., & Brown, K. A. (2006). Randomised trial of infant sleep location on the postnatal ward. *Archives of Disease in Childhood, 91*(8), 1005–1010.

Baumgarder, D. J., Muehl, P., Fischer, M., & Pribbenow, B. (2003). Effect of labor epidural anesthesia on breast-feeding of healthy full-term newborns delivered vaginally. *Journal of the American Board of Family Practice, 16*(1), 7–13.

Beilin, Y., Bodian, C. A., Weiser, J., Hossain, S., Ittamar, A., & Feierman, D. (2005). Effect of labor epidural analgesia with and without fentanyl on infant breast-feeding: A prospective, randomized, double-blind study. *Anesthesiology, 103*(6), 1211–1217.

Bergman, N. J., Linley, L. L., & Fawcus, S. R. (2004). Randomized controlled trial of skin-to-skin contact from birth versus conventional incubator for physiological stabilization in 1200- to 2199-gram newborns. *Acta Paediatrica, 93*(6), 779–785.

Boies, E., Chantry, C. J., Howard, C. R., & Vaucher, Y. (2004). *Clinical protocol #10: Breastfeeding the near-term infant (35 to 37 weeks gestation).* New Rochelle, NY: Academy of Breastfeeding Medicine.

Bullough, C. H., Msuku, R. S., & Karonde, L. (1989). Early suckling and postpartum haemorrhage: Controlled trial in deliveries by traditional birth attendants. *Lancet, 2*(8662), 522–525.

Caton, D., Frolich, M. A., & Euliano, T. Y. (2002). Anesthesia for childbirth: Controversy and change. *American Journal of Obstetrics and Gynecology, 186*(5 Suppl.), S25–S30.

Cheng, Y. W., Shaffer, B. L., & Caughey, A. B. (2006). Associated factors and outcomes of persistent occiput posterior position: A retrospective cohort study from 1976 to 2001. *Journal of Maternal-Fetal & Neonatal Medicine, 19*(9), 563–568.

Christensson, K., Siles, C., Moreno, L., Belaustequi, A., De La Fuente, P., Lagercrantz, H., et al. (1992). Temperature, metabolic adaptation and crying in healthy full-term newborns cared for skin-to-skin or in a cot. *Acta Paediatrica, 81,* 488–493.

Coalition for Improving Maternity Services. (2003). *Problems and hazards of induction of labor: A CIMS fact sheet.* Ponte Vedra Beach, FL: Coalition for Improving Maternity Services. Retrieved April 9, 2007, from: http://motherfriendly.org/Downloads/induct-fact-sheet.pdf

Cotterman, K. J. (2004). Reverse pressure softening: A simple tool to prepare areola for easier latching during engorgement. *Journal of Human Lactation, 20*(2), 227–237.

Cotton, D. B., Gonik, B., Spillman, T., & Dorman, K. F. (1984). Intrapartum to postpartum changes in colloid osmotic pressure. *American Journal of Obstetrics and Gynecology, 149*(2), 174–177.

Davies, D. P., Gomersall, R., Robertson, R., Gray, O. P., & Turnbull, A. C. (1973). Neonatal jaundice and maternal oxytocin infusion. *British Medical Journal, 3*(5878), 476–477.

DeCarvalho, M., Robertson, S., Friedman, A., & Klaus, M. (1983). Effect of frequent breastfeeding on early milk production and infant weight gain. *Pediatrics, 72*(3), 307–311, .

Emde, R. N., Swedberg, J., & Suzuki, B. (1975). Human wakefulness and biological rhythms after birth. *Archives of General Psychiatry, 32*(6), 780–783.

Evans, K. C., Evans, R. G., Royal, R., Esterman, A. J., & James, S. L. (2003). Effect of caesarean section on breast milk transfer to the normal term newborn over the first week of life. *Archives of Disease in Childhood (Fetal and Neonatal Edition), 88*(5), F380–F382.

Fraser, W. D., Turcot, L., Krauss I., & Brisson-Carrol, G. (1999). Amniotomy for shortening spontaneous labor. *Cochrane Database of Syntematic Reviews, 4,* CD000015.

Fraval, M. P. R. (1998). A pilot study: Osteopathic treatment of infants with a sucking dysfunction. *Journal of the American Academy of Osteopathy, 8*(2), 25–33.

Fryman, V. M. (1966). Relation of disturbances of craniosacral mechanism to symptomatology of the newborn: Study of 1250 infants. *Journal of the American Osteopathic Association, 65,* 1059–1075.

Gartner, L. M., Morton, J., Lawrence, R. A., Naylor, A. J., O'Hare, D., Schanler, R. J., et al. (2005). Breastfeeding and the use of human milk. *Pediatrics, 115*(2), 496–506.

Goland, R. S., Wardlaw, S. L., Stark, R. I., & Frantz, A. G. (1981). Human plasma beta-endorphin during pregnancy, labor, and delivery. *Journal of Clinical Endocrinology and Metabolism, 52*(1), 74–78.

Gonik, B., Cotton, D., Spillman, T., Abouleish, E., & Zavisca, F. (1985). Peripartum colloid osmotic pressure changes: Effects of controlled fluid management. *American Journal of Obstetrics and Gynecology, 151*(6), 812–815.

Gray, L., Miller, L. W., Philipp, B. L., & Blass, E. M. (2002). Breastfeeding is analgesic in healthy newborns. *Pediatrics, 109*(4), 590–593.

Gray, L., Watt, L., & Blass, E. M. (2000). Skin-to-skin contact is analgesic in healthy newborns. *Pediatrics, 105*(1), e14.

Hall, R. T., Mercer, A. M., Teasley, S. L., McPherson, D. M., Simon, S. D., Sanots, S. R., et al. (2002). A breastfeeding assessment score to evaluate the risk for cessation of breastfeeding by 7 to 10 days of age. *Journal of Pediatrics, 141,* 659–664.

Heinrichs, M., Neumann, I., & Ehlert, U. (2002). Lactation and stress: Protective effects of breastfeeding in humans. *Stress, 5*(3), 195–203.

Howard, C. R., Howard, F. M., & Weitzman, M. L. (1994). Acetaminophen analgesia in neonatal circumcision: The effect on pain. *Pediatrics, 93*(4), 641–646.

Jacobson, B., & Bygdeman, M. (1998). Obstetric care and proneness of offspring to suicide as adults: Case-control study. *British Medical Journal, 317*(7169), 1346–1349.

Jawalekar, S., & Marx, G. F. (1980). Effect of IV fluids on maternal and fetal blood glucose. *Anesthesiology, 53*(3), 311S.

Jordan, S., Emery, S., Bradshaw, C., Watkins, A., & Friswell, W. (2005). The impact of intrapartum analgesia on infant feeding. *BJOG: An International Journal of Obstetrics and Gynecology, 112*(7), 927–934.

Kaul, B., Vallejo, M. C., Ramanathan, S., Mandell, G., Phelps, A. L., & Daftary, A. R. (2004). Induction of labor with oxytocin increases cesarean section rate as compared with oxytocin for augmentation of spontaneous labor in nulliparous parturients controlled for lumbar epidural analgesia. *Journal of Clinical Anesthesia, 16*(6), 411–414.

Kent, J. C., Mitoulas, L. R., Cregan, M. D., Ramsay, D. T., Doherty, D. A., & Hartmann, P. E. (2006). Volume and frequency of breastfeedings and fat content of breast milk throughout the day. *Pediatrics, 117*(3), e387–e395.

Keren, R., Bhutani, V. K., Luan, X., Nihtianova, S., Cnaan, A., & Schwartz, J. S. (2005). Identifying newborns at risk of significant hyperbilirubinaemia: A comparison of two recommended approaches. *Archives of Disease in Childhood, 90*(4), 415–421.

Kroeger, M., & Smith, L. J. (2004). *Impact of birthing practices on breastfeeding: Protecting the mother and baby continuum.* Sudbury, MA: Jones & Bartlett.

Lapeer, R. J., Prager, R. W. (2001). Fetal head moulding: finite element analysis of a fetal skull subjected to uterine pressures during the first stage of labour. *Journal of Biomechanics, 34*(9), 1125–1133.

Lamaze International. (2006). *The Lamaze Institute for Normal Birth.* Retrieved April 9, 2007, from: www.lamaze.org/institute

Lieberman, E. (2004). Epidemiology of epidural analgesia and cesarean delivery. *Clinical Obstetrics and Gynecology, 47*(2), 317–331.

Lieberman, E., Davidson, K., Lee-Parritz, A., & Shearer, E. (2005). Changes in fetal position during labor and their association with epidural analgesia. *Obstetrics and Gynecology, 105*(5 Pt. 1), 974–982.

Loftus, J. R., Hill, H., & Cohen, S. E. (1995). Placental transfer and neonatal effects of epidural sufentanil and fentanyl administered with bupivacaine during labor. *Anesthesiology, 83*(2), 300–308.

Lucas, A., Adrain, T. E., & Aynsley-Green, A. (1980). Iatrogenic hyperinsulinism at birth. *Lancet, 1*(8160), 144–145.

Ludka, L. M., & Roberts, C. C. (1993). Eating and drinking in labor: A literature review. *Journal of Nurse-Midwifery, 38*(4), 199–201.

McKenna, J. J., & McDade, T. (2005). Why babies should never sleep alone: A review of the co-sleeping controversy in relation to SIDS, bedsharing and breast feeding. *Paediatric Respiratory Reviews, 6*(2), 134–152.

Montagu, A. (1986). *Touching: The human significance of the skin* (3rd ed.). New York: Harper & Row.

Morrison, B., Ludington-Hoe, S., & Anderson, G. C. (2006). Interruptions to breastfeeding dyads on postpartum day 1 in a university hospital. *Journal of Obstetric, Gynecologic, & Neonatal Nursing, 35*(6), 709–716.

Netter, F. H. (1989). *Atlas of human anatomy.* Summit, NJ: CIBA-Geigy Corporation.

Nissen, E., Lilja, G., Matthiesen, A. S., Ransjo-Arvidsson, A. B., Uvnas-Moberg, K., & Widstrom, A. M. (1995). Effects of maternal pethidine on infants' developing breast feeding behaviour. *Acta Paediatrica, 84*(2), 140–145.

Peitsch, W. K., Keefer, C. H., LaBrie, R. A., & Mulliken, J. B. (2002). Incidence of cranial asymmetry in healthy newborns. *Pediatrics, 110*(6).

Quillin, S. I., & Glenn, L. L. (2004). Interaction between feeding method and co-sleeping on maternal-newborn sleep. *Journal of Obstetric, Gynecologic, and Neonatal Nursing, 33*(5), 580–588.

Radzyminski, S. (2005). Neurobehavioral functioning and breastfeeding behavior in the newborn. *Journal of Obstetric, Gynecologic, and Neonatal Nursing, 34*(3), 335–341.

Ransjo-Arvidson, A. B., Matthiesen, A. S., Lilja, G., Nissen, E., Widstrom, A. M., & Uvnas-Moberg, K. (2001). Maternal analgesia during labor disturbs newborn behavior: Effects on breastfeeding, temperature, and crying. *Birth, 28*(1), 5–12.

Righard, L., & Alade, M. O. (1990). Effect of delivery room routines on success of first breast-feed. *Lancet, 336*(8723), 1105–1107.

Righard, L., & Alade, M. O. (1992). Sucking technique and its effect on success of breastfeeding. *Birth, 19*(4), 185–189.

Riordan, J., Gill-Hopple, K., & Angeron, J. (2005). Indicators of effective breastfeeding and estimates of breast milk intake. *Journal of Human Lactation, 21*(4), 406–412.

Sepkoski, C. M., Lester, B. M., Ostheimer, G. W., & Brazelton, T. B. (1992). The effects of maternal epidural anesthesia on neonatal behavior during the first month. *Developmental Medicine and Child Neurology, 34*(12), 1072–1080.

Singhi, S. (1988). Effect of maternal intrapartum glucose therapy on neonatal blood glucose levels and neurobehavioral status of hypoglycemia term newborn infants. *Journal of Perinatal Medicine, 16*, 217–224.

Singhi, S., Chookang, E., Hall, J., & Kalghatgi, S. (1985). Iatrogenic neonatal and maternal hyponatremia following oxytocin and aqueous glucose infusion during labor. *British Journal of Gynecology, 92*, 356–363.

Singhi, S., Kang, E. C., & Hall, J. (1982). Hazards of maternal hydration with 5% dextrose. *Lancet, 2*(8293), 335–336.

Tappero, E. P., & Honeyfield, M. E. (1993). *Physical assessment of the newborn.* Petaluma, CA: NICULink.

U.S. Food and Drug Administration. (May 2005). *Misoprostol (marketed as Cytotec).* Retrieved April 9, 2007, from: www.fda.gov/cder/drug/InfoSheets/patient/MisoprostolPIS.pdf

U.S. Food and Drug Administration. (1998). *Public health advisory: Need for caution when using vacuum assisted delivery devices.* Retrieved April 9, 2007, from: www.fda.gov/cdrh/feta1598.html

Vain, N. E., Szyld, E. G., Prudent, L. M., Wiswell, T. E., Aguilar, A. M., & Vivas, N. I. (2004). Oropharyngeal and nasopharyngeal suctioning of meconium-stained neonates before delivery of their shoulders: Multicentre, randomised controlled trial. *Lancet, 364*(9434), 597–602.

Wall, V., & Glass, R. (2006). Mandibular asymmetry and breastfeeding problems: Experience from 11 cases. *Journal of Human Lactation, 22*(3), 328–334.

Ward, R. C. (Ed.). (2003). *Foundations for osteopathic medicine* (2nd ed.). Philadelphia: Lippincott Williams and Wilkins.

World Health Organization, & United Nations Children's Fund. (2003). *Global strategy for infant and young child feeding.* Geneva: World Health Organization.

World Health Organization, & United Nations Children's Fund. (2006). *WHO/UNICEF baby-friendly hospital initiative: Revised, updated and expanded for integrated care.* Geneva: World Health Organization.

Zanardo, V., Nicolussi, S., Carlo, G., Marzari, F., Faggian, D., Favaro, F., et al. (2001). Beta endorphin concentrations in human milk. *Journal of Pediatric Gastroenterology and Nutrition, 33*(2), 160–164.

Zanardo, V., Nicolussi, S., Giacomin, C., Faggian, D., Favaro, F., & Plebani, M. (2001). Labor pain effects on colostral milk: Beta-endorphin concentrations of lactating mothers. *Biology of the Neonate, 79*(2), 87–90.

Chapter 4

How Infants Learn to Feed: A Neurobehavioral Model

Christina M. Smillie

When a healthy hungry human infant is with his mother, whether on her abdomen, in her arms, on her chest, or up on her shoulder, the infant will begin to make certain predictable movements, bobbing his head, "pecking" with his open mouth, moving his head and neck, flexing his arms and legs, squirming, and attempting to propel himself in one direction or another toward the breast.

This behavior has many variants, but it is a behavior we have all seen, as parents or professionals, in newborns only a half hour old, in infants days and weeks and months old, and even in babies of a year or more. We see it in experienced breastfed infants, in newborns who have never been at breast, and even in those unfortunate infants who have had only trouble at the breast, and who will cry and fret as soon as they reach the breast. We even see this pecking and twisting behavior in older artificially fed infants, completely inexperienced with the breast, when hungry and in their mother's or father's arms.

However, we do not see this breast-seeking behavior in deeply sleeping babies, nor in frantically crying babies. The full-blown behavioral sequence of bobbing and pecking and twisting is seen only in alert and hungry babies, and, occasionally, in more muted form, in mildly sleepy but mildly hungry infants.

Such behaviors are often termed "rooting" responses or "feeding cues." An inexperienced new mother, confused by her newborn's bobbing behavior, might ask, "What is he doing?" but most mothers appear to quickly learn to recognize this behavior at least as a sign of hunger.

And some mothers, confident in their infant's competence, will even explain, "He's trying to get to the breast."

Those mothers are right, of course. These behaviors are not mere reflex responses or even simply signs of hunger, they are full-fledged and purposeful feeding behaviors, which, if recognized and not thwarted, can initiate a cascade of behaviors that not only take the baby to the breast, but allow him to find the nipple and begin suckling. If his mother responds to his pecking and twisting, and supports rather than restrains his movement, even the naïve and inexperienced infant will then bob, bounce, gently fall, or throw his body down toward the breast. Once there, under a variety of specific facilitating circumstances that I will describe later in this chapter, the infant then has the opportunity to initiate a feed, reaching his wide open mouth over the nipple to orally grasp the breast, and begin to suckle.

However, western culture has not prepared either mothers or professionals to expect such infant competence. On the contrary, the newborn is usually understood to be quite incompetent, his behavior restricted by unpredictable and intrusive reflex responses, insatiable drives, and neurological disorganization.

From this viewpoint, if the infant begins, apparently randomly, to peck and squirm, his mother will restrain her infant, protect the head and neck, and interfere with his movement. Without an expectation of competence, she will not see what her infant is trying to do.

It is the expectation of incompetence in the human infant that has kept us from seeing this ordinary mammalian behavior, a behavior consistent with what we know about other mammalian infants, and the evolutionary roots of adaptive animal behavior.

Innate Mammalian Newborn Feeding Behaviors

Biologists have long recognized that mammalian behavior is both genetically scripted and environmentally adaptive. The human newborn, like all mammalian infants, is a biological organism uniquely adapted to the developmentally specific environmental habitat for which evolutionary forces have prepared him—the interactive environment of his mother's care.

This evolutionary preparation includes a rich repertoire of innate physiologic and neurobehavioral responses that allow the infant to adapt to, interact with, learn from, and even alter his environment, to meet the infant's primary tasks of survival and growth. This is discussed in more detail in Chapter 2.

Innate Infant Feeding Behaviors in Nonhuman Mammals

From species to species, the immediate postnatal behaviors of all mammalian newborns are remarkably similar: After a short period of recovery, the newborn of each species, using a series of neurosensory cues to guide it, searches for and independently finds its mother's teat, grasps it with its mouth, and initiates feeding. A tiny kitten, eyes still sealed closed, nuzzles in, finds a teat, and begins to feed. The still wet fawn struggles to its feet, reaches up to find a soft hairless area, follows its nose, finds a teat, and begins feeding (Wiessinger, personal communication, 2003). The baby rat twists to turn itself over so that it can crawl along its mother's underside, probes and scans to find the nipple, grasps it, attaches, and begins to suckle (Eilam & Smotherman, 1998). The tiny Australian marsupial, the Tamar wallaby, after just a month's gestation, looking more embryonic than fetal, its epidermis still translucent and red, nevertheless crawls the long distance from its mother's perineum up her abdomen and up into her pouch, and back down to attach to her teat, which looks almost as big as the neonate itself (Bergman, 2003).

All of this is done without maternal assistance. Nonprimate mammals do not have arms, and so most mammalian mothers cannot easily assist their young with this first task even if they had the neuroendocrine priming to do so.

However, even in our primate cousin, the monkey, the newborn apparently receives no help from its mother's arms as it seeks out its first meal. The mother macaque monkey, once she has physically pulled her infant from her birth canal, leaves it on her belly to rest. From there, the newborn monkey, independently and completely without its mother's assistance, climbs over her abdomen on up to her chest, searches for and finds the nipple, and grasps it with its mouth to begin its first feeding (Rosenblum & Youngstein, 1974).

Innate Newborn Feeding Behavior in the Human Infant

It is only quite recently in western medical literature that this same innate mammalian newborn behavioral sequence has been described in the human neonate. In 1987, in a seminal study, Swedish midwife Ann-Marie Widström and her research team described the ability of the human newborn, in the first hour of life, to find and grasp the nipple and begin suckling, all without the active participation of the mother (Widström et al., 1987). A few years later, another Swedish research team, Lennart Righard and Margaret Alade, also described and videotaped the very young infant, in the first hour of life, using first the stepping response to crawl up the mother's abdomen to find the breast, and then the rooting response to locate the nipple, grasp it, attach, and begin suckling, a complex behavior they termed infant "self-attachment" (Righard & Alade, 1990).

Both Widström et al. and Righard and Alade emphasized the fragility of what was then felt to be a fleeting behavior, easily disrupted by common western delivery room routines, and best seen in the undisturbed first hour of life. Righard has, however, since suggested that this behavior might be seen at least for a few weeks, or as long as the crawling or stepping reflex persists (Righard & Frantz, 2005).

Infant-Initiated Feeding Behaviors: Persistence Beyond the First Days of Life

A few years after these pioneering Swedish studies, Australian midwife and lactation consultant Heather Harris (1994) described several infants of a few weeks of age, who had not yet learned to breastfeed, and who had had significant prior trouble at the breast. She found that when mother and baby were put together in a bathtub, mother pouring warm water over the infant's back, these infants would move toward the breast and initiate breastfeeding on their own. Harris described this "co-bathing" as a technique to calm and relax both infant and mother, to facilitate the behavioral sequence. However, at the time, this technique became popularized as "rebirthing." That term probably stemmed from the belief that the infant's behavior was facilitated by the association of the bath water with the infant's earlier experience with amniotic fluid, suggesting perhaps a re-creation of those first 24 hours. Harris, however, does not sees the water as requisite, and has seen infants of various ages, in a variety of circumstances, who, when calmed, were able to take themselves to breast, grasp the nipple and a mouthful of breast, and feed (Harris, personal communication, 2003).

Kathryn Meyer, while a nursing student at Case Western under Gene Cranston Anderson, described in 1999 her accidental discovery of the value of "kangaroo care" to full-term infants who were experiencing difficulty learning to feed in the first days of life. During her rotation through the maternity floor, she discovered that if she simply left such a newborn infant alone, skin on skin, on his mother's chest, the infant would find the breast on his own and be feeding comfortably when she returned a short time later (Meyer & Anderson, 1999).

In my breastfeeding medicine practice, both full-term and pre-term infants have demonstrated that this instinct is not limited to the first weeks of life; indeed, my clinical experience suggests that this innate capability probably persists for at least a year or much longer (Smillie, 2001).

Karleen Gribble, an Australian researcher, has compiled 32 cases from adoptive mothers who reported that their postinstitutionalized adopted children spontaneously initiated breastfeeding-seeking behaviors without maternal invitation (Gribble, 2005). This unsolicited behavior was described in children of various ages, ranging from 8 months to 12 years.

In addition, many individual mothers, nurses, and lactation consultants have described anecdotal and seemingly chance experiences with infant "self-attachment," in infants of various ages.

Despite these observations, I have found no literature suggesting universality or persistence to this infant capability, nor any neurobehavioral explanation for these observations. What follows, then, are my best descriptions of what I have seen in my breastfeeding medicine practice, over the past 10 years.

That this remarkable innate competence of the infant to "self-attach" has so long gone unrecognized has allowed many to believe that it is an uncommon and unpredictable occurrence. But my observations (Smillie, 2001) demonstrate that, when understood and nurtured, these infant capabilities are quite robust, persistent, universal, and of important clinical significance. Indeed, my clinical experiences have demonstrated that this wonderful neonatal capability is not limited to the first 24 hours of life or to the bathtub, and that, when recognized, this innate competence can help infants avoid or overcome a wide variety of difficulties encountered as they learn to breastfeed.

Baby-Led Learning

I term this behavior *baby-led learning, baby-led latching,* or *baby-led feeding,* rather than infant self-attachment, to acknowledge the interactive nature of the process, which involves the mother supporting the infant's state regulation, reading her infant's communications, and following her baby's cues.

Observations from My Practice: The Neurobehavioral Cascade

In my clinical experience, the infant cuddled vertically upright between his mother's breasts calms and relaxes. The vertical position stabilizes the infant's vestibular system, while the midline ventral position allows the baby a stabilizing symmetric posture, minimizing intrusive postural reflexes (Morris & Klein, 2000). With her baby upright on her chest, even a very insecure and unsure mother will usually begin stroking her infant, apparently instinctively, vocalizing and often attempting to make eye contact with her baby. Eye contact and the mother's voice help the infant remain calm and focused, and enhances motor control. Neck support helps prevent intrusive reflex motor movements. A sequence of neurosensory cues will, in this context, direct the infant toward the breast. The smell of the milk apparently helps orient the baby (Porter & Winberg, 1999; Varendi & Porter, 2001; Varendi, Porter, & Winberg, 2002), directing the baby to crawl in the direction of the breast (i.e., from the mother's abdomen upward or from the mother's shoulder or upper chest downward). The sensation of the infant's upper chest against his mother, skin against skin, appears to promote a searching response in the vertically positioned, hungry, quiet alert infant. The infant who is curled up, so that his chest is no longer in contact with the mother's skin, is less likely to initiate a move toward the breast, and yet as soon as his mother helps him straighten his torso, allowing him to feel his chest against her chest, the infant will begin or resume his searching.

The stepping or crawling reflex described by Righard and Alade (1990) is but one of many ways that infants can take themselves to the breast. I have observed that when the mother is sitting or standing upright, the infant can also use his arms and trunk to bob, bounce, throw himself, or gently fall toward the breast. I differentiate this innate gross motor behavior from the classic rooting behavior, which involves primarily the head and neck, by terming it the *searching response*.

It appears that part of what stimulates the infant to begin the behaviors that will initiate feeding is the momentum begun by this searching behavior itself. If the searching baby is interrupted, shuts down, falls asleep, or becomes distressed, that momentum can be disturbed and attempts cease. However, if his mother brings him back to that neutral midline position, changing both his body position and his behavioral state, he may suddenly reinitiate his search, find the breast, and begin feeding.

What in the past was termed the *rooting reflex* is now called the *rooting response,* to acknowledge the complexity of this neurobehavior. My observations reinforce the view that the rooting response is not stereotypical but varies, with a choice of movements depending upon the infant's state, body position, and the sensory cues received.

Once the baby has moved himself closer to the nipple and into a feeding position, the mother's intuitive support of the infant's pelvis against her body allows the positional stability necessary for organization for feeding (Glover, 2004; Morris & Klein, 2000). Comfortable and relaxed pelvic, trunk, and neck support to the infant's body gives the infant the positional stability for optimal motor control.

With his neck slightly extended, head slightly back, the infant approaches the breast with his chin leading, rather than his mouth or nose, a position that allows him to open his mouth widely. In this way, his nose is floating over the nipple in a "sniffing" position, and his chin, lower lip, and tongue are firmly on the breast, away from the nipple, when the pressure of the chin on the breast stimulates him to reach his upper lip up and over the nipple, to grasp a mouthful of breast, and begin to suckle.

However, if, before he is able to finish this behavioral sequence, the infant's face loses contact with the mother's skin, I've observed that the infant behaves as if he has been separated from his mother—he becomes anxious, distressed, tenses, and arches. His mouth may be only a half centimeter away from the nipple, and his eyes may be closed or wide open, but if his face is not in contact with her skin, he will behave as if the breast has been removed. Because the very distressed infant often arches, the mother may misinterpret this behavior as the infant trying to "get away" from the breast. In actuality, however, the arching is not purposeful, but a sign of distress. The perceived separation has put him in the sympathetic or adrenergic state, disorganizing his behavior and making voluntary motor activity difficult. If his mother can calm him, as she helps his face or mouth resume contact with her breast (not shoving mouth to nipple, but permitting face to touch the breast), the baby may relax and resume his rooting behavior. If his neurobehavioral state has been sufficiently disrupted, she may need to use specific comfort measures, for example, letting him suck on his own hand or her finger as she talks to him, or moving him away from the nipple and even back to an upright position, before he can reorganize and resume the sequence.

Once at the breast, the infant's hand may brush the nipple, which in turn becomes erect. The infant's face, in contact with the mother's skin, turns towards the smell of her nipple, and the classically described rooting behavior is seen. Repeated observations suggest to me that it is the firm pressure of the chin against the breast that then organizes the gape, stimulating the infant to open his mouth wide, reach down with his tongue, and grasp a mouthful of breast. It is then the infant's oral sensation, the breast filling infant's oral cavity, with palate, buccal, and lingual surfaces all in full contact with the breast that stimulates the infant to begin suckling. Although some enthusiastic infants will begin suckling with only the smallest amount of breast in their mouths, or none at all, many infants will come off the breast if they do not get that big mouthful of breast that provides the significant intraoral contact that will initiate suckling. The nipple, firmed by contact with the infant's hand or mouth, when felt against the palate, provides the neurosensory stimulus to help sustain suckling.

All of these are most likely instinctive, hard-wired behavioral sequences, which occur under specific circumstances. The association of sensorimotor feedback, the provision of milk, and the mother's relaxed demeanor probably provide the positive reinforcement for infant learning. The feeding process moves from an instinctively driven behavior to a learned behavior, from an innate situational response to the learned associations that make breastfeeding easy.

Why Haven't We Noticed This Before?

Most of the searching behaviors I've described are probably quite familiar to the reader. Those of us who work with breastfeeding dyads often call many of these behaviors *feeding cues*. However, I would contend that they are more than just a behavioral form of communication. If not obstructed, these movements initiate a cascade of behaviors that lead the baby to feed. When we view these behaviors as mere cues, we don't give the infant the opportunity to follow through and finish the full sequence.

As an infant tries to twist downward toward the breast, I've observed that parents and health professionals unfamiliar with infant competence typically respond by restraining the infant. This cultural inclination to restrain and protect newborn head movements has kept many of us from noticing or utilizing this infant capability. This restraining of the beginning of the feeding sequence while attempting to force the end of the sequence (latch) can potentially cause infant anxiety, stress, neurobehavioral disorganization, and breast refusal.

Explaining Infant Competence: The Neurobehavioral Literature

To understand both the neurological basis for this infant competence and the many variations of this infant behavior, we need to look to infant and animal neurobehavioral literature.

Reflex Responses

Righard and Alade (1990) demonstrated that the "stepping" or "crawling" response is not merely a residual and useless "primitive" reflex, but is a vital behavior, just as the rooting response is. Although the pediatric neurology literature does not address how other infant reflexes might also help the infant feed, animal studies describe similar searching behaviors.

We know that the mother herself has reflexes that facilitate infant feeding. Nipple erection occurs in response to infant touch as well as to specific sensory and psychosocial signals (Uvnäs-Moberg & Ericksson, 1996). When infants are held skin to skin, maternal breast skin temperature changes quickly via vasodilation or constriction, rapidly responding to infant skin temperature, to maintain it within narrow euthermic limits (Ludington-Hoe, Nguyen, Swinth, & Satyshur, 2000; Ludington-Hoe et al., 2006). Somatosensory stimuli cause the release of pituitary oxytocin to initiate milk ejection, and the release of a variety of gastrointestinal hormones in both mother and infant (Uvnäs-Moberg, Widström, Marchini, & Winberg, 1987; Widström et al., 1990). The reflex release of oxytocin elicits a variety of complex maternal physiologic, emotional, and behavioral responses (Matthiesen, Ransjo-Arvidson, Nissen, & Uvnäs-Moberg, 2001; Uvnäs-Moberg & Eriksson, 1996; Uvnäs-Moberg, Johansson, Lupoli, & Svennersten-Sjaunja, 2001).

Instinctive or Hardwired Neuroendocrine Programs for Behavior

Beyond simple reflex behaviors are far more complex patterns of instinctive behaviors for both mother and baby. A slight drop in blood sugar may cause the infant to initiate a searching response (Marchini, Persson, & Uvnäs-Moberg, 1993), but a wide variety of searching behaviors occur in that context. These are far too complex to be merely reflexive, but they are, nevertheless, "hardwired" innate behaviors. Such instinctive patterns of behavior can be understood as neuroendocrine programs for behavior, which occur in specific environmental (autonomic and social) circumstances (Marchini et al.). If the baby is hungry and in his calm mother's arms, he will be in a calm parasympathetic state, which allows him to look for the breast, and facilitates both learning and feeding. If separated from his mother, the hungry baby experiences stress and enters a sympathetic or adrenergic state characterized by a rise in catecholamines and serum cortisol. He will squirm and cry, behaviors that help him get back to his mother (Bergman, 2003; Christensson, Cabrera, Christensson, Uvnäs-Moberg, & Winberg, 1995).

These instinctive behaviors can be disrupted. State regulation is important to permit organized feeding responses, even in the physical presence of the mother. Even when the infant is chest against chest in his mother's arms, if he is overly hungry and so distressed that his mother is unable to return him to the calm, quiet, alert state, the infant may be unable to organize his behavior. His own hunger, his instincts to feed, and the insistent sensory cues from his mother's chest may overstimulate him, creating a clash between the distress of his hunger and the behavioral state necessary to relieve that distress. Once calmed, for example by sucking on his father's finger, the baby may now have the state regulation necessary to organize his motor behavior to search for the breast. Widström and Thingström-Paulsson (1993) demonstrated that when the newborn infant is permitted to initiate feeding on his own, he approaches the breast making licking movements, with tongue down in a position that makes it easy to grasp the breast. However, when infants cry, they lift their tongues to their palates, making it impossible to grasp the breast. Infants forced to the breast likewise fail to drop their tongues.

The mother also has hardwired neuroendocrine patterns of behavior, her "maternal instincts," which, like her baby's instincts, can be disrupted if she is unable to achieve her own state regulation. In the presence of her infant, the self-confident mother demonstrates a variety of predictable instinctive behaviors as she seeks to calm and communicate with her infant. Usually even the inexperienced mother will actively and spontaneously seek eye-to-eye contact with her infant, stroke him in specific ways, vocalize, and demonstrate a predictable repertoire of responses to her infant's behaviors (Kjellmer & Winberg, 1994; Uvnäs-Moberg, 1994). These oxytocin-mediated patterns of behavior can calm her infant, and permit him to follow his own instincts.

The Importance of Social Interaction to Infant State Regulation

Over 50 years ago, British pediatrician and psychoanalyst Donald Winnicott observed that "There is no such thing as a baby, there is a baby and someone" (Winnicott, 1960). That is, he explained, it is only within the context of the infant's interaction with the mother, or with another, that the baby can be understood. Since then, American pediatricians T. Berry Brazelton (1979) and John Kennell and Marshall Klaus and psychotherapist Phyllis Klaus (Klaus, Kennell, & Klaus, 1995; Klaus & Klaus, 1998), and others have observed and chronicled the neurobehavioral competence of the infant, as facilitated by interaction with either the mother or an examiner.

Over the past several decades research in a wide variety of disciplines has helped us better understand the neurophysiologic basis for these newborn behaviors.

The American neuropsychoanalyst Allan Schore, in work integrating research from the neurosciences, psychology, behavioral pediatrics, and psychiatry, offers a compelling theoretical model that describes the right-brained communication between mother and infant as central both to the infant's psychophysiologic state regulation and to his ongoing psychoneurodevelopment (Schore, 2001). It is in episodes of "affective synchrony" with his mother, involving interactive resonance between the amygdalae, limbic systems, and right brains of both infant and mother, that the infant achieves the state regulation necessary for such important life-preserving functions as feeding.

This resonance between the nervous systems of mother and infant is achieved through direct sensory communication—eye-to-eye contact, skin-on-skin contact, and vocal/auditory communication, permitting what Schore describes as direct right-brain-to-right-brain communication. Thus connected, the mother-baby dyad exists as a single psychoneurobiological organism. In that context, connected to her infant via their right brains, the mother is able to help her infant with state regulation, first as her right brain resonates in tune with his, and much later as this experience of attachment helps him to develop his own abilities for state regulation, autonomic regulation, and the regulation of his emotions.

For the mother to communicate with her infant, she, too, must let her right brain lead. When the mother herself is in a calm and relaxed state, she is open to subtle communication with her newborn, she can connect and respond to his state, and she can transfer that calm state regulation to her infant.

It has been said that in the postpartum period women tend to demonstrate a "cognitive deficit" (Eidelman, Hoffmann, & Kaitz, 1993). They can be quite daunted by such tasks as following verbal instructions, remembering dates or their baby's weights, paying attention to time, or counting diapers. I believe that this is probably not so much a total global "cognitive deficit," but rather, the effect of the mother's left brain taking a bit of a back seat to the right brain, making it easier for her to connect with her baby. When a mother can allow her left brain to step back, she can make room for more of the right brain's holistic, intuitive, attentive, in-the-moment, emotionally based thinking. This permits the mother to think more like her baby does, to empathize with her baby, that is, to "connect" with him, in both the colloquial sense, and, as Schore (2001) would say, right brain to right brain, thus allowing the mother to better understand her baby's moment-to-moment needs and be attentive to his moment-to-moment communication.

I think the reason these newborn abilities have been so long overlooked in the western world is that mothers and newborns are so rarely left together, just to relax and connect, without a "left-brained" agenda for what the infant was supposed to do. Only in that first hour of life, or later, sitting together in a warm bathtub, could mothers and babies just relax and enjoy each other *not* feeding. When the mother leaves her left brain's agenda behind, and follows her right-brained instincts to simply calm and relax her infant, only then can her feelings coincide with his, and the two right brains begin to resonate as one. Thus I believe that the key to what we are seeing, when an infant can search and find the breast to feed, is the state regulation made possible by this right-brain-to-right-brain maternal-infant communication, which Schore has so elegantly explained.

Nearly twenty years before Schore proposed this model, French pediatric neurologists Claudine Amiel-Tison and Albert Grenier (1983) described an alert newborn state that they distinguished from Prechtl's (1974) simple "quiet alert" state, a state they termed the "communicative state." These neurologists noted that when a young baby, in the first months of life, was in this more socially interactive alert state, they were able to elicit more advanced and organized infant neurobehavior than would otherwise be seen at that age.

This was very useful in the neurologic examination of the very young infant, so they wanted a technique for facilitating this alert behavioral state by transiently "liberating" the newborn from the intrusive reflex motor activity that usually inhibits the infant's voluntary movement. They hypothesized that neck instability was the primary trigger for most of these intrusive neonatal "primitive" motor reflexes. They noted that when the examiner supported the infant's neck and shoulders, rocking the infant while making eye contact and socializing verbally with the infant, after a few minutes the infant would attempt to vocalize responsively, fixing on the examiner's eyes and making social facial expressions. In this "communicative" state, a 2- or 3-week-old infant could be transiently "liberated" from intrusive obligatory reflex motor movements, and could even support his own head and neck with minimal examiner intervention.

Although Amiel-Tison and Grenier (1983) focused their attention on the stabilized neck, their monograph describes the adjunct use of eye-to-eye contact, rocking, and social vocalization. These interactions with the infant create precisely the right-brained interactions that Schore (2001) later conceptualized as key to infant state regulation.

These two pediatric neurologists devised this technique specifically to aid their neurologic exam of the newborn, with no discussion of the broader implications for their findings. Nevertheless, their method demonstrates for us how new parents get to know their newborns—"charming" the infant with eye contact and social verbalization, thus stabilizing the infant's autonomic regulation and permitting better motor control. No wonder so many mothers tell us that their babies held their heads up all by themselves at but a few days of age, when our developmental texts tell us it should not happen for another couple months! And, of course, it is that same liberated motor control that I believe permits the infant to follow his sense of smell, search for the breast, find the nipple, grasp the breast, and suckle.

Neuroendocrine Correlates of Behavior

Over the past few decades a large literature has developed demonstrating how skin-to-skin care facilitates both newborn autonomic stability and breastfeeding behaviors (Anderson et al., 2003a; Bergman, Linley, & Fawcus, 2004). At the same time, much research, both in Sweden and throughout the world, has further helped us understand the neuroendocrine correlates of both maternal (Matthiesen et al., 2001; Pedersen, 1997; Uvnäs-Moberg, 1994; Uvnäs-Moberg & Eriksson, 1996) and infant (Christensson et al., 1992, 1995; Luddington-Hoe, Cong, & Hashemi, 2002; Marchini et al., 1993) behavior, and their interaction (Kjellmer & Winberg, 1994; Nelson & Panksepp, 1998; Rosenblatt, 1994). A physiologic drop in blood sugar will trigger hunger (Marchini et al., 1993), or a minute rise in serum osmolality can trigger vasopressin release (Marchini & Stock, 1997), and either will then cause the initiation of infant feeding behaviors. A variety of tactile, visual, olfactory, and auditory sensory cues will, in the context of hunger, direct the infant's feeding behaviors toward the breast.

Infant Learning

Many studies have shown us that infants learn quite quickly by making associations between certain somatosensory experiences (Klaus & Klaus, 1998). Milk transfer can quickly "teach" a baby how to suckle as the infant makes an association between milk flow and a particular oral-motor sensory pattern and a particular autonomic state.

Maternal-Infant Interactions

The interactive behavior between mother and baby constitutes a continuous neuropsychological and neurobehavioral dance. A variety of neurosensory mediators are involved in these mutually reinforcing maternal and infant neuroendocrine responses, which affect the state regulation of both mother and baby, as well as physiologic and social processes necessary for infant survival.

These interactions may be positive or negative, and mutual reinforcement may promote or disturb homeostasis. The infant's calm responsive behavior may aid maternal learning just as much as maternal state regulation aids infant learning. Conversely, infant distress provokes maternal distress, evoking physical tension, which in turn can interfere with her ability to calm her baby, listen to her instincts, or make use of verbal instructions she may have been given.

On the other hand, when mothers are able to see their babies searching for the breast, they are usually quite impressed by their infant's spontaneous movements. The mother's positive response to seeing her infant's competent behavior helps calm both mother and baby further, so that the mother's arms, if tensed, often begin to relax, and her body language encourages her infant on his mission, allowing him to maintain the neurobehavioral organization needed to follow through with the complex cascade of behaviors necessary to initiate feeding.

Baby-Led Learning: From Theory to Practice

The infant's feeding behaviors described here are not rare or idiosyncratic. Since I started using this approach in 1996, I have witnessed no exceptions to the healthy hungry infant's primary inclination to search for the breast. Predictable factors affect the infant's ability to maintain the organized neurobehavioral state that enables the cascade of innate behaviors to trigger the final moves that end in feeding. The infant's ability to remain organized, his mother's ability to facilitate his neurobehavioral organization, past experiences at the breast—all of these affect whether or not the searching behavior will conclude in an actual feed. However, whether or not the infant is able to complete the behavior, the search itself appears to be quite universal, and appears far more complex and varied than the simple "rooting reflex" that begins with a brush to the cheek.

How Babies Can Learn to Feed: An Alternative Approach

The key to seeing these infant-initiated seeking and feeding behaviors is to permit both mother and baby to be calm, relaxed, and interacting with each other, with no other agenda. The process of learning to feed can be facilitated by protecting mother and infant from stress, and by allowing the infant to lead the process.

I do not ask the mother to make her infant learn to feed all by himself—I think it would be unphysiologic to ask a mother not to respond to her baby—but I do suggest that she follow her baby's lead, and let her own intuition (i.e., her right brain) guide her to help her baby stay comfortable.

1. First, We Start with a Calm Baby

We don't force a baby to learn to feed, we allow him to follow his instincts. The baby, not the mother, initiates the process. The mother simply follows her baby's lead, and allows the successful transfer of milk to teach the infant. It is then that the infant moves from an instinctive process to a learned process.

2. Skin on Skin in Any Comfortable Position

The mother starts by simply holding her baby, skin on skin, with the baby's body and the mother's body in continuous contact along the length of the baby's torso. The mother might begin by placing her baby chest against chest, in a neutral vertical position, or any other position they both find cuddly and comfortable. The mother might be sitting, lying down, or even standing, and the infant's face will not necessarily be near the breast at all. The mother will probably be talking to her baby, making eye contact if possible, so that they are communicating, socializing, and enjoying each other's company, with no other agenda, on baby time.

3. Mother Keeps Infant Calm, and Follows Baby's Lead

As her baby begins to move toward one breast, the mother follows her baby's lead, helping him as he moves his upper torso in the direction of one breast or the other, perhaps by stabilizing his hips at her waist. If he takes a position across her lap, his body will likely take something close to a 45-degree angle, with his hips snugly below her opposite breast. If she holds him under her arm, his body may end up wrapped around her waist, hips near her back. If she is standing, her lap will be gone, so her natural instinct to give support to her baby's hips and shoulders will be reinforced.

The mother helps her infant along as she instinctively speaks to him, calming and encouraging him with her voice, stroking him, or perhaps making eye contact. It's important that she follow her instincts to keep her baby calm and happy. If her baby shows any tension, she may want to move the baby away from the breast/nipple if necessary to calm him.

As the baby moves toward one breast, she can follow his lead, helping him maintain physical contact with the breast, allowing his face and cheek to touch the breast. Her support to his hips gives his body the stability to let him search. Her support of his shoulders allows him to tilt his head back, with his chin firmly against her breast. When he approaches the breast from underneath, it allows his chin contact with the full underside of the breast, which encourages him to open his mouth wide. If the baby's hands get "in the way," allowing him to suck on them will usually calm him so that he can resume his search, particularly if his mother reassures him with her voice and body language. The mother's hand, cupped under her breast, also can get in the infant's way, particularly if the mother is doing this because it has been taught, rather than as a momentary and transient instinctive movement. When left to their instincts, mothers often raise the breast if needed by placing their flat hands palm side down on the upper breast, briefly raising the breast by pulling the skin from above, as needed, so that the breast still hangs comfortably, undistorted by her hands, allowing the infant's chin to make full and firm contact with the full curved underside of the breast. The feel of that breast fullness on his chin will stimulate him to open widely, and then, reaching his upper lip upwards over the top of the nipple, he can then grasp a mouthful of breast, and begin suckling.

No One Correct Way

There will be many variations on how this is done, because babies and mothers come in many sizes, shapes, and personalities. Women can have short and long torsos, larger and smaller breasts, and babies can be smaller and larger, longer or shorter. So, mothers and babies will not all fit together in the same way. The large breasted woman whose nipple points down may find that her baby moves down low below where her breasts naturally fall and may end up nearly on his back, his eyes and face looking up at her, chin under the breast. On the other hand, the small breasted woman whose nipples point straight out may well find her baby in a more "tummy to tummy" position, and may or may not find it more comfortable for her baby to nurse in a more vertical position, his hips down by her waist, as he also looks up at her.

When we cease giving the mother specific rules as to what she "should" do, she is free to follow her own hardwired maternal instincts, as they are facilitated by the confidence she gets from watching her infant's competent behavior.

How Babies Can Relearn to Feed: An Approach to Breast Refusal

In my practice, I use this "baby-led" approach not only for initial mother-infant learning, but also for the wide variety of feeding problems that can be seen when these innate processes have been impeded. Premature or ill infants who have been long separated from their mothers' arms may need a long period of skin-on-skin reacquaintance before they are ready to learn.

Babies who have been repeatedly pushed forcefully to the breast, bypassing their instincts, may learn to associate distress with the breast. Thus, when placed skin on skin, these babies will usually still search for the breast and move toward the nipple, but when they get close to the breast they can suddenly become disorganized, their tongues rise to their palates, and they become so tense and distressed that they are unable to follow through to grasp the breast. They may even arch, cry, or pull away from the breast. Fortunately, this problem is easily addressed.

Such babies simply need the opportunity to regain trust and a positive association with the breast. This can be done by stopping all attempts to "make" the baby breastfeed. The baby will need to be fed expressed breast milk via an alternative means, usually for a day or two, but occasionally for as long as a week or more, depending primarily on the level of the baby's distress. During this time of exclusively alternative feeds, the mother and baby can reestablish trust via repeated periods of safe, quiet, skin-on-skin time, after alternative feedings, when the infant is not hungry, so that the baby has no impulse to search for the breast.

Once trust has been re-established, the baby forgets his negative associations, and he will be able to again follow his natural instincts to the breast. I usually advise mothers that the first several times that she permits the baby to go to the breast should only be on her maternal instinctive (right-brained) "impulse"—so that she only gives the baby the opportunity to search for the breast when the baby is displaying one of those "golden moments" when he seems particularly alert and social, that is, when he is in the "communicative state."

Even older babies who have never been to breast can learn to feed in this manner. Although I have seen babies as old as 10 months learn to feed for the first time in this manner, it is much easier in the first 3 months of life. Once infants reach 4 or 5 months of age, when developmentally they are more and more distractible, their curiosity and high activity can interfere with the behavioral state that allows them to follow through on their instincts for the breast.

Our Role in Helping Mothers and Babies As They Learn to Breastfeed

Our role, as healthcare professionals, is to convey this information in a calm, relaxed way, allowing each mother to feel comfortable and confident, so that she can help her baby be comfortable and competent. That often means we offer this information with more visual and physical demonstration than verbal instruction, so that we show her what we mean by speaking to her right brain, without using the kind of left-brained language that can often sound more complicated and technical than the mother's postpartum brain is prepared to handle.

We certainly need not use the language of this chapter; a woman need not become a lactation consultant herself to feed her baby.

What we want to convey with our demeanor, and our emotional connection with the mother, is our confidence in her and in her baby. We let her know that we believe in her, that of course she will be able to do this, that any negative experiences up to this point were not her fault. In this way, she can, as she begins to trust the process, convey those same right-brained messages to help her infant feel relaxed, calm, and competent.

I like to encourage the mother to talk to her infant. I don't usually "instruct" her to do so, but simply model the conversation, by talking to the infant myself. And when the mother spontaneously speaks to her infant, and she usually does, I will comment on how the infant calms to her speech, or remark on how the infant paused to listen, or sped up his suckling in response.

We want to encourage the mother to enjoy the process of learning, to recognize that this can take time, just like learning to walk or dance or ride a bike. We want to emphasize that this is all part of mothering—that the problems that brought her to us don't mean that she's incompetent.

It is helpful to interpret her baby's behavior, to show her how competent her infant is. If he gets on the breast and immediately comes off, only to try again, she may be confused and think he is doing something wrong. I tell her how smart he is, how he didn't get on quite far enough or didn't get the flow just right, and he wants to try again. Or if he comes off and quits, that's fine, too, he knows his limits and "needs to chill" a bit. Whatever is going on, it is instinct at work, so I reinterpret it for the mother as normal, as positive. As I do this, I see the mom relax over time. And after awhile, I can point out to her how much more relaxed she is, and how that too is helping her baby.

I tell the mother that her job is not to learn to breastfeed, nor to make her baby learn. Her job is simply to keep her infant calm and relaxed and comfortable so that he can learn. I will often quote Nils Bergman, who tells his students, "Mothers don't breastfeed, babies breastfeed," to let her know that it is her baby who is doing the learning, to take the pressure off of her and encourage her own self-confidence.

There is no one right way to do this. The key is to use right-brain techniques to give the mothers the confidence they need to keep their babies calm, which in turn promotes the infant behavior that then reinforces the mother's confidence. By modeling patience and calm, the healthcare professional can elicit in the mother the autonomic and emotional state that she needs to help her baby. It is through helping her baby be relaxed, alert, and calm, and in the parasympathetic state, that the mother can allow her infant to follow his instincts to search, root, grasp the breast, and learn to feed. And then, as she watches his innate behavior, her own confidence increases, and in this way the two help each other as they begin their journey.

References

Amiel-Tison, C., & Grenier, A. (1983). Expression of liberated motor activity (LMA) following manual immobilization of the head. In C. Amiel-Tison & A. Grenier (Eds.), *Neurologic evaluation of the newborn and the infant* (pp. 87–109). (J. Steichen, P. Steichen-Asch, & C. P. Braun, Trans.) New York: Masson Publishing USA.

Anderson, G. C., Moore, E., Hepworth, J., & Bergman, N. (2003a). Early skin-to-skin contact for mothers and their healthy newborn infants. *Birth, 30*(3), 206–207.

Anderson, G. C., Moore, E., Hepworth, J., & Bergman, N. (2003b). Early skin-to-skin contact for mothers and their healthy newborn infants. *Cochrane Database System Review, 2,* CD003519.

Bergman, N. J. (2003). *Humans and kangaroos—A biological perspective.* In: Conference syllabus, International Lactation Consultants Association, Sydney, Australia.

Bergman, N. J., Linley, L. L., & Fawcus, S. R. (2004). Randomized controlled trial of skin-to-skin contact from birth versus conventional incubator for physiological stabilization in 1200- to 2199-gram newborns. *Acta Paediatrica, 93*(6), 779–785.

Brazelton, T. (1979). Behavioral competence of the newborn infant. *Seminars in Perinatology, 3,* 35–44.

Christensson, K., Cabrera, T., Christensson, E., Uvnäs-Moberg, K., & Winberg, J. (1995). Separation distress call in the human neonate in the absence of maternal body contact. *Acta Paediatrica, 84,* 468–473.

Christensson, K., Siles, C., Moreno, L., et al. (1992). Temperature, metabolic adaptation and crying in healthy full-term newborns cared for skin-to-skin or in a cot. *Acta Paediatrica, 81,* 488–493.

Eidelman, A. I., Hoffmann, N. W., & Kaitz, M. (1993). Cognitive deficits in women after childbirth. *Obstetrics and Gynecology, 81*(5 Pt 1), 764–767.

Eilam, D., & Smotherman, W. P. (1998). How the neonatal rat gets to the nipple: Common motor modules and their involvement in the expression of early motor behavior. *Developmental Psychobiology, 32,* 57–66.

Glover, R. (2004). *Lessons from innate feeding abilities transforms breastfeeding outcomes.* In: Conference syllabus, International Lactation Consultants Association, Scottsdale, Arizona.

Gribble, K. D. (2005). Post-institutionalized adopted children who seek breastfeeding from their new mothers. *Journal of Prenatal and Perinatal Psychology and Health, 19*(3), 217–234.

Harris, H. (1994). Remedial co-bathing for breastfeeding difficulties. *Breastfeeding Review, 11*(10), 465–468.

Kjellmer, I., & Winberg, J. (1994). The neurobiology of infant–parent interaction in the newborn: An introduction. *Acta Paediatrica, 397*(Suppl.), 1–2.

Klaus, M. H., Kennell, J. H., & Klaus, P. H. (1995). *Bonding: Building the foundations of secure attachment and independence.* New York: Addison-Wesley.

Klaus, M., & Klaus, P. (1998). *Your amazing newborn.* Reading, MA: Perseus Books.

Ludington-Hoe, S. M., Cong, X., & Hashemi, F. (2002). Infant crying: Nature, physiologic consequences, and select interventions. *Neonatal Network, 21*(2), 29–36.

Ludington-Hoe, S. M., Lewis, T., Morgan, K., Cong, X., Anderson, L., & Reese, S. (2006). Breast and infant temperatures with twins during shared kangaroo care. *Journal of Obstetric, Gynecologic, and Neonatal Nursing, 35*(2), 223–231.

Ludington-Hoe, S. M., Nguyen, N., Swinth, J. Y., & Satyshur, R. D. (2000). Kangaroo care compared to incubators in maintaining body warmth in preterm infants. *Biological Research for Nursing, 2*(1), 60–73.

Marchini, G., Persson, B., & Uvnäs-Moberg, K. (1993). Metabolic correlates of behaviour in the newborn infant. *Physiology & Behavior, 54,* 1021–1023.

Marchini, G., & Stock, S. (1997). Thirst and vasopressin secretion counteract dehydration in newborn infants. *Journal of Pediatrics, 130*(5), 736–739.

Matthiesen, A. S., Ransjo-Arvidson, A. B., Nissen, E., & Uvnäs-Moberg, K. (2001). Postpartum maternal oxytocin release by newborns: Effects of infant hand massage and sucking. *Birth, 28*(1), 13–19.

Meyer, K., & Anderson, G. C. (1999). Using kangaroo care in a clinical setting with fullterm infants having breastfeeding difficulties. *MCN. The American Journal of Maternal Child Nursing, 24*(4), 190–192.

Morris, S. E., & Klein, M. D. (2000). *Pre-feeding skills: A comprehensive resource for mealtime development* (2nd ed.). Tucson, AZ: Therapy Skill Builders.

Nelson, E., & Panksepp, J. (1998). Brain substrates of infant–mother attachment: Contributions of opioids, oxytocin, and norepinephrine. *Neuroscience and Biobehavioral Reviews, 22,* 437–452.

Pedersen, C. (1997). Oxytocin control of maternal behavior: Regulation by sex steroids and offspring stimuli. *Annals of the New York Academy of Sciences, 807,* 126–145.

Porter, R. H., & Winberg, J. (1999). Unique salience of maternal breast odors for newborn infants. *Neuroscience and Biobehavioral Review, 23,* 439–449.

Prechtl, H. F. (1974). The behavioural states of the newborn infant (a review). *Brain Research.* Aug 16;76(2):185–212.

Righard, L., & Alade, M. (1990). Effect of delivery room routines on success of first breast-feed. *Lancet, 336,* 1105–1107.

Righard, L., & Frantz, K. (2005). *Delivery self-attachment* [DVD]. Los Angeles: Geddes Productions.

Rosenblatt, J. S. (1994). Psychobiology of maternal-behavior: Contribution to the clinical understanding of maternal behavior among humans. *Acta Paediatrica, 83*(Suppl. 397), 3–8.

Rosenblum, L. A., & Youngstein, K. P. (1974). Developmental changes in compensatory dyadic response in mother and infant monkeys. In M. Lewis & L. A. Rosenblum (Eds.), *The effect of the infant on its caregiver* (pp. 141–161). New York: John Wiley.

Schore, A. N. (2001). The effects of a secure attachment relationship on right brain development, affect regulation, and infant mental health. *Infant Mental Health Journal, 22,* 7–66.

Smillie, C. M. (2001). How newborns learn to latch: A neurobehavioral model for self-attachment in infancy. [Abstract PL9]. *Academy of Breastfeeding Medicine News and Views, 7,* 23.

Uvnäs-Moberg, K. (1994). Oxytocin and behaviour. *Annals of Medicine, 26*(5), 315–317.

Uvnäs-Moberg, K., & Eriksson, M. (1996). Breastfeeding: Physiological, endocrine and behavioural adaptations caused by oxytocin and local neurogenic activity in the nipple and mammary gland. *Acta Paediatrica, 85,* 525–530.

Uvnäs-Moberg, K., Johansson, B., Lupoli, B., & Svennersten-Sjaunja, K. (2001). Oxytocin facilitates behavioural, metabolic and physiological adaptations during lactation. *Applied Animal Behaviour Science, 72*(3), 225–234.

Uvnäs-Moberg, K., Widström, A.-M., Marchini, G., & Winberg, J. (1987). Release of GI hormones in mother and infant by sensory stimulation. *Acta Paediatrica Scandinavia, 76,* 851–860.

Varendi, H., & Porter, R. H. (2001). Breast odour as the only maternal stimulus elicits crawling towards the odour source. *Acta Paediatrica, 90,* 372–375.

Varendi, H., Porter, R. H., & Winberg, J. (2002). The effect of labor on olfactory exposure learning within the first postnatal hour. *Behavioral Neuroscience, 116*(2), 206–211.

Widström, A.-M., Ransiö-Arvidson, A. B., Christensson, K., Matthiesen, A.-S., Winberg, J., & Uvnäs-Moberg, K. (1987). Gastric suction in healthy newborn infants: Effects on circulation and developing feeding behaviour. *Acta Paediatrica Scandinavia, 76,* 566–572.

Widström, A.-M., & Thingström-Paulsson, J. (1993). The position of the tongue during rooting reflexes elicited in newborn infants before the first suckle. *Acta Paediatrica, 82,* 281–283.

Widström, A.-M., Wahlberg, V., Matthiesen, A.-S., et al. (1990). Short-term effects of early suckling and touch of the nipple on maternal behavior. *Early Human Development, 21,* 153–163.

Winnicott, D. W. (1960). The theory of the parent-child relationship. *International Journal of Psychoanalysis, 41,* 585–595.

Chapter 5

The Infant–Maternal Breastfeeding Conversation: Helping When They Lose the Thread

Rebecca Glover

Diane Wiessinger

We are the only mammals who could write—or want to read—a chapter like this one. For all other mammals whose behaviors have not been altered by domestication, lactation is an uneventful stage between umbilical cord and solids. Mammals spend a significant portion of their lives *in utero,* and produce very low numbers of total offspring during a lifetime; it makes no biological sense for newborn starvation to be a common follow-up to mammalian birth. Yet in the United States, if we assume that bottle feeding represents failed lactation, one human in three would not survive to 1 month of age (National Center for Health Statistics, 2005).

Our problems began because we are social primates. Infant feeding proceeds uneventfully for the mouse or raccoon who has never seen it before. For higher primate mothers, however, there is a learned component. We would have learned to breastfeed first by breastfeeding into childhood, then by observing it frequently and at close range for many more years. That generation-to-generation learning had largely vanished by the middle of the 20th century, when we began trying to re-create the feeding conversation between mother and baby from scratch. We found ourselves without role models, observing those few mothers who breastfed successfully, making assumptions based on our familiarity with bottle feeding. We tried to break breastfeeding into its component pieces, creating a series of awkward, disjointed, often ineffective phrases in a mother–baby dialogue that had lost all grace and flow. Many of our early assumptions and approaches were wrong. Many of them may still be. However, what follows here seems to work better than other approaches of the past 50 years. This chapter is a work in progress; every mother or assistant who finds it helpful or unhelpful is a chance for all of us to learn still more.

Preparation for the Breastfeeding Conversation

Sensory Readiness

Preparation for breastfeeding in the newborn involves both physiological and reflex responses.

Physiological Response: The Oxytocin Effect

The release of oxytocin during breastfeeding triggers the milk ejection reflex, or milk release, but oxytocin is also released—by both mother and baby—when a baby is simply held skin-to-skin or is in firm contact with his mother's clothed body and breast. Indeed, oxytocin is sometimes called the "love, labor, and lactation hormone." It stimulates mother and baby to interact with each other; makes them feel calm and "in love"; increases blood flow to the skin on the mother's chest and breast, which helps to keep the baby warm; and triggers the release of digestive hormones in both mother and baby (Uvnäs-Moberg & Eriksson, 1996). Suzanne Colson calls these mutual responses biological nurturing: "Biologically it is the suckling baby who takes the initiative in feeding. The baby's body on or closely wrapped around the mother's body seems to trigger breastfeeding reflexes [in the infant], while infant cues elicit maternal responses in a reciprocal manner" (Colson, 2002, p. 15).

Reflex Response

For the first 3 to 4 months of life, babies' breastfeeding movements are largely the result of automatic, reflex movements that only occur when the baby is given the right physical contact (sensory input), not unlike the patellar tendon (knee jerk) reflex, which responds *only* if tapped in exactly the right spot.

Firm, frontal contact with the mother's body and breast provides the infant with the most powerful sensory input for breastfeeding. The position of the mother and baby, and later the feel of the breast and nipple in the mouth, affects the type and range of movements the infant will execute for attachment and breastfeeding (Morris & Klein, 1987). In particular, to attach well, the infant's chest, chin, and lips need to feel firm physical contact with his mother's body and breast in order for him to lift his chin and mouth reflexively, to seek the breast and nipple with a wide-open mouth, and to "scoop" a large enough portion of breast and nipple into the mouth. Once the breast fills the baby's mouth, the physical sensation of the breast touching all the inner surfaces of the mouth gives the infant the sensory stimuli and feedback he requires to support the suck-swallow-breathe cycle (Millar, 2002).

Beginning at approximately 3 to 4 months, breastfeeding gradually becomes less reflexive and more voluntary, and the infant gradually becomes less dependent on his mother for physical stability and tactile cues. But in the early weeks, breastfeeding is not a visual behavior for babies. They may see the nipple in front of them and yet fail to respond. Because their mothers are extremely visual, this lack of response can seem especially frustrating. "It's right there, dear one! Don't you see it?" He does see it, but only the appropriate physical sensations will trigger feeding behavior.

Positional Stability

Positional vs. Postural Stability

All newborn mammals are uneasy when they are placed on their backs. They struggle to "right themselves"—to feel the ground or nest or mother's body against their chest and belly. Even aquatic mammals want to be "right side up," as if they could gather their limbs under them and travel. Indeed, all newborn mammals *are* able to travel, provided they are in a stable position. Left on their backs, every one of them gives a strong impression of instability and helplessness. Flip newborns onto their chests, and there is a clear sense that the infant has regained some measure of control. Human infants, like all other mammals, are calmer when their chest and belly are against a firm support—preferably against an adult body. We calm a baby instinctively by picking him up, putting his chest and belly against our shoulder, and shushing and patting him. The Moro reflex, or startle response, does not occur when the baby's ventrum is held firmly against an adult body. The human baby who rides on his mother's hip, the gorilla baby who clings to his mother's back, the premature infant in kangaroo care, even the baby in a "colic hold"—facing away from the adult but with firm pressure from the adult's forearm along his chest and belly—all these babies are stabilized by the position in which they are held. This externally controlled stability is called *positional stability* (Morris & Klein, 1987).

An adult horse may roll on its back pleasurably, an adult dog may enjoy being belly-up for a scratch, and an adult human can nap comfortably on his or her back. But these adult mammals are capable of internally generated stability, or *postural stability* (Morris & Klein, 1987). Their mature nervous systems allow them to be in control of their bodies no matter what position they choose to assume. Many mammal infants can make themselves comfortable in other positions as well, provided they are hugged, or swaddled, or cuddled. In order to encourage separate, supine sleep, we find ourselves swaddling our babies or at least clothing them, to allow them the illusion of the firm, continuous frontal contact.

What does positional stability have to do with suckling? Imagine being offered a sandwich while you're walking on a narrow beam. "Not now," you say. "Wait until I'm more stable." It's difficult to think about lunch when you're fighting to keep your balance. One thing at a time, please! Newborns to 3- or 4-month-old infants are totally reliant on positional stability; they develop postural stability only with increasing maturity. For smooth, calm execution of the complex sequence of movements required for attachment and the suck-swallow-breathe cycle, an infant must be provided with good positional stability.

Principles of Positional Stability

To understand how important this stability is for the infant and how it applies to breastfeeding we need to look at some of the key principles that govern stability, function, and mobility.

A Stable Base. A stable base is fundamental to easy movement; remember the person balancing on the beam who focuses on the beam instead of on lunch. All human movement and functional skills require a stable base. "Without stability, our function or mobility is less controlled or even impossible" (Morris & Klein, 1987, p. 14). Creating this stable base for an infant involves both midline and proximal stability.

Midline Stability. Optimal function of the neck, head, and oral area is dependent on the symmetrical movement of the muscles on *both* sides of the infant's body (Freeman, 2000). *Midline stability*—the stabilization of an imaginary line down the center of the infant's body— provides the breastfeeding infant with a stable base from which to perform the symmetrical movements of breastfeeding. It is especially important for the infant's upper body to be well-supported and straight, but midline stability involves the baby's body from tip to toe. Our emphasis in the past has been on having the baby's entire body facing the mother, but not on having it well-stabilized. The baby who lies in his mother's arms with a gap between his ventrum and her body may be in a straight line but he is not well-supported; ask the mother who holds her baby this way to stand up, and you will see a shift in how she holds the baby. She must stabilize him as she moves, or he wobbles and sways. In contrast, if her infant lies snug against her body, arms forward and flexed at the elbow, no gaps between his torso and hers, she can sit, stand, even run without distressing him.

Midline stability gives the baby "a sense of center," helping the infant to focus his attention on the breast in front of him.

> The sense of center, whether it is developed in the trunk, hand, foot, or mouth, is important for helping children focus attention. If a child's energies move away from the center or if there is no sense of midline it becomes extremely difficult to obtain and maintain focused attention to tasks. Eating is an activity that requires attention and concentration and the developed sense of midline can help both. (Morris & Klein, 1987, p. 18)

Proximal Stability. Physical and occupational therapists point out that "proximal stability promotes distal mobility." When we stabilize a part of our body closer to our core, we are better able to move a related body part that is farther away from that point of stability. Our hand moves a computer mouse more accurately when our forearm rests on a firm surface. We have a steadier hand for the finer motion of placing the cursor when our wrist is braced on the desktop. In each case, we use *proximal stability* in order to allow more controlled motion distal to the stabilized point. In the same way, stabilizing a baby's shoulders gives proximal stability to his head and neck, allowing him much better mobility and control.

The concept of proximal-to-distal control is highly relevant when discussing functions of the oral area.... [T]he head is distal and the neck and shoulders are proximal to it. You could imagine that the head and neck sit on the floor of the shoulders. If that floor is unstable, then all distal functions are influenced ... [but] from a controlled proximal base of stability, [the shoulder girdle], the infant can have the possibility of greater mobility and more refined distal control. (Morris & Klein, 1987, p. 14)

Babies older than 3 to 4 months have acquired enough postural stability, muscle control, and experience to breastfeed easily in many positions. However, "[i]n the newborn oral stability is dependent on the development of neck and shoulder girdle stability *which are in turn* dependent upon trunk and pelvic stability" (Morris & Klein, 1987, p. 15). It is remarkable how careful attention to stability—especially of the shoulders—helps a hungry baby lift his head and seek the breast (see **Figure 5-1**).

The "Instinctive Feeding Position"

Head-lifting requires considerable strength in the neck's extensor muscles—a strength that many parents assume a newborn lacks. But remember that a baby operating from a stable base operates best. Parents may say, proudly, "He could lift his head up when he was only a week old." In fact, that ability is utterly normal and exists in healthy babies from day one. Provided he is allowed to operate from a stable base, a normal infant shows "a tendency towards active movements of the extensor muscles of the neck," especially during the first 3 months (Morris & Klein, 1987, p. 16).

Figure 5-1
A positionally stable baby.

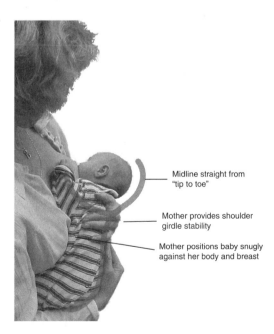

Midline straight from "tip to toe"

Mother provides shoulder girdle stability

Mother positions baby snugly against her body and breast

A Stable Baby

Baby's whole body faces mother, midline straight, positioned firmly against her body.

- *Infant's response:* Release of oxytocin and gastric hormones; becomes calm and begins seeking behaviors.
- *Mother's response:* Release of oxytocin and gastric hormones; becomes calm and attentive to her baby.

Baby is held firmly against his mother behind the shoulders. This should "uncurl" baby, pushing the baby's chest against the mother's chest and the side of her breast.

- *Infant's response:* Baby is physically able to carry out his reflexive feeding behaviors.
- *Mother's response:* Mother follows her baby's cues, working with her baby, and helping him attach if necessary.

When he begins his innate feeding behaviors, the human infant uses those extensor muscles to adopt a distinctive posture—head lifted and tilting back—so that the baby approaches the breast with the chin and mouth leading. This is the infant's "instinctive feeding position" (Glover, 2004). Bringing a newborn to 3- to 4-month-old baby to the breast in this position automatically works with his anatomy, reflexes, and physical capabilities.

The Hyoid Bone and Muscles: Optimizing Strength and Function

Lifting the baby's head into the instinctive feeding position is not entirely the work of the extensor muscles in the neck, however.

> There are numerous muscular connections between the structures of the mouth, pharynx, larynx, skull and shoulder girdle. These structural connections are the basis for reciprocal influences between feeding, swallowing and breathing, and *head and neck posture.* The hyoid bone and the muscles that attach to it play a key role in this relationship. (Wolf & Glass, 1992, p. 7)

The hyoid bone is a U-shaped bone in the neck, located between the mandible and the larynx (see **Figure 5-2**). It is the only bone in the body that does not articulate with other bones, but it is the attachment site for a number of muscles involved in breastfeeding's large and small motor skills. Some of these muscles connect to the clavicle, scapula, and cervical vertebrae (the shoulder girdle). Others connect to the skull, mandible, pharynx, and larynx; still more control and support the tongue. Collectively, the muscles attaching to the hyoid bone are responsible for most of a baby's seeking, attaching, and suckling behaviors, and their ability to function is directly affected by the position of the infant's head and neck. A stable shoulder girdle thus stabilizes a host of muscles that give the baby the strength, leverage, and control not only to lift his head, but also to open his jaw wide, move his tongue forward, and "scoop" in a large mouthful of breast.

Figure 5-2
Schematic of hyoid bone and its muscle attachments to other bones.

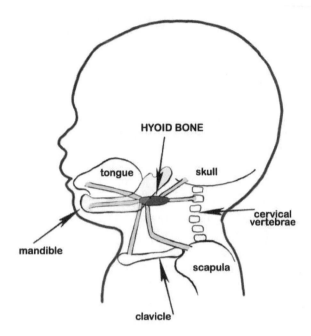

The Optimal Position for Oral Stability and Oral-Motor Function

The Optimal Position for Oral Stability and Oral-Motor Function

All muscles have an optimal position for strength and function (Freeman, 2000). For example, to pick up an object, we hold our arm neither fully extended nor fully flexed, but bent in the mid-range. This maximizes our strength and manipulative options, whether we are picking up a pen or a brick. Try it! When an infant is in the instinctive feeding position, his head is neither flexed nor fully extended. He maintains it in a comfortable mid-range, optimizing both his strength and his control.

The Instinctive Feeding Position Makes Good Attachment Physically Possible

Woolridge (1986) stated that for the infant to take the critical area of breast, "the region below the nipple" (from the baby's perspective), it is "essential to ensure that the baby is held in the correct posture relative to the mother's body" (p. 175). He describes "supporting the baby across the shoulders and bringing baby to the breast with the head tilted slightly backward to ensure that baby approaches the breast with the chin and mouth forward" (p. 176).

When a baby assumes his instinctive feeding position, important changes take place not only in the placement of his jaws, but also inside his mouth. You will understand this most easily by using yourself as a model.

Drop your chin down toward your chest, open your mouth wide, and notice the position of your tongue. The tongue retracts from the lower gum and humps at the back of the mouth near the junction of the hard and soft palate, *blocking the space where the nipple needs to go.* Now let your head drop back into the instinctive feeding position, and open your mouth wide. You can open your mouth much wider, and your tongue now lies flat on the floor of your mouth. Indeed, you will find it difficult to retract or curl your tongue back; tilting the head back has the overall effect of dramatically increasing the size of the oral cavity.

The gag reflex is also less sensitive with your head in the instinctive feeding position. Try touching your soft palate with your finger, first with your mouth wide open and your chin down, then with your mouth wide open and your head in the instinctive feeding position, and you will experience the difference.

Finally, try taking several large, quick swallows from a full glass of water, first with your chin down, then with your chin raised. Drinking is more comfortable, for both adults and babies, when the head is in the instinctive feeding position.

Woolridge's (1986) ultrasound studies demonstrate that, when attachment is good, a baby takes enough breast to fill the mouth. The nipple comes to rest close to the junction of the hard and soft palate and the infant's bottom lip, tongue, jaw, and chin lie deeply and securely under the breast tissue (see **Figure 5-3**). With this essential mouthful in place, the infant can breastfeed comfortably and effectively. To enable mother and baby to achieve this essential mouthful, Woolridge also defines a "critical area for attachment" as the "region below the nipple [from the baby's perspective], apposed to the baby's lower jaw and tongue" (p. 175). He describes, in essence, a bite from a very large sandwich.

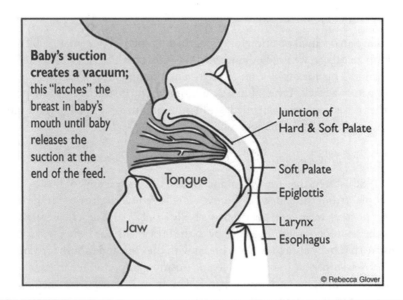

Figure 5-3 The essential mouthful.

Source: Reprinted with permission by Rebecca Glover, IBCLC

Mouth Mechanics and the Breastfeeding Infant

Imagine that you are trying to eat a very thick sandwich with the top slice of bread vertical and facing you. You cannot take a bite out of it because you have been presented with a wall; no place to put your jaws. Next, try turning the sandwich perpendicular to your lips, with vertical slices of bread to your left and right. There is still no place to put your jaws because you are unable to get your maxilla (upper jaw) and mandible (lower jaw) above and below the sandwich. Now hold the sandwich horizontal and parallel to your lips, but with the edge of the sandwich directly in front of your lips. Although this probably allows you to take a bite, and sounds optimal, it is actually an ineffective way to achieve the largest possible mouthful. Let's look at this third scenario more closely.

If our mouths were symmetrically constructed, we would be able to take the largest possible bite out of a sandwich presented to the center of our mouths. However, mammalian mouths are never symmetrical. Our maxilla is a fixed part of our skull and projects slightly beyond our mandible; only the mandible is capable of moving. This means that we take the largest bite of a sandwich by ensuring that the largest possible amount of the lower side of the sandwich fits into our mouth and onto our tongue, giving our mandible maximum access to it. Our maxilla then rests passively on top.

When you bring a thick sandwich to your mouth, you first hold it parallel to your lips. You may squeeze it slightly, to present yourself with a narrower oval. You do not worry about the placement of the fingers near your upper jaw, but you make sure to keep your lower jaw fingers (your thumbs, in this case) well out of the way.

You open wide, bring the bottom of the sandwich to your mouth, and lay it well back on your tongue. The more deeply you position your jaw under the sandwich the bigger the mouthful you are able to take. The rocking motion that follows rolls additional sandwich into your mouth, landing it first on your lips, then on the front of the tongue, then still farther back as our stationary maxilla lands on top. Our upper-jaw fingers tend to stay near our upper lip; we may use them to tuck a bit more of the sandwich into our mouth at the last minute.

If we hold the sandwich directly in front of our closed mouth to start, when we open our mouth our maxilla remains in place, and our mandible swings down … and away from the sandwich. When a mother's nipple is placed directly in front of her baby's mouth, the simple act of opening the mouth results in the baby's bottom lip and chin losing good contact with it, especially if his head is prevented from tilting back.

If the sandwich begins directly in front of our closed mouth and it is stationary in space, the only way to bring our opened mouth back into contact with the sandwich is to bend our knees slightly so that the sandwich is above our top lip. We then tip our head back, which thrusts our chin forward. *In order to bring our open mouth into the deepest possible contact with the sandwich, we have assumed the instinctive feeding position.* When a baby is positioned and stabilized well, the mother's nipple will usually be above the baby's top lip just before the baby initiates a latch, as Woolridge (1986) describes and as your own experiments with a sandwich suggest.

Assuming a stationary sandwich, as above (mimicking a stationary breast for a baby), you will be able to take the largest, most comfortable bite if you keep the sandwich above your top lip to begin with. To reach the sandwich, you rock your head back slightly, thrusting your mandible forward and underneath the sandwich. You keep your lower-jaw fingers well back on the bottom slice of bread, because that's where your mandible will land. You needn't worry about the fingers on the upper slice until the last moment; indeed, as your maxilla lands on the sandwich, you can even use those fingers to tuck a bit more sandwich into your mouth, provided that you have kept them close to where your maxilla will land. In other words, you hold the sandwich asymmetrically—mandible fingers well away, maxilla fingers close to your upper lip. Remember these finger placements; we will revisit them later, when a mother helps her baby onto the breast.

Now suppose that, instead, you hold the sandwich parallel to your lips but below the level of your mouth, near your chin. You will have to tuck your chin in order to take a bite. As you tuck your chin, your mandible will swing away from the sandwich, not toward it, and your nose will likely become buried in the top slice of bread.

When a baby is held too far to the side of the mother's body, he must tuck his chin in order to reach her nipple. His nose swings into her breast and his mandible swings away, rather than his nose lifting free and his mandible digging in. If the mother's nipple is long enough, the baby who tucks his chin will probably be able to reach it with his lower jaw, but the nipple must stretch, the latch is likely to be painful, and the lack of breast tissue over the tongue may compromise milk intake. If the nipple shank is short, he may have difficulty latching at all. The more a baby's chin is tucked, the more difficult effective attachment becomes.

Your own experiments with a sandwich may make it easier for you to understand why certain common approaches to positioning are likely to result in painful nipples, difficult or failed latches, a buried nose, or a reluctant baby (Wiessinger, 1998).

Common Miscommunications

- If the mother supports her breast in the "C-hold" that is sometimes taught, with a baby completely horizontal in her arms, the baby is being asked to grasp a "breast sandwich" that is oriented perpendicular to his mouth, and may not achieve a deep enough attachment. If a mother chooses to hold or shape her breast, it makes more sense to do so in such a way that the "sandwich" she creates matches the direction of the baby's lips—vertical if the baby's mouth is vertical, angled if the baby's mouth is angled. It can be difficult, at first, for a mother to "see through her baby's eyes" and recognize when her hand position is appropriate. Barbara Boston (personal communication, 2003) suggests that the mother think in terms of creating a mustache for the baby with the fingers closest to the baby's upper jaw, similar to laying a finger between the baby's nose and upper lip in imitation of a mustache, but with the finger on the breast rather than on the baby's lip. Any time a mother shapes her breast with that "upper-jaw finger" in the position of a mustache, she is probably creating an appropriately angled "sandwich" for the baby.

- If the mother holds her breast with some of her fingers near the baby's chin, she is likely to crowd his mandible's access to the breast, forcing him into a shallow latch.

- If the mother holds her baby completely horizontal across her torso, with his mouth at her nipple, his lower body will be draped across the other breast. This position, also common when a breastfeeding pillow is used, can make it difficult for the baby to assume his instinctive feeding position. Held across both breasts, he is, in essence, reaching across from one mountain top to another, with less need to extend his head. If, however, he is snuggled in to the base of his mother's breast, with his body below the opposite breast, he finds himself looking up the mountain, and the instinctive feeding position brings his mouth toward and over the mountain peak, or nipple.

The physical position and posture of the baby in relation to his mother's body and breast are fundamental to resolving any attachment or latch difficulty, from the most simple to the most difficult, and to enabling the baby to enjoy a smooth breastfeeding conversation with his mother.

The Breastfeeding Conversation: Baby-Led Self-Attachment

Feeding Sequence

Every mother knows that she has to support her newborn's body and head if she holds him over her shoulder. And every mother quickly learns that her baby is untrustworthy there. He may wobble, bobble, curl, or lunge if she does not prevent it. For decades, we assumed that this was part of an incompetent baby's mindless movement. Thanks to Christina Smillie's observations in her breastfeeding medicine practice, we now know better.

Every mammal is born with the ability to move instinctively to its mother's nipple. This *feeding sequence*—a series of predictable and standardized moves that culminates in suckling—often involves some minor maternal assistance such as nudging the newborn with her nose or making her teats more available, but it is essentially the baby's perform-ance. In some mammal newborns, the feeding sequence is so rigidly preset that if they are placed directly at a teat they are unable to feed. In humans the sequence is less rigid. Nonetheless, the baby who seems confused or angry when offered the breast directly will often latch eagerly when allowed to perform the entire sequence, especially if he does so in skin-to-skin contact with his mother.

During his first 3 to 4 months, *any* normal, hungry infant who is held in a stable posi-tion by his mother will begin to move toward her breast (Smillie, 2001). In response, the mother who is urged simply to follow her baby's lead will generally offer instinctive, gentle assistance, moving his legs under the opposite breast and supporting his shoulders and head as he moves to the base or side of the mountain that is her breast. Her hands and arms will likely assume constantly shifting arrangements as she supports his ever-changing posi-tions. Because she does not focus on head support, however, he is able to extend his head into the instinctive feeding position, seeking the nipple with a widely gaping mouth. His neck may be supported by her wrist or forearm, or perhaps by the webbing between thumb and forefinger. This is the opening dialogue in their breastfeeding conversation: mother holds the baby in a stable position, baby begins to move toward her breast, mother responds by supporting his movements.

As the baby searches for the nipple, he may bob repeatedly or "peck" at her breast. His touch on her breast is likely to cause her nipple to become more firm and thus more obvious. And the feel of her breast on his lower face tends to result in a very focused baby and the instinctive feeding position—mouth open, chin thrust forward. As his tongue "scoops" in ample breast tissue, and his upper lip clears the nipple, he sweeps his mandible closed, draws the breast deeply into his mouth, and begins to suckle. In this final part of their dialogue, the mother may make small adjustments, lifting or shifting her breast slightly to accommodate either the baby's apparent desires or her own comfort but always firmly supporting the baby's shoulder girdle.

Summary of the Baby-Led Attachment Conversation

Mother: Holds baby skin-to-skin against her body and breast, and stabilizes him firmly across the shoulders.

Baby: Becomes calm and focused, and begins moving toward the breast, lifting the chin and mouth up, which tilts the head back.

Mother: Works with the baby, revising her support as his position shifts.

Baby: Lips and chin make firm contact with the breast; attachment reflexes are triggered, and baby opens the mouth wide with the tongue down.

Mother: Works with baby, presenting the portion of her breast below the nipple.

Baby: "Scoops" the breast in over the tongue, using deep jaw movement and suction.

Mother: Brings baby fully onto the breast.

Baby: Forms a vacuum, which fixes the breast in the mouth until he releases it at the end of the feed; breast tissue touches virtually all surfaces in the baby's mouth, stimulating further suckling.

Mother: Makes small adjustments for her own comfort and for her baby's apparent comfort.

This completely baby-led breastfeeding conversation is unnecessarily time-consuming once mother and baby are familiar with their roles. Even during the learning phase, the mother may need or want to direct the conversation a bit, either to interject a phrase that the baby seems to be hesitating over, or simply to skip much of the opening dialogue. As the mother and baby gain skill, either one may initiate the conversation, but it is the mother—lifting her shirt and putting her baby smoothly and absent-mindedly to breast—who determines just when attachment occurs.

The Quick Breastfeeding Conversation: Mother-Sped Self-Attachment

When a mother wishes or needs to take the lead in dialogues with her baby, the most important thing you can teach her is how to continue to stimulate, observe, and work with her infant's instinctive feeding abilities and responses. Mother-led self-attachment represents a continuum from the mother simply *wanting* to speed up the natural easy process by bringing the baby directly to breast, to her *having* to step in and take a more active role, when circumstances require some help from the mother for the baby to put his natural process into action. This can occur when there are such physical factors as a mother with very large breasts or a baby with a very receding chin. Long ago, a mother could have learned from the women of her community how to cope with a range of physical variations. Today, she may need to cope not only with physical variations but with a baby whose responses are temporarily altered by birth interventions, or even with infant psychological factors, such as a baby whose head has been forced toward the breast repeatedly.

If her baby needs assistance, here is one effective mother-sped breastfeeding technique, described as if the baby will be feeding at the mother's left breast. As with all techniques, its effectiveness for a given mother and baby is judged by only two criteria: the comfort mother and baby experience during attachment and feeding, and the efficiency with which the baby removes the milk.

Mother-Sped Technique

To start, the mother uses one hand to support the baby's back and shoulders. His head rests on her left wrist or, if she uses her right hand to support him, his skull base rests in the webbing between her right thumb and forefinger. She checks to see that his chest is snuggled into the base of her breast so that as he lifts his head in the instinctive position, he looks "up the mountain" toward her nipple. His body will generally be angled down, so that gravity helps him maintain midline stability; his hip may rest on her thigh. The mother then places the tip of her free finger or thumb just above her nipple, running parallel to her baby's upper lip. This will position her nipple above baby's top lip, opposite baby's nose; it also will flatten the top of her breast; and will tilt or lift her nipple so that she offers the baby the breast below the nipple first (see **Figures 5-4** and **5-5**).

In response to his stable hold with the nipple above his top lip, the baby assumes the instinctive feeding position, his bottom lip well under the breast. The farther the bottom lip is under the breast, the bigger the mouthful the baby will ultimately take and the farther back the nipple will go in the baby's mouth. Because her top finger is very close to the base of her nipple, she can use that finger, if needed, to help guide the portion of breast that is below the nipple into the baby's mouth as she brings him onto the breast. The key is to encourage the baby to take a large portion of *breast* into his mouth. The nipple is attached; it will follow!

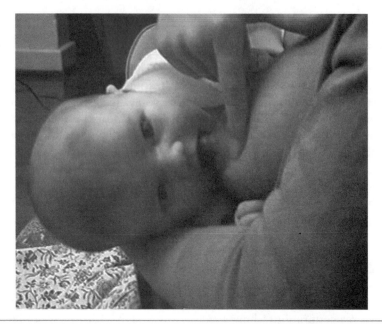

Figure 5-4   Mother using index finger of opposite hand to keep nipple above baby's top lip.

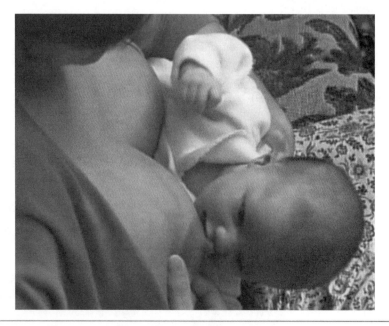

Figure 5-5   Mother using thumb to keep nipple above baby's top lip.

The baby's wide mouth is the mother's cue to hug the baby's shoulders quickly and firmly into closer contact with her body. The baby's bottom lip, jaw, and chin then sink into the breast, making it possible for the baby to scoop the breast into his mouth and sweep his mandible closed on a good mouthful of breast. As the baby scoops the breast into his mouth, the nipple brushes or folds under baby's top lip and rolls back near the junction of the hard and soft palate. Remember that it is how the infant *feels* his environment that matters; he responds to the tactile cues in this conversation, not to the visual ones. The mother's guiding finger near the nipple is of less importance than the stable position in which she holds him and the hug that helps him to complete his mouthful.

Most mothers eventually hold the baby with the arm on the same side as the breast. They may briefly shape the breast between the index and middle fingers, or middle and fourth fingers of the opposite hand. Using the opposite hand allows a mother to shape her breast without inserting her arm between her baby and herself. This "scissor hold" and its more subtle variations appear in artwork and statuary across cultures and through time.

Once the baby has attached to the breast, the mother can use either or both hands to support him against her, focusing on his shoulder girdle. Because the baby's body is typically angled down, rather than lying straight across the mother, his hip may rest on the seated mother's thigh. Because of her close hold—baby held *against* her comfortably seated body rather than hanging *from* her hunched torso—most of the remainder of his weight is distributed on her body. Her arms and shoulders are in a relaxed position (see **Figure 5-6**).

Figure 5-6
A relaxed hold; mother's torso helping to support baby's weight.

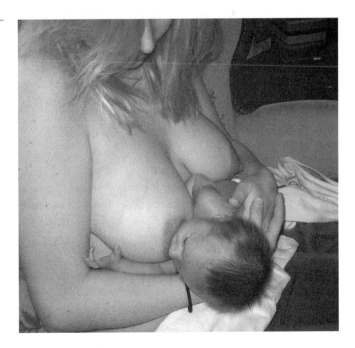

These variations are simple conversations that develop most readily if the baby is born alert and unmedicated, and is kept in skin contact with his mother. They are simple conversations that develop most readily if the mother has already watched many other mothers and babies initiate attachment. However, because this normal birth and breastfeeding continuum so seldom happens today, a translator is often needed—someone with a much larger vocabulary than either baby or mother, someone who can introduce the right word or phrase at the right moment for mother or baby, to help them continue to focus on their simple conversation together.

Stepping in to Translate: When Mother or Baby Loses the Conversational Thread

When nipple pain or poor milk transfer is a result of simple "miscommunication," our first approach as translators is to review the mother's and baby's basic grammar. The most common miscommunications seem to relate to our history of bottle feeding, and of wearing bras that lift the breasts from their natural position.

- The new mother often holds the baby too far to the side of her body, in imitation of the familiar sunny side up, crook of the elbow bottle-feeding hold that keeps the unnecessary breast away from the baby's face. Using a bottle-feeding hold for breastfeeding results in having the nipple well below the baby's upper lip instead of above it, so that the baby must tuck his chin to reach it. Moving him toward midline and providing good chest contact and stability can change an apathetic feeder to an eager one.

- The mother may focus on supporting the baby's head and bottom, curling the baby into a comma with his head in the crook of the arm and her hand supporting his bottom, and creating a gap between their bodies. Often, simply closing the gap and focusing on stabilizing his shoulder girdle will move a baby abruptly from fretfulness to breast-seeking and gaping, especially if his lower face is touched to the breast as a tactile reminder to him.

- She may feel that her nipple should be in front of her baby's mouth. This causes him to tuck his chin and drop his lower jaw away from the breast, rather than tipping his head back, lifting his chin into her breast, and "looking up the mountain." Help her to focus on having the breast below the nipple become the mouthful. Keep the baby close enough for the nipple to rest above his top lip so that his bottom lip and chin make firm contact with the breast below the nipple. Chin and lower lip contact with the breast help stimulate the baby to extend his head and gape.

- She may have been told to hold the baby's neck tightly or to push on the baby's head when he gapes. Pushing on the back of the head not only upsets the baby, it pushes his chin toward his chest, preventing normal head extension.

- Perhaps because a bra lifts both breasts unnaturally high, women in this culture tend to want to lift the breast from its normal position, when it has been released from the bra for feeding. Having done so, often using a hold that creates a poorly aligned "sandwich" for the baby, they must then lift the baby to match the lifted breast, and they find themselves unable to release their hold on the breast until the end of the feed. Breastfeeding pillows tend to encourage this unnecessarily high placement of breast and baby, and are usually both undesirable and unnecessary. Starting the feed where the nipple is—which is surprisingly low for many women—can give the mother a free hand and a much more comfortable feeding.

Variations on the above miscommunications between mother and baby account for most of the attachment difficulties that are not baby-based. Physical anomalies that can interfere with attachment are discussed elsewhere in this book. Within every mammalian species, however, there are normal variations of shape and size. Physical variations are less likely to be a problem when positioning supports a baby's natural abilities.

Even if the mother "speaks clearly" to her healthy, full-term infant, the baby may not "hear clearly."

- The baby's instincts and abilities may have been blunted by birth medications and procedures, so that he is temporarily unable to respond normally.
- Early feeding from an alternative sucking source—typically a bottle or finger—may have taught him where and how to expect food. When the breast does not deliver food in the same manner, he may reject it as a reliable food source.
- A seriously underfed baby may lack the energy to breastfeed normally until he approaches his expected place on the growth curve.

The mother spending all or much of each day in skin contact with her baby is one of the fastest, most pleasurable routes toward improved breastfeeding. In addition, if a baby's instinctive responses are not working well or need to be reawakened, the mother can help by bringing her baby to the breast in the instinctive feeding position, positioning the chin and bottom lip deep below the nipple, and finally using the top finger to help guide the breast below the nipple into baby's mouth as she brings baby quickly and firmly onto the breast. These steps are simply those that have been discussed previously, and will help many mothers and babies achieve comfortable, effective latches.

However, many babies may already have spent their early hours, days, or weeks failing to latch. They come to us with a history of poor communication. Presented here is a series of options to consider, from the straightforward to the more interventionist, in assisting a mother and baby with attachment for breastfeeding.

Conversation Starters: When a Baby from 1 Week to 3 Months Does Not Latch

Baby-Led Self-Attachment

The mother sits, topless, holding her topless baby vertically between her breasts and following her baby's lead. The healthy baby *will*, if he is hungry but calm, move toward a breast.

The mother assists him by keeping his chest and body in firm contact with her body and, once he starts to move, gently shifting his hips and legs under the opposite breast. If he begins to fuss, she checks to make sure his chest is in good contact with her. If he continues to fuss, she can arrange for some part of her breast to touch his lower face as a reminder to him, or, if fussing continues, bring him back to vertical, calm him, and let him begin again. As he latches, she may want to give his back and shoulders an extra (but gentle) hug, to help him bring his mouth deeply onto the breast, and make any adjustments that seem appropriate to her. Christina Smillie discusses this approach further in Chapter 4.

Key concepts for this approach:

- *Offer the baby a normal experience:* He needs good physical contact, good positional support, and a large mouthful of breast. With a normalized experience, other interventions are often unnecessary (Bovey, Noble, & Noble, 1999).

- *Positional stability:* The baby is much more likely to seek the breast, attach, and suckle if he begins from a stable position and maintains ventral contact with his mother. If a gap occurs between his torso and his mother's, the baby will not receive the sensory information and stability he needs to continue his innate behavior. He may lose focus or become tense.

- *Focus on the baby's back and shoulders:* The mother's hand and wrist should support his back and shoulders, with his head allowed to fall back off her wrist or fingers. Gravity can assist in stabilizing him, if he is angled down rather than across her. Depending on the height of her nipple above her lap, her second hand may give secondary support to his hip, or his hip may rest on her thigh (see **Figure 5-7**).

- *Babies expect to reach for the nipple:* Some babies will have learned to reach down, rather than up, for the nipple. If the mother keeps her nipple above his top lip, rather than chasing his mouth with it, he will begin to look for it above him. Rushing him or trying to bring the nipple to his mouth may confuse him.

- *Babies cannot go backwards:* If the baby, in his eagerness, "overshoots" the nipple, the mother can bring him back toward her midline so that he can try again.

- *No head pushing:* Pushing on the baby's head is *never* helpful!

- *Babies rely on touch and smell, not sight:* If he loses his focus, touching his lower face to the breast often refocuses him. Visual cues are not enough.

- *Leaning forward creates instability:* The mother who leans forward will cause her nipples to point downward, her breast to jiggle, and her baby to lose solid contact with her body. With good lumbar support she can settle into a comfortable upright position and the baby becomes stable against her body, much of his weight is transferred to her torso, and she creates more space below her breasts, allowing his body to angle down toward her lap.

Figure 5-7
Conversation starters 1: baby-led self-attachment, baby's hip rests on mother's thigh.

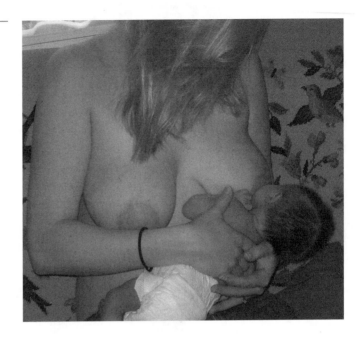

Baby-Led with Mother Standing

This approach is the same as above, but the mother stands up. Standing can help remind her to hold her baby against her rather than relying on her lap. She will tend automatically to focus on holding the baby's back and shoulders, supporting the rest of his body secondarily but generally maintaining a straight midline for him (see **Figure 5-8**). She may achieve a more relaxed, spontaneous hold standing than she is able to achieve while sitting.

Key concepts for this approach:

- *See the key concepts for the previous section:* With the mom standing, these concepts may come more naturally; she focuses on keeping him from falling instead of focusing on the actual attachment.

- *Keep baby stabilized; no gaps:* This is an old line by now, but worth repeating.

- *Avoid the unhelpful hitch:* If the mother holds her baby with the arm opposite the breast she plans to use, she may hitch his bottom up under her arm. Tucking the baby's bottom up under the mother's forearm transfers the emphasis to holding his bottom against her body, instead of holding baby's chest and shoulders against her chest and breast. Try it; you can't do both at the same time. When other higher primates feed their babies, they usually hold the baby more vertically

Figure 5-8
Conversation starters 2:
baby-led self-attachment,
mother standing.

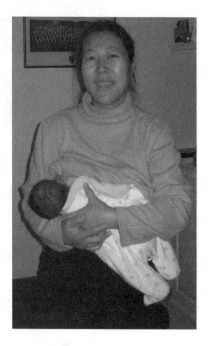

than horizontally. One of the most helpful hints you can give a mother who is having some attachment difficulty is to let her baby's body drop more vertically, to let gravity help keep his body in alignment so that she can focus on his back and shoulders. Standing allows her to do so without the complications of a lap.

- *Add the baby bounce:* Some mothers have found it helpful to add a gentle bounce to the standing approach. Walking while breastfeeding is a common way to end a "nursing strike," and the same distraction technique may be helpful in some cases of reluctant latching.

Baby-Led with Nipple-Tilting By Mother

This is probably the single most effective technique to use in helping a normal infant who has not had successful experiences at breast and who now shows breast aversion. It proceeds exactly like the previous two methods. The mother may be either sitting or standing, but she provides a little latching "boost" for the baby, as described in the "mother-sped conversation" earlier in the chapter. Using the tip of a finger or thumb placed just above her nipple and running parallel to her baby's lips she can tilt or lift her nipple to position it above baby's top lip, opposite baby's nose, and offer the breast below the nipple towards baby (see **Figure 5-9**). The baby will lift his chin and mouth, tilting his head back to open his mouth wide and positioning his bottom lip, jaw, and chin well under the breast. Positioned thus, a mother can assist the innate conversation and help her baby to latch deeply by

Figure 5-9
Conversation starters 3: mother tilts the nipple to keep it above baby's top lip; baby lifts his chin and mouth to take a good mouthful of breast below the nipple.

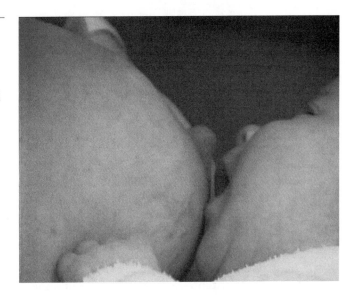

"catching" a good amount of breast below the nipple and then using her finger or thumb to "feed" the breast into her baby's mouth as she hugs baby's shoulders closer, bringing baby's chin, bottom lip, and mouth onto the breast. The aim is to fill baby's mouth with breast to maximize oral sensory input which is "[t]he least invasive means of applying appropriate orofacial stimuli" for infants with suck problems (Bovey et al., 1999, p. 26).

Key concepts for this approach:

- *The lower lip lands first and far:* The farther the bottom lip is under the breast the bigger the mouthful baby will be able to take and the farther back the nipple will go in baby's mouth. Expect the baby's lower lip to land at least 4 cm from the tip of the nipple.

- *Follow baby's cues and wait for the widest open mouth:* It is worth waiting for that wide mouth. The mother may notice that there seems to be a moment for the baby when he suddenly understands and offers an animated, searching mouth, perhaps with a brief and subtle head shake—not of confusion but of eagerness.

- *With baby's mouth open wide, hug him extra close:* This involves a *clear* ("Now, dear") push between baby's shoulder blades, to bring the baby deeply onto the breast—chest, chin, and mouth forward, head tilted back—and to ensure that baby's bottom lip and chin sink into the breast first. The nipple is attached; it will follow.

- *She who hesitates is lost:* How big a mouthful the baby takes depends on how wide the baby's mouth is when his lips close on the breast. Wherever the lips touch the breast, *all* the breast and nipple tissue between the lips goes into baby's mouth. If the mother holds the baby too far from the breast or hesitates at the crucial moment, the baby will have begun to close his mouth before his lips reach the breast and he will take a smaller portion of breast into the mouth. A too-small mouthful is not only likely to be painful, but may not stimulate the baby to begin sucking.

- *Move baby to breast, not breast to baby:* If the mother tries to put the nipple in the baby's mouth first, the bottom lip usually slides up toward the nipple and attachment will be shallow and painful.
- *Avoid moving the baby to cover the nipple:* This has the effect of sliding the bottom lip and chin toward the nipple, resulting in shallow, painful attachment.
- *Avoid moving the breast toward the baby's mouth:* You may see a mother pushing her breast toward her cleavage and her baby in the opposite direction, with frustrating results for both. Even when a baby needs help to attach well, any movement of the breast into the mouth must be secondary to the bottom lip and chin sinking firmly into the breast.
- *The breast can nonetheless help to "catch" the mouth and hold it open:* The idea is not to put the breast into the baby's mouth, but rather to catch the lower lip of the baby's open mouth with that portion of breast below the nipple, holding his mouth open fractionally longer as the baby is brought onto the breast.

Try this sitting or standing, whichever seems to work better.

Mother-Led with Exaggerated Breast-Shaping

This may be useful for the baby who does not respond normally to the assistance offered above. The baby starts, skin-to-skin, upright between his mother's breasts as above. As he approaches the breast, she uses one hand to help "narrow the sandwich" for him, tilting the nipple as above but also using that hand to shape the entire breast. One digit presses near the base of the nipple, parallel to the baby's lips; the rest of her fingers create a "sandwich" shape—an oval that also runs parallel to the baby's lips (see **Figure 5-10**). These lower-jaw fingers must be far from the nipple—usually well off the areola and perhaps even kept as far away as the breastbone. The mother may find this works best if she shapes her left breast with her left hand, or right breast with her right hand. The hand comes from below the breast in this case, not from above.

Key concepts for this approach:

- *The lower jaw needs ample room:* If the mother's fingers are anywhere near where the baby's jaw needs to land, the latch will be shallow. It is much better to have those fingers too far away than to have them too close. Fingers may be very close to the upper lip, but not to the lower lip.
- *Shape the breast rather than supporting it:* For most mother-baby pairs, the mother need only shape the breast. If she also lifts it from its normal position, she will

Figure 5-10
Conversation starters 4: mother-led with exaggerated breast shaping.

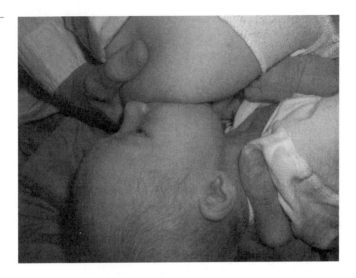

find she must continue to hold it throughout the feed; releasing it will cause it to drop out of the baby's mouth. If, however, she simply shapes it where it rests naturally, after the baby begins active suckling she can slowly relax and remove her hand, provided she makes sure that the baby moves closer to her body as her breast eases toward her. Some babies will require that the breast be held throughout the feed, in order for them to maintain an adequate mouthful. A long-breasted woman with downward-pointing nipples may need to lift her breast for effective positioning.

- *Present the breast, not the nipple, to the baby:* As always, the nipple should be tilted away from the baby's mouth, toward his nose, so that it is the last part of the breast to enter his mouth. If the nipple is presented directly to his mouth, he will probably respond with forward-reaching lips rather than with a wide-angled mouth. Shaping the breast also firms it, increasing sensory input to the baby and preventing the breast and nipple from slipping away from the baby if he needs time to investigate before attaching. See all of the suggestions for previous approaches.

Side-Lying

The mother lies on her side on a firm mattress (not a waterbed). She makes herself comfortable and balanced, rolling neither toward her front nor toward her back. She lifts her lower breast and sets it back down on the bed, so that her nipple is a "baby's cheek height" above the mattress. She rolls the baby onto his side, facing her, and moves him toward the foot of the bed so that his lower shoulder is below her breast, probably with her nipple near his eye. In this position, if he rocks his head back, his mouth will usually reach her nipple nicely (see **Figure 5-11**). When he rocks back, gapes, and covers her nipple, she presses the middle of his back in slightly more to help him finish the latch. His body will usually arch slightly backward and he will be looking up at his mother's face as he latches.

Key concepts for this approach:

- *Active babies move upward:* A baby cannot move back down the bed on his own. Unless he latches fairly quickly, the mother may find that he has crawled up past her nipple. She can pull him back down for another try. She may need to do this several times.

- *Support the middle of his back, not his shoulders:* In this side-lying position, the baby is reasonably stable without maternal support. Pressing his shoulders toward her may cause his face to burrow into the breast instead of encouraging the instinctive feeding position. Pressing the middle of his back toward her tends to encourage a slight arch, with head extended.

- *Tilting the nipple and shaping the breast may be helpful, but remember the angle:* The mother is now sideways, and so is the baby's mouth. The "breast sandwich," if it is used, should run floor to ceiling in order to run parallel to the baby's lips.

- *Catch the lower lip if needed:* Occasionally, it may be helpful not only to shape the sandwich and tilt the nipple, but also to catch the lower lip of the open mouth with the breast, helping the nipple to brush or fold under the baby's upper lip at the end and bringing the middle of the baby's back closer as he attaches.

- *Respect some babies' need for distance:* One of the advantages of lying down is that it allows the infant both stability and space. The infant who has had his head forced into the breast repeatedly or who has been otherwise traumatized at breast may prefer some distance between himself and his mother at first. Depending on her breast size, she may be able to achieve comfortable positioning with the baby some distance from her torso. There is no need to bring him closer if he prefers this arrangement.

Figure 5-11
Conversation starters 5:
side-lying attachment,
in this case using upper
breast.

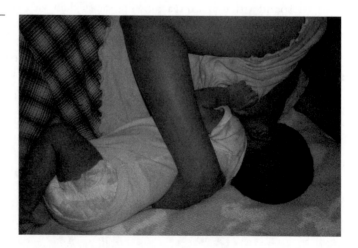

- *Fast milk flow is handled more easily by a baby with an extended head:* A large mouthful of breast and a slightly extended head can help the baby cope with fast milk flow. One of the reasons a baby may be wary of an in-arms breastfeeding position is that he has tried to cope with a rapid milk flow with his chin slightly tucked. As in all the options presented in this section, the instinctive feeding position makes both latching and swallowing easier.

Mother-Led with Baby's Body at an Angle to Mother's

If the baby has a painful neck or shoulder, if the mother has been stretching his lower arm too far around her breast, or if the mother has large or heavy breasts, mother and baby may do better with a technique used by Barbara Wilson-Clay (see **Figure 5–12**):

> Begin with the infant cradled in a supine position. Draw the infant's lower shoulder and lower hip under mother's breasts, against her rib cage, before slightly rotating the baby's body towards the mother. The mother's arms securely support the baby. The baby's body becomes a shelf that supports the weight of the breasts. The baby's upper shoulder and hip will angle away from the mother. Their two bodies touch along the edges like the side of a relaxed, open V. In side-lying position, the lower shoulder is placed up against the rib cage under the breast, and the lower hip is placed under the "over-hang" of the mother's belly. The mother uses her hand placed on the baby's back to rotate the baby just slightly towards her body. Their bodies touch along their edges and their body positions mirror each other. Rather than looking like two parallel lines (unstable knife blades on edge) both are three-quarters on their backs. This is very relaxed, and if either falls asleep, they roll onto their backs, which is safest for the baby. (Wilson-Clay, personal communication, 2006)

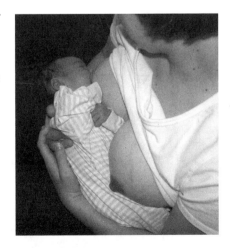

Figure 5-12
Conversation starters 6: baby's body angled away from mother's, in this case with mother sitting up. Note baby's lower arm across his body rather than hugging the breast.

Key concept for this approach:

- *Bringing one of baby's hands to midline brings both to midline:* Angling the baby against the mother, with the baby's arms on his chest, reduces stress to the baby's arms and shoulders. The baby's arm is essentially positioned at mid-line by the weight of the breast on the lower shoulder. This helps to calm frantic arm movement. If one arm is comfortably positioned in the center of the baby's torso, the other arm will seek it, creating a flexed shoulder position that is not stressful for the baby. Once the positioning feels secure to both mother and baby, the baby can concentrate on latching. (Wilson-Clay, personal correspondence, 2006)

Supporting Breast and Baby When Breasts Are Large or Heavy

Some breasts are so long that there is little room for the baby beneath them. The nipple may point down, which means stabilizing the baby's chest against the mother's body puts the baby in the wrong place. The mother lifts her breast and rests it on the baby's chest. She does not lift her breast so high that its full weight falls on the baby in her arms, but high enough that the baby's support prevents breast movement. This closes the gap between baby and breast. If the mother's breast is especially long or if she cannot see her nipple, she can use the palm of one hand above her breast to lift and hold the entire breast and angle the nipple slightly more forward (**Figure 5-13**).

Key concepts for this approach:

- *Baby supports the breast like an "underwire bra":* The mother may, over the course of several feeds, begin to lower the baby, forgetting that the baby is her breast's support. It may help her to think in terms of breast support.

Figure 5-13
Conversation starters 7: supporting breast and baby when breasts are large, long, or heavy, using one hand to lift breast slightly from above.

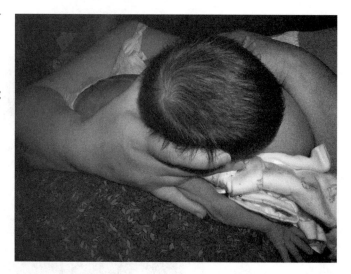

- *The breast supports the baby:* The baby's stability comes not from her torso but from the breast itself. Remember, babies can feel secure in any position, provided they have firm pressure on their ventrum and midline stability. Because breast and baby become a unit, the breast is less likely to slip from the baby's mouth.

Choosing a Technique

There is no immutable order to these approaches, and not every approach makes sense for every mother and baby. If you know that the baby has had numerous bad experiences at breast, you might want to move straight to lying down, so that he has a completely new experience from the start. If you know that the baby has developed an aversion to the breast, you might want to encourage a few days or a week of shared skin and an alternate feeding method before going further. If you know that others have tried without success to help a mother and baby, you might move more quickly to an artificial aid—perhaps one of the ones described in the next section.

The mother's instincts and her sensitivity to her baby are the best guides in knowing when and even whether to offer the breast. Follow her lead as she follows her baby's lead. Sometimes an office visit is simply ill-timed. If mother and baby are not likely to "converse" well, use the session to describe and demonstrate techniques she can use at home when she feels her baby is interested, offer encouragement, and express confidence in the baby's innate abilities. One mother reported that there came a day when "my baby just looked different to me," and breastfeeding proceeded uneventfully from that point. We can suggest "conversation starters," but it is the mother and baby who must gauge each other's moods and begin talking.

When Technique Is Not Enough

Jumping through a fiery hoop is an unnatural act for a tiger, yet he can be encouraged to do so by a combination of patience, mutual trust, technique . . . and tools. Breastfeeding is an entirely natural act for a baby. When patience, trust, and technique are insufficient to help a normal baby breastfeed, there are some tools that may be helpful.

Dripped Enticement

Simply dribbling a bit of sterile water, expressed colostrum, or milk on the nipple with an eyedropper or syringe can sometimes encourage a baby to begin licking, tasting, and showing interest. Tucking a dropper, syringe, or periodontal syringe into the corner of the baby's mouth after an unenthusiastic latch, and adding a few drops of milk, may cause him to swallow, draw in a bit more breast, and perhaps begin sucking. If he is truly hungry, however, he may need to take in significant calories before he is able to breastfeed effectively.

Reverse Pressure Softening

Initial engorgement can make it difficult for a baby to attach. One of the best tools in this situation is the mother's own fingers. All five fingertips of one hand can be pressed around the base of her nipple for approximately a minute, or about as long as it takes her to hum a lullaby. The pressure moves fluids more deeply into the breast, softening and indenting the area that the baby needs for attachment just as a fingertip pressed into any other tissue with pitting edema creates a soft, temporary dent. The mother can also press with the sides of two or more fingers, perhaps laying an index finger at the nipple base where the baby's upper lip will be, and two fingers from the opposite hand where his lower jaw will land, fingers running parallel to where his lips will be (Cotterman, 2004).

Inverted Syringe

Necessity is the mother of invention. An Indian physician wanted a quick, inexpensive aid for babies who were unable to attach to inverted nipples. He chose a syringe whose diameter was roughly the same as the mother's nipple diameter, removed the piston, and cut off the needle. He then slid the piston into the cut end, so that he had a small suction device with a smooth open end. The mother places the smooth end over her nipple, and draws back the piston until her nipple everts, but not so far that she causes discomfort. If the syringe loses suction because it fills with milk, she simply withdraws the piston further. After about a minute, she releases the suction by depressing the piston, and offers her breast to the baby before the nipple inverts. Most babies who require this temporary aid learn quickly to attach to their mothers' less-than-prominent nipples without preliminaries (Kesaree, 1993). A commercial version of this device is sold in the United States under the name Evert-it.

Bottle Feeding as a Prelude to Offering the Breast

The baby may be more receptive to breastfeeding if he has taken at least part of a meal first. If the mother likes, the bottle can be tucked under her arm so that the baby can be held against her as if for breastfeeding, with the bottle teat close to her own. Another way to feed the baby and offer breastfeeding practice at the same time is to alternate between the two, as described in the following section.

Bait and Switch

The mother holds the baby as if for breastfeeding, but in such a way that she can also offer a bottle. Holding the bottle under her arm is one such position. Holding him along her side, with him looking up at her, is another. She offers several swallows from the bottle, then quickly removes the bottle and offers her breast. Most likely he will refuse. She immediately offers several more swallows from the bottle, then offers the breast again. After several such back-and-forth offerings, the baby may have gained enough energy and interest to attach to the breast and begin feeding. The shorter the time between removing the bottle and offering the breast, the more likely the baby is to shift his suckling behavior to the breast. In the end, even if he does not attach to the breast, the baby will have been fed. For a full discussion and photos of paced bottle-feeding technique, see Chapter 11.

Nipple Shield

The human nipple is soft, is sometimes very short or attached to a very firm breast, and tends to retreat from a baby if he mouths it before latching. In contrast, a nipple shield stays very assertively *there,* allowing the baby to feel it, play with it, grasp it correctly or incorrectly, even push it away with his tongue. Its unchanging shape can make it a very helpful "bridging tool" for the baby who is suspicious of the breast, who is accustomed to a bottle teat, or who has decided that there is no reason to try. Premature infants may actually increase their milk intake with the help of a shield; it keeps the mother's nipple from sliding away from a weaker baby with thinner buccal fat pads during the pauses between suckling bursts (Meier et al., 2000).

Modern silicone nipple shields have a stiff nipple section and very soft rim. They come in several nipple diameters and nipple lengths. Although the nipple shield chosen needs to accommodate the mother's nipple comfortably, it must also match the infant's palate length. Barbara Wilson-Clay and Kay Hoover (2005) suggest selecting the shield with the shortest possible nipple length and smallest possible diameter at the nipple base. When a baby latches deeply onto a well-fitted shield, the thin and flexible rim usually allows him to milk the breast with near-normal efficiency. This level of efficiency was not possible with the old latex shields.

To attach the shield, the mother can grasp the rim of the shield between thumb and fingers, with fingers curled at the base of the nipple section, nipple facing away from her. She stretches the base of the teat open as if she is trying to turn the teat inside out, and brings the lower edge of the nipple section onto the breast, beginning well below her own nipple and stretching the shield over the nipple, centering the shield's nipple over her own. This brings a good portion of her breast and nipple into the shield, with slightly more tissue below her nipple, helping to ensure that her baby will take more breast into the mouth with the shield. Because the base of the nipple section has been stretched onto the breast it grips the breast and is not readily dislodged. The mother brings the baby onto the breast and shield, with his head tilted back and mouth open wide. As his bottom lip and chin sink into the rim of the shield, well below the nipple, his top lip will glide over the upper surface of the shield's nipple section, facilitating a deep asymmetrical latch. A baby who is able to attach well can take a truly effective mouthful of breast and suckle almost as if the nipple shield does not exist.

Some nipple shields have a portion of the rim cut away to remove any barrier between the baby's nose and the mother's skin. They can be difficult to apply to the breast using the method previously described. An alternate approach with either type of shield is for the mother to hold the shield on opposite sides at the outside edge using the thumb and index finger of each hand, nipple section facing away from her. With her middle fingers, she gently applies pressure to the tip of the shield's nipple portion until it begins to collapse, pushing until the nipple section is just a little longer than her own nipple. She places the partially inverted shield over her nipple, the rim curling away from her breast. Using the first two fingers from each hand, she slides the backs of her fingernails down the slope of the shield's nipple. When her fingertips touch the bottom of the "moat" around it and the pads of her fingers touch the outer edge of the "moat," she stops sliding her fingernails and uses the pads of her fingers to stretch the "moat" out onto the areola. Her nipple tip is drawn into the shield as the "moat" disappears (Pohl, personal communication, 2006).

The shield's rim may curl over the baby's nose while he feeds; this is merely a cosmetic issue. The nipple section stays in the baby's mouth and the rim will not interfere with the baby's breathing. If the baby repeatedly dislodges the shield, a piece of tape along the upper edge can help to hold it in place. Moistening the underside may also help it to adhere.

As with most breastfeeding tools, breastfeeding specialists are still discovering ways to use a nipple shield. The cut-away style, for instance, can be positioned with the cut-out portion at the side, rotated 90 degrees from the suggested position, giving the mother more room to hold the shield on the opposite side, as the baby comes to breast (Shenk, personal communication, 2006). Different practitioners prefer different sizes, and have different approaches for choosing the best size. It matters only that both mother and baby are comfortable and that milk transfer is effective.

At times, a baby's inability to breastfeed effectively with a shield simply mirrors his inability to breastfeed effectively without it; these mother-baby pairs will need additional support in the form of milk expression and an alternate feeding method. However, the nipple shield has helped many babies learn to latch and to associate the breast with food, and often gives the mother of a nonlatching baby a way to enjoy her baby at breast while they learn to breastfeed.

Most babies relinquish the shield without difficulty once they gain some competence and confidence; an occasional baby continues to rely on a nipple shield for months or, rarely, for the duration of the breastfeeding relationship. Breastfeeding with a shield is still breastfeeding. Until a baby using a shield has demonstrated a normal feeding pattern and normal pattern of weight gain, his progress should be followed closely. Babies can use a nipple shield ineffectively, spending long periods of time at breast without significant intake.

Pillow

Pillows can cause breastfeeding problems as well as solve them. Pillows are not helpful if they raise the baby above the natural level of the mother's nipple, create a crevice into which the baby rolls, force the baby's body to lie across the other breast instead of below it, or allow the baby's body to drift away from the mother's. However, a firm, flat pillow can be very helpful to a mother who must breastfeed two babies simultaneously, and it can allow some distance for the baby who resists close contact. It can serve as a "bait and switch" platform, perhaps even with a nipple shield in place so that the baby can approach the breast with only the lightest maternal touch, allowing him to explore the shield at will.

Feeding Tube

Although feeding tubes are normally used to supplement a baby who latches, they can occasionally help a baby attach to a very flat-nippled breast, by providing a focal point for his efforts. Held or taped so that the tubing runs along the underside of the breast (on top of the baby's tongue when he is suckling) and extending slightly beyond the nipple tip, the added stimulus can make a nearly featureless breast less confusing. Beware of letting a baby learn to suck on the tube, rather than the tube helping baby to learn to attach and suckle effectively at the breast. Unless an anomaly of mother or baby prevents normal breastfeeding, keep in mind that the goal is normalization. Any at-breast aid like a feeding tube or nipple shield can allow suboptimal breastfeeding behavior to masquerade as normal. Maximizing normal interactions with the mother's body and breast is more desirable and more effective than allowing a baby to suckle ineffectively and indefinitely on an appliance.

Conclusion

When any fluid act is broken into discrete components—when a right-brained, "body sense" activity like dancing, tennis, walking, or bicycling is taught in left-brained steps—fluidity is lost and instinct bows to instruction. And yet many of the lessons we have learned from our decades of disruptive, left-brained breastfeeding analysis can serve certain mothers and babies. As translators, we now have a much greater vocabulary than before. Our new job is to learn when it is *not* needed. If we can facilitate the smooth, instinctive, right-brained process with little more than a nudge or a better presentation of the breast, most of the time we can drop into the background of a conversation in which we do not rightly belong.

When aids are used, remind the mother that the basics are still of primary importance and ensure that any lactation aid used will help to move the mother and infant toward normal and effective breastfeeding.

Encourage her to begin as many feeds as possible with skin-to-skin time, using artificial aids as supports when needed. Learning to breastfeed can take time. Simply encouraging the mother to enjoy ample skin-to-skin time with her baby and to follow her baby's lead are the most important steps of all. With time, with repeated positive experiences, and with a mother who respects and works with the baby's innate abilities, the great majority of normal babies will eventually begin to feed normally.

Helping the mother of a nonlatching baby requires more than an understanding of positioning, tools, and techniques. It requires an understanding of one's own limitations and of the mother's and baby's limits for the day and for the future. It requires a knowledge of other helping resources that may be available. And it requires confidence in the breastfeeding process. This is, after all, nothing more than the normal feeding process of all mammalian infants.

It is possible to exhaust a mother and baby with attempts and experiments, so that breastfeeding fails before it begins. Instead, be ready to find more experienced help *before* the mother's emotional well runs dry. The goal is not to have the baby latch today, or to reach the bottom of one's bag of tricks, or to "be the one who made it work," but to help ensure that mother and baby will be a happy breastfeeding pair at some point in the future. Is there someone else who might help her more efficiently? Then refer the mother, go with her, and add to your skills by observing. For all our texts, tools, and techniques, the mothers and babies themselves are our best and most effective teachers.

It may be that our enlarged vocabulary will help us invent and improve breastfeeding aids. There is room for supplemental feeding tube devices that are simpler to clean, easier to use, and more durable. Nipple shields and pumps may undergo substantial redesign. No doubt simple "bridging tools" that help a baby make the transition from bottle to shield, or shield to breast, have yet to be invented. All these changes will come from an ongoing dissection of the breastfeeding process. But we know enough, now, to proceed carefully with that dissection. Our interventions can harm as easily as they can heal, and far too many mothers today find themselves pumping for months because "he just never latched."

Today we have a clearer understanding of the "cascade of events" that leads to so many stumbling or halted conversations: inadequate maternal support during and after the birth, a medicalized approach to the perinatal process, our cultural insistence on unnecessary birth medications, our desire for immediate baths for mother and baby, and most of all our failure at the simple act of putting mother and baby skin-to-skin for hours and hours and hours, so that they can talk to each other as long and as often as they like, and learn from each other as they talk.

References

Bovey, A., Noble, R., & Noble, M. (1999). Orofacial exercises for babies with breastfeeding problems. *Breastfeeding Review, 7*(1), 23–28.

Colson, S. (2002). Womb to world: A metabolic perspective. *Midwifery Today, 61,* 12–17.

Cotterman, K. J. (2004). Reverse pressure softening: A simple tool to prepare areolae for easier latching during engorgement. *Journal of Human Lactation, 20*(2), 227–237.

Freeman, G. (2000). Poor Feeders Workshop, Melbourne, Australia.

Glover, R. (2004). Lessons from innate feeding abilities transform breastfeeding outcomes. *ILCA Conference Syllabus,* Scottsdale, Arizona, p. 87.

Kesaree, N. (1993). Treatment of inverted nipples using a disposable syringe. *Journal of Human Lactation, 9*(1), 27–29.

Meier, P. P., Brown, L. P., Hurst, N. M., Spatz, D. L., Engstrom, J. L., Borucki, L. C., & Krouse, A. M. (2000). Nipple shields for preterm infants: Effect on milk transfer and duration of breastfeeding. *Journal of Human Lactation, 16*(2), 106–114; quiz 129–131.

Millar, A. J. (2002). Oral and pharyngeal reflexes in the mammalian nervous system: Their diverse range in complexity and the pivotal role of the tongue. *Critical Reviews in Oral Biology and Medicine, 13*(5), 400–425.

Morris, S. E., & Klein, M. D. (1987). *Pre-feeding skills.* San Antonio, TX: Therapy Skills Builders.

National Center for Health Statistics. (2005). *Health, United States, 2005, with chartbook on trends in the health of Americans.* Hyattsville, MD: U.S. Department of Health and Human Services.

Uvnäs-Moberg, K., & Eriksson, M. (1996). Breastfeeding: Physiological, endocrine and behavioural adaptations caused by oxytocin and local neurogenic activity in the nipple and mammary gland. *Acta Paediatrica, 84,* 525–530.

Wiessinger, D. (1998). A breastfeeding teaching tool using a sandwich analogy for latch-on. *Journal of Human Lactation, 14*(1), 51–56.

Wilson-Clay, B., & Hoover, K. (2005). *The breastfeeding atlas* (3rd ed.). Manchaca, TX: Lactnews Press.

Wolf, L. S., & Glass, R. P. (1992). *Feeding and swallowing disorders in infancy: Assessment and management.* San Antonio, TX: Therapy Skills Builders.

Woolridge, M. W. (1986). The "anatomy" of infant sucking & aetiology of sore nipples. *Midwifery, 2,* 164–176.

Chapter 6

The Goldilocks Problem: Milk Flow That Is Not Too Fast, Not Too Slow, but *Just* Right

Or, Why Milk Flow Matters and What to Do About It

Lynn S. Wolf
Robin P. Glass

Introduction

Successful breastfeeding is one of the first achievements of the newborn infant. Immediately after birth the baby is able to root, grasp the breast, and begin to suckle. The ease with which this occurs leads many to think of newborn feeding as a simple skill. Infant feeding, however, is a very complex activity that requires exquisite coordination of three foundation processes—sucking, swallowing, and breathing. The coordination of these processes, and thus the success of the baby's feeding, is easily influenced by the flow rate of the liquid the baby is ingesting. A high flow rate can lead to significant discoordination, aspiration, and/or feeding refusal. A slow flow rate might help a baby with respiratory illness return to feeding, but in another case may lead to poor weight gain. This chapter will provide an overview of sucking, swallowing, and breathing; their coordination; and how flow rate impacts the success or difficulty of breastfeeding. The assessment of flow rate during breastfeeding will be discussed, along with management of feeding problems related to flow rate.

Foundations of Infant Feeding: A Triad of Skills

Thoroughly understanding the skills that form the foundation for infant feeding provides the framework to identify feeding problems. This triad of skills includes sucking, swallowing, and breathing. It is important to have a working knowledge of each skill, and an appreciation of their coordination during infant feeding.

Sucking

This skill establishes flow rate and determines how sucking, swallowing, and breathing are coordinated. Infant sucking is organized into bursts of sucks, interspersed with pauses (**Figure 6-1**). At the beginning of a feeding, the bursts are long with infrequent and short pauses. Over the course of the feeding, the sucking bursts gradually become shorter, and pauses are longer, until at the end of the feeding the young baby is sucking occasionally with long pauses between sucks (Chetwynd, Diggle, Drewett, & Young, 1998; Mathew, Clark, Pronske, Luna-Solarzano, & Peterson, 1985). If the infant is fed on both breasts (paired feeding) this pattern is typically repeated on each breast, though duration of active sucking and milk intake is typically less on the second breast (Drewett & Woolridge, 1979, 1981). Flow rate during sucking bursts will vary depending on the availability of milk in the breast and the competence and strength of the baby's suck.

During nutritive sucking bursts (when there is active fluid flow), infants suck at a rate of approximately one suck per second. This is in contrast to non-nutritive sucking (such as on a finger or pacifier) when the baby sucks more rapidly, at about two sucks per second (Wolff, 1968). Fluid flow is the reason for this difference. During nutritive sucking, the baby's sucking rate is slower to accommodate swallowing.

The strength of the suck is also a factor influencing flow rate. Sucking strength is developed as the baby creates two types of pressure—positive pressure, or compression, and negative pressure, or suction. The healthy term baby has some control over the type and amount of pressure that is generated (Sameroff, 1968). At the breast, the interaction of pressure components is complex. Suction is necessary for the baby to latch to the breast; to draw the breast deeply into the mouth, and to maintain latch appropriately. Once the baby is latched, we understand less about how pressure is used to release mother's milk, though there is evidence that milk flows from the human nipple when the infant exerts negative pressure (Ramsay & Hartmann, 2005). (See Chapter 1.) Although mothers can obtain milk flow through compression (manual expression) or suction (standard breast pumps), it is likely that each baby determines the relative amount of compression vs. suction to use with their own mother to create optimal milk flow. It is also likely that the mother's breast "learns" to respond to the particular characteristics of a baby's sucking pattern, modifying the milk release pattern over time. Developing synchrony between mother and baby to

NUTRITIVE SUCKING (NS)

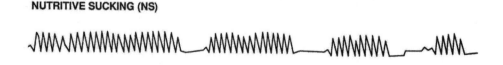

Figure 6-1   Nutritive sucking burst pause pattern.

establish functional milk flow is often one of the challenges of early breastfeeding. If abnormal oral structures or movements, or maternal factors, interfere with this process, the baby may have trouble latching, or appear to be latched yet not create adequate milk flow.

Sucking movements are seen in utero starting at 14–16 weeks, and they progressively mature in terms of pressure components and coordination. Thus sucking is immature in premature infants, especially those babies born at less than 36 weeks gestation. Lau and colleagues (Lau, Alagugurusamy, Schanler, Smith, & Shulman, 2000) have used pressure monitoring during early bottle feeding to demonstrate that in the premature infant compression develops first, though it initially lacks organization into clear sucking bursts. This compressive force begins to form rhythmic bursts around 34 weeks gestation. Suction begins to emerge at this point but is not coordinated with compression until 36–38 weeks gestation. Additionally, premature infants feeding on a bottle show an immature pattern of bursts and pauses, with shorter bursts, longer pauses, and less rhythmicity (**Figure 6-2**). Each of these factors impacts the rate of milk flow the baby is able to create. The developmental progression of these skills has important implications for the premature infant who is trying to latch and maintain latch during breastfeeding. Although maturation of feeding skills follows a fairly typical sequence, each infant will mature at his or her own rate.

Swallowing

Swallowing is a complex task involving precise timing and coordination of the many muscles within the mouth, pharynx, larynx, and esophagus, and controlled by the activity of cranial nerves. A swallow occurs when enough milk is present in the mouth to stimulate the numerous sensory receptors in the posterior oral cavity. The swallow carries milk through the pharynx, while protecting the airway, into the esophagus and stomach. In newborn infants, one nutritive suck usually produces a quantity of milk (bolus) that fills the oral cavity and initiates a swallow. This creates a suck to swallow ratio of 1:1 (Bu'Lock, Woolridge, & Baum, 1990; Weber, Woolridge, & Baum, 1986). If the flow rate is very low, more sucks will be needed to fill the oral cavity and trigger a swallow. The suck to swallow ratio might be three or more sucks to one swallow. The older infant has a larger oral cavity, so two or three normal volume sucks may be taken before a swallow is required; however, if the flow rate is very rapid the infant may need to swallow after each suck. Fluid flow is the key to determining the ratio of sucks to swallows (Mathew & Bhatia, 1989).

An important function of the swallowing process is airway protection. During initiation of swallow the soft palate elevates to close the nasal passages, and fluid flows into the pharynx by movement of the tongue. To protect the airway, the larynx then elevates, the epiglottis moves downward to cover the laryngeal opening tightly, and the vocal cords adduct (pull together). Next, the upper esophageal sphincter relaxes and the bolus moves into the esophagus. Finally, the structures return to their resting positions—the soft palate sits on the base of the tongue with nasal passages open, the epiglottis has uncovered the larynx, and the upper esophageal sphincter is closed. All of this has occurred in about 0.1 seconds (Tuchman, 1993).

Stage	Sample Tracings	Suction/Expression Amplitude Range of Tracings (mm Hg)	Description
1A and 1B	Suction	Absent	No Suction
	Expression	+0.5 to +1.0 mm Hg	Arrhythmic Expression
	Time (sec)		and
	Suction	−2.5 to −12.5 mm Hg	
	Expression	+0.5 to +1.0 mm Hg	Arrhythmic alteration Suction/Expression
2A and 2B	Suction	Absent	No Suction
	Expression	+0.2 to +0.4 mm Hg	Arrhythmic Expression
	Time (sec)		and
	Suction	−7.5 to −15.0 mm Hg	
	Expression	−+0.2 mm Hg	Arrhythmic alteration Suction/Expression
3A and 3B	Suction	Absent	No Suction
	Expression	+0.8 to +1.0	Rhythmic Expression
	Time (sec)		and
	Suction	−15 to −75	Rhythmic Suction/Expression:
	Expression	+0.5 to +0.7	• Suction amplitude increases • Wide amplitude range • Prolonged sucking bursts
4	Suction	−50 to −75	Rhythmic suction/expression
	Time (sec)		• Suction well defined • Decreased amplitude range
	Expression	+0.5 to +0.7	
5	Suction	−110 to −160	Rhythmic/well defined suction/expression
	Time (sec)		• Suction amplitude increases
	Expression	+0.6 to +0.75	• Sucking pattern similar to that of fullterm infant

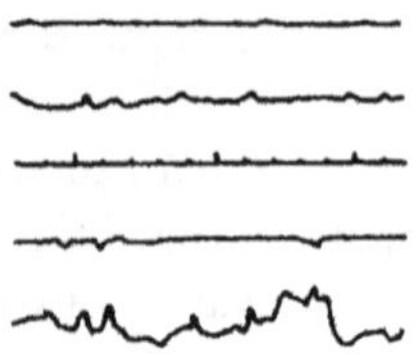

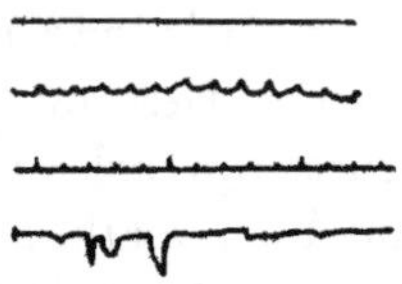

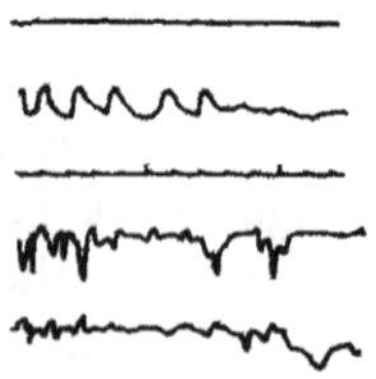

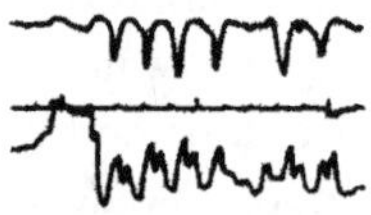

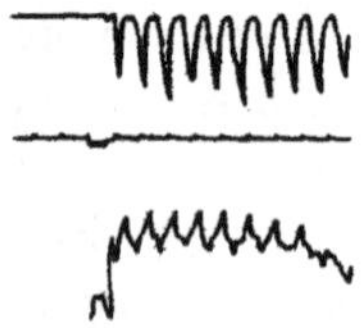

Figure 6-2 Maturation of expression and suction in premature infants.

If the airway is not fully protected during swallowing, milk can be aspirated into the lungs. This can happen before, during, or after the swallow. If timing of the initiation of swallow is delayed, milk moves into the pharynx before the airway is protected, and can then enter the airway *before* the swallow has been initiated. Once the swallow sequence has been initiated, if the airway is not fully "sealed," fluid can be aspirated *during* the swallow. If a safe swallow occurs, but food is not fully cleared from the pharynx, it can be aspirated into the airway during breathing, leading to aspiration *after* the swallow (Wolf & Glass, 1992). The amount of material aspirated can vary from occasional microaspiration to consistent frank aspiration. Some infants may cough or choke with aspiration; however, many do not. An immature infant may stop breathing and become apneic to prevent further food coming into the lungs (Mortola & Fischer, 1988). In infants of all ages, aspiration can also be silent, with no apparent external response.

Flow has an important relationship to swallowing function. If flow is very low, multiple sucks may occur before a swallow is necessary. This slower rate of swallowing also allows more time for the baby to organize the initiation of each swallow. If the bolus is very large, or moving at a very fast speed (high flow), timing of the initiation of swallow, as well as the swallow itself, may be compromised. This can lead to poor protection of the airway as the bolus passes through the pharynx, and can result in aspiration.

Breathing

Breathing is a critical process for the success of infant feeding. Although less obvious when observing feeding than sucking and swallowing, it has a strong relationship to flow rate. For the baby, feeding is "work," not unlike exercise for adults. This requires adaptability of the respiratory system. During sucking and swallowing, opportunities to breathe are reduced, so the baby must have respiratory reserve to compensate for these ventilatory reductions. The baby needs to be able to adjust the rate and depth of breathing, in order to integrate breathing into the sucking/swallowing sequence. During nutritive sucking bursts, breaths are short and less frequent. During pauses they may be more rapid and deeper (**Figure 6-3**).

NORMAL COORDINATION OF SUCKING, SWALLOWING & BREATHING

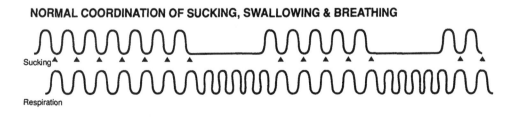

Figure 6-3   Breathing coordinated with sucking and swallowing.

Medical conditions that impact breathing affect the baby's respiratory adaptability (**Table 6-1**). Feeding problems are frequently associated with these conditions, and it is often the respiratory portion of the feeding process that underlies the problem. Flow rate plays a significant role in determining how much time the baby has available to breathe during feeding. In general, the higher the flow rate, the less time available for breathing, so the greater the respiratory challenges for the baby (Wolf & Glass, 1992). Altering the flow rate can sometimes improve feeding in babies with respiratory compromise.

Coordination of Sucking, Swallowing, and Breathing

In infants, as in adults, breathing ceases during swallowing. The pharynx is the centerpiece of this activity, serving as a conduit to move air from the nose/mouth to the lungs, and to move food from the mouth to the stomach (**Figure 6-4**). At rest the structures are arranged for breathing, and alterations are made during swallow. It is this dual role that creates the need for coordination of sucking, swallowing, and breathing, and leads to many of the challenges of infant feeding. If air moves into the stomach, the baby may be gassy. More significantly, if milk moves into the lungs, aspiration occurs, which can lead to a variety of secondary symptoms such as respiratory illness or feeding refusal.

Multiple studies confirm that during infant feeding breathing stops during each swallow. This presents a unique challenge for the infant who swallows after each suck, and must rapidly switch between swallowing and breathing. Selley and associates (Selley, Ellis, Flack, & Brooks, 1990) have depicted this clearly, showing exquisite rhythmic coordination of

TABLE 6-1 Medical Conditions Affecting Respiratory Function

Central Nervous System	Upper Airway	Lower Airway	Lung Parenchyma	Thoracic
Central apnea	Micrognathia	Respiratory distress syndrome	Collapsed lung	Diaphragmatic hernia
Periodic breathing	Choanal atresia	RSV (respiratory syncytial virus)	Pulmonary hemorrhage	Paralyzed diaphragm
Tumors	Tracheo-laryngo-malacia	Meconium aspiration	Pulmonary hypertension	Rib anomalies
HIE (hypoxic ischemic encephalopathy)	Paralyzed vocal cords	Primary alveolar collapse		Cardiac anomalies
	Hemangiomas			

Figure 6-4
Dual role of the pharynx.

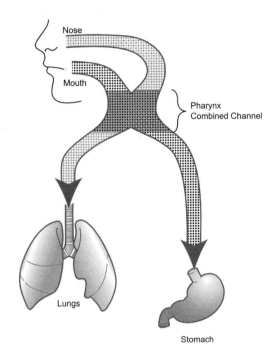

these processes for the mature newborn. While feeding, the baby sucks, stops breathing to swallow, then starts breathing again. This cycle repeats approximately once each second during the sucking burst. The need to frequently stop breathing causes the infant to draw on their respiratory reserves during sucking bursts. During a sucking pause, breaths are rapid and deep, allowing some "catch up" in breathing (see Figure 6-3). Similar to other aspects of feeding, the coordination of sucking, swallowing, and breathing shows a maturational sequence. Although term infants can have incoordination of sucking, swallowing, and breathing, it is more common in premature babies. Flow rate can have a significant effect on this process, with premature infants particularly vulnerable; this will be discussed in detail in the following section.

The Relationship Between Flow Rate and Coordination of Sucking, Swallowing, and Breathing

In addition to the sequential organization of sucking, swallowing, and breathing during infant feeding, there is also an interrelationship among these components. Each can affect the others, and thus further impact the baby's feeding performance. Flow plays an important role in these relationships. High flow, whether it is actually high or just perceived by the baby as high, can upset the delicate balance of sucking, swallowing, and breathing coordination.

Flow and the Relationship Between Swallowing and Breathing

Whether at the breast or simply managing saliva, every time the baby swallows breathing must pause momentarily. The higher the swallowing rate, the more often breathing will be interrupted. During a vigorous nutritive sucking burst, the young baby swallows after each suck, thus pausing breathing enough to lower the respiratory rate, tidal volume (size of each breath), and minute ventilation (amount of air inhaled per minute). This lowers the amount of available oxygen and leads to a slight, but measurable, decrease in oxygen saturation, even if it remains in the normal range (Mathew et al., 1985). The longer the nutritive sucking burst lasts, the greater the reductions in ventilation.

High flow leads to a higher swallowing rate and even less time for breathing. In some cases when flow is too high for the baby, swallowing will be favored and there will not be sufficient time to breathe. This results in feeding-induced apnea, which is characterized by a vigorous and rhythmic sucking burst, with swallows to clear the food, but no breathing. These apneic pauses can lead to falling oxygen saturations, bradycardia, coughing/choking, and/or lethargy (Gewolb et al., 2001). This pattern is more prevalent in premature infants but can be seen occasionally in term infants (Hanlon et al., 1997).

In other cases, high flow affects the integrity of the swallow. If the baby is swallowing rapidly there may not be time to adequately protect the airway before the bolus moves through the pharynx. This can lead to aspiration. Typically, swallowing will be followed by exhalation, possibly affording the baby some protection (Gewolb & Vice, 2006).

Flow at the breast is variable throughout the feeding. As the baby latches to the breast there is very little flow, until the mother's milk ejection reflex (MER). During the MER the flow may be steady and then flow may taper as the MER subsides. This natural reduction in flow allows the baby the opportunity to continue sucking with less frequent swallowing, thus having more time to breathe until the next MER is stimulated. Many babies with an elevated respiratory rate are most comfortable with lower flow. This variability in flow pattern during breastfeeding provides more opportunity for breathing than during bottle feeding, unless the mother's flow is excessive.

Flow and the Relationship Between Sucking and Breathing

Milk flow is typically high during sucking bursts and when sucking is strong. Milk flow is typically low or absent when sucking strength is poor and during sucking pauses. When there is little or no flow the baby doesn't need to swallow, allowing for an increase in respiratory rate, tidal volume, and minute ventilation. During times of low flow or during a sucking pause, an actively feeding baby may actually seem to "pant" as they catch up on breathing.

If high flow overwhelms breathing, the baby can exert some control over this situation through their sucking pattern. One example is to take short sucking bursts. This allows more pause time, where catch-up breathing can occur. Another strategy, when mother's milk is flowing faster than the baby can handle it or continues to flow as the baby tries to stop sucking, is to use prolonged compression to try to stop the flow and allow breathing.

In some cases, babies may refuse to suck if they perceive the breathing adjustments as too stressful. Other babies learn to suck with very little pressure as a way to reduce flow rate. These same babies may love non-nutritive sucking on a finger or a pacifier, because it gives them the comfort of sucking without the stress of handling flow and making breathing adjustments. Although we may be tempted to look for ways to increase flow for these "inefficient" feeders, if respiratory difficulties underlie their sucking patterns, this strategy can make the situation worse (Wolf & Glass, 1992).

Flow and the Relationship Between Sucking and Swallowing

Sucking sets up the initiation and timing of swallowing, so it has a very direct impact on swallowing performance. If the baby is sucking at a fast rate and each bolus requires a swallow, the swallowing rate will be high. During fast flow, the swallowing structures need to move and recover quickly, with little time for breathing, or for timing errors. Regardless of the sucking rate, milk flow can be high and bolus size large if the baby's sucking is strong or mother's milk flow is very abundant. This may lead to premature spillage of the bolus into the pharynx, poor timing of the swallow, and possibly aspiration.

When a baby has a primary swallowing dysfunction they may be reluctant to create any fluid flow, in an effort to avoid swallowing. This baby may refuse to suck nutritively, though they may be eager to suck non-nutritively and/or may show significant stress cues during nutritive sucking (Wolf & Glass, 1992).

Factors to Consider in Assessing Flow Rate

When flow rate is optimal for a baby, breastfeeding performance and nutrition are supported. The baby can take the amount of food needed in a reasonable amount of time, without distress. When flow is too fast, the baby can show physiologic compromise and behavioral stress, and may become a reluctant feeder or even refuse to feed. If the flow rate is too slow, the baby will spend excessive time and energy feeding, and/or have inadequate intake. The appropriate flow rate for any baby is individual and based on that baby's physical skills, temperament, and medical condition. Before flow is adjusted, the clinician must consider a variety of factors. The questions in each of the following sections can be used to guide assessment of flow rate and its impact on the infant.

Sucking

Evaluating various characteristics of sucking can help determine the reasons that flow rate may be too high or too low.

- Is the baby able to create suction? Compression?
- Can the baby alternate between suction and compression?
- What is the strength of the baby's suction?

- How long is the sucking burst?
- What is the rate of sucking—non-nutritive and nutritive?
- Is the baby able to latch effectively to the breast?
- Are the baby's sucking mechanics and abilities similar in all situations, or do they vary among breast, non-nutritive sucking, and bottle or other alternate feeding method?
- Could the strength or rate of suck be creating flow that is too high?
- Could the strength of suck or quality of latch be leading to poor milk transfer and low flow?

When milk flow at the breast is low, we must determine whether the underlying issue is poor milk supply or the baby's inability to transfer milk. If milk is present but the baby is not able to obtain it, irregularities in latching and/or sucking are often present. We must then determine whether these are primary problems for the baby or if the latch/suck problems are the baby's attempt to keep the flow low to compensate for another problem.

Swallowing

There is a strong relationship between flow rate and swallowing function. Understanding the signs of swallowing dysfunction helps the clinician evaluate the infant's performance in this area.

- Does the baby have signs or symptoms of swallowing dysfunction?
  - History of pneumonia or frequent respiratory illness
  - Coughing/choking frequently during feeding
  - Apnea during feeding
  - Rattley, wet-sounding breathing
  - Preference for non-nutritive sucking
  - Pulling away at the start of the MER

Although swallowing dysfunction (dysphagia) is not common, it may be seen in former premature infants, babies post heart surgery, those with neurologic or anatomic problems, and even occasionally in healthy infants. Breastfeeding does not protect a baby from swallowing dysfunction or aspiration. Aspiration of breastmilk, however, is more likely to be silent, and may be less likely to lead to respiratory infections. In the breastfeeding baby, coughing/choking and reluctance to nurse are frequently attributed to overactive MER or hyperlactation. In this situation the baby should be carefully evaluated for swallowing dysfunction, including a trial with controlled flow at a lower rate ("emptied" breast, or bottle if necessary). Babies with a true swallowing dysfunction will usually also have problems in a "normal" flow situation.

If it appears the baby may have a primary swallowing problem, a more detailed evaluation by an experienced health professional is indicated. This may include clinical evaluation of swallowing and/or a videofluoroscopic swallowing study (also known as a modified barium swallow). This test can assess swallowing function and safety, and explore treatment options. Based on the results of this test, interventions that may be considered include providing a controlled, low flow rate, or using thickened liquid. These treatments may require feeding away from the breast, and in some cases oral feeding of any kind may not be safe. Human milk can still be supplied, and pacification at the freshly pumped breast may be possible, depending on the severity of the infant's dysphagia. See Chapter 11 for more information.

Breathing

While often overlooked during a feeding assessment, careful evaluation of breathing status during feeding can help to uncover the reason for many infant feeding problems.

- What is the baby's respiratory rate before, during, and after feeding?
- Is the baby showing increased work of breathing?
- Does the baby have stridor?
- How is the baby's energy/endurance?
- How often and how long are the breathing pauses?
- Does the baby have any diagnosis that would affect breathing?

Breathing issues are often overlooked in evaluating feeding problems, but in infants they can be a key component of a feeding problem. It is important to appreciate the baby's baseline respiratory status, and how it changes during feeding, in order to gauge the impact of respiratory issues. If a baby with breathing problems is also having feeding problems, reducing flow is often helpful. Although some babies will modify sucking patterns to reduce flow on their own, others eagerly generate high flow, only to become stressed or overwhelmed by the flow.

Listening to the quality of breathing helps identify the location of the difficulty. The presence of stridorous, high-pitched, noisy respiration suggests some type of airway obstruction (see Table 6-1 earlier in the chapter), which will make it hard for the baby to breathe adequately during feeding. Hearing wet or rattley breathing suggests swallowing problems.

Coordination of Sucking, Breathing, and Swallowing

Rhythmicity is a hallmark of infant feeding that results from normal coordination of sucking, swallowing, and breathing. Clinicians should have an understanding of normal, as well as atypical, patterns of coordination.

- What is the baby's pattern of coordination?
  - *Normal:* In the beginning of feeding, swallowing and breathing are smoothly integrated into bursts of at least 20–30 sucks.
  - *Short sucking bursts:* Sucking bursts early in the feeding last only 3–5 sucks, with frequent and perhaps lengthy breathing pauses.
  - *Feeding-induced apnea:* During sucking bursts the baby swallows, but does not breathe. This may lead to oxygen desaturation, coughing or choking, or pulling away from the milk flow.

When poor coordination of sucking, swallowing, and breathing is noted, it is important to investigate the underlying reasons for the pattern that is observed. Short sucking bursts may be seen in the baby who is premature or weak, and lacks stamina to sustain sucking. The baby who has respiratory or swallowing problems may use short sucking bursts to limit milk flow. This pattern may also be seen if the mother has little milk, or the baby is not able to transfer the milk. If feeding-induced apnea is observed, it may be a primary problem of coordination for the baby due to maturational or neurologic issues, or it could be related to high milk flow.

Assessing Flow Rate During Breastfeeding

Determining flow rate during breastfeeding is done by direct and indirect methods of observation.

Sucking Rate

Observing sucking rate is a quick and simple method to screen for rate of flow during breastfeeding.

- How fast is the baby sucking?
  - Two or more sucks / second = non-nutritive sucking
  - One suck / second = nutritive sucking
- Does it change throughout the feeding?
- When do changes occur?

If the baby is sucking at two sucks per second or faster, they are probably sucking non-nutritively and flow is low. This faster sucking rate is typical of the first 10–60 seconds at the breast, before the MER. When milk flow begins, the baby's sucking rate should slow down to about one suck per second. This is characterized by a pause in jaw movement when the jaw is at its lowest point during the sucking cycle. Much of the feeding should be characterized by sustained active sucking at this nutritive sucking rate. If the baby shows only small portions of the feeding with this type of nutritive sucking activity, overall flow is probably low. Total length of time at each breast does not correlate with amount of milk transferred.

Swallowing Rate

The swallowing rate reflects flow rate, and is an excellent method of estimating flow. Assessment of swallowing rate is enhanced by using a stethoscope to amplify the swallow sounds.

- How many sucks occur before each swallow?

A ratio of one to three sucks per swallow should indicate normal flow as long as this is sustained over the majority of the feeding. If clear swallows are heard less frequently, flow may be low. Typically, swallowing has been determined by listening for soft swallow sounds. This method may miss the more subtle swallows that are not always evident to the naked ear. A more precise method is cervical auscultation. This method uses a neonatal size stethoscope, placed laterally on the baby's throat to distinctly hear swallowing and breathing sounds (Vice, Heinz, Giuriati, Hood, & Bosma, 1990; see **Figure 6-5**).

Behavioral Cues

While decidedly "low tech," a baby's behavior, in conjunction with other observations, can provide the clinician with information about flow rate.

- How wakeful is the baby before and during feeding?
- Does the baby quickly fall asleep at the breast?
- Is the baby content at the breast but cries when taken off?
- Does the baby pull away from the breast or look distressed during feeding?
- Is the baby fussy while feeding?
- Does the baby resist going to the breast?

Figure 6-5
Cervical auscultation.

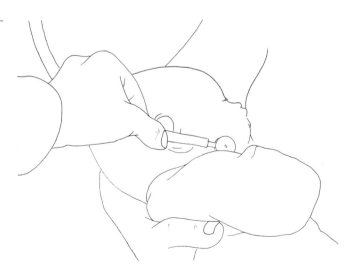

The baby's behavior can give important information about flow rate and how they cope with it. Babies getting milk at a rate they can handle generally have open eyes and an intent look. Babies who are getting inadequate flow often become sleepy early in the feeding, seem to fall asleep, or act uninterested. The content baby who cries when taken off the breast also may not be getting adequate milk transfer. Babies who receive very high flow rate will often show stress cues. One baby might generate high flow and momentarily show stress, but then settle into a pattern of rapid but comfortable feeding. Another baby in the same situation may show stress in their eyes, turn their head away, or stop sucking.

Test Weights

Test weights are a definitive measure of intake. When compared to feeding time, it provides information on flow rate.

- How much milk has the baby taken?
  - On each breast?
  - Cumulatively?
- How long has it taken?

By weighing the baby before and after breastfeeding with a digital scale accurate to +/− 1 gram, overall flow rate can be objectively determined (Meier, Lysakowski, & Engstrom, 1990). This method is accurate and often gives surprising results. The mother who is worried that her baby only stays at the breast for 5 minutes and won't nurse often, learns that her baby gets 3 ounces in 5 minutes—a very high flow rate. Another mother with good milk supply and a baby who nurses constantly learns that her baby is eliciting a very low flow rate, only getting 0.5 ounces in 15 minutes.

Milk Production

The amount of milk mother has available, and the ease with which it is transferred to the baby during the MER, can be highly correlated with flow rate. The clinician should consider the following information about milk production when assessing flow.

- Is it adequate, low, or abundant?
- How has milk production been determined?
- Are there signs of overactive let-down?
- Is mother exclusively breastfeeding?
- Is mother pumping?

When there are problems related to flow, it should be determined if they are related to the mother's milk supply or baby-sided issues. Assessing the baby's performance without accurate information on the mother's supply may lead to an inaccurate understanding of the problem.

- A mother can have normal flow, but the baby perceives it as too high and may have inadequate intake or other feeding problems.

- A mother can have abundant milk production, yet believe that she has little milk when her baby feeds quickly and is unsettled.

- A mother can truly have an oversupply and/or robust MER, which causes the baby to pull away, cough/choke, or become resistant to eating.

- The mother has adequate supply, yet the baby generates little flow, indicating a baby-sided feeding problem. Milk production will decrease rapidly if milk is not removed from the breast.

- The mother truly has low production, thus the baby generates low flow.

Simply observing the baby at the breast may give an inaccurate indication of the mother's milk supply. Objective measurements, such as doing test weights and then having the mother pump any residual milk, are more accurate. The total that the baby transferred plus the pumped milk would be her potential supply for that feeding. If the baby is not feeding at the breast, pumping with a high quality breast pump will determine the mother's milk supply. Keep in mind that when using a pump, the mother may not transfer milk in the same way that she does for her baby.

Common Diagnoses Related to Flow Issues

Prematurity

Many premature babies struggle with breastfeeding, and flow issues may contribute to these difficulties. The following information can help focus the assessment of feeding problems.

- At what gestational age was the baby born and what is the current corrected age?

- What is the baby's respiratory status, including respiratory rate, need for oxygen, work of breathing, and endurance?

- Can the premature baby sustain suck adequately (length of burst and suction pressure) at the breast to create necessary flow?

- What is the pattern of suck/swallow/breath control?

- Is there any evidence of feeding-induced apnea?

- If the baby is struggling with feeding, has there been a trial with controlled low flow?

Premature infants often have medical and/or maturational issues that lead to sensitivity to high flow during feeding. Respiratory distress syndrome and chronic lung disease are often seen in premature infants and are associated with a high resting respiratory rate, increased work of breathing, poor respiratory reserve, and low endurance. High flow, or even "normal" flow, may not be tolerated by these babies who often prefer non-nutritive sucking or very low flow. Due to immaturity, preterm babies are prone to feeding-induced apnea, which is exacerbated by high flow. Also due to immaturity, sucking bursts are short, with suction strength emerging. This may lead to trouble maintaining latch and creating adequate milk flow at the breast. How preterm infants are cared for, how early they initiate breastfeeding, and their individual medical conditions help determine their feeding competence. See Chapter 7 for more information on breastfeeding preterm infants.

Oral-Facial Anomalies

Feeding problems are common among babies with oral-facial anomalies such as cleft lip and/or palate, Pierre Robin sequence, hemifacial microsomia, and macroglossia. When assessing babies with these diagnoses, the clinician should consider the following:

- Can the baby create suction during sucking?
- What is the suction strength?
- Are there associated breathing issues?
- Is there airway obstruction (stenosis, malacia, glossoptosis, etc.)?
- Is there evidence of swallowing dysfunction?

The baby with oral anomalies, including any oral cleft, is often unable to create suction. For an isolated cleft lip, the soft breast tissue may fill the "gap" and allow the baby to create suction and latch effectively to the breast. For a cleft palate, it is not possible to create suction, so latch is inadequate, milk flow is limited, and supplementation is required.

When an oral-facial anomaly, such as micrognathia (small lower jaw) with glossoptosis (a posteriorly placed tongue that intermittently occludes the airway), causes intermittent airway obstruction, feeding will be limited by difficulty breathing and coordinating breathing with sucking and swallowing. Reducing flow may be helpful, but intake may still be inadequate. Babies with oral-facial anomalies are also at increased risk for swallowing disorders, so it is important to observe for signs of swallowing dysfunction. See Chapter 8 for more on this issue.

Respiratory Compromise

Because respiration plays such an important role in infant feeding, the clinician should pay particular attention to respiratory issues when assessing feeding problems.

- Does the baby have a medical diagnosis that could impact respiratory function? (See Table 6-1)
- What is the baby's respiratory status prior to feeding?
    - Respiratory rate
    - Need for additional oxygen

- ▪ Need for breathing treatments or medications
- ▪ Work of breathing
- ▪ Energy
- ▪ Signs of obstruction (stuffy nose, wheezing, stridor, breathing pauses)
- How do respiratory parameters change with feeding?
- If the baby is struggling to breathe during feeding, has there been a trial in a controlled low flow situation?
- Are the oral feeding expectations appropriate for the baby's respiratory status?

The baby with compromised respiratory status will often require ongoing intervention such as oxygen or breathing treatments, or have a high respiratory rate and/or work of breathing. All of these issues make handling the ventilatory reductions associated with feeding and coordinating sucking, swallowing, and breathing much more challenging. High flow exacerbates this and further reduces opportunities for breathing. The baby may use a pattern of short sucking bursts, or suck with less pressure to try to limit flow. Even when the baby uses normal feeding patterns, energy and endurance may be limited due to the increased "work" required during feeding. Because the baby often takes in less than expected and feeds slowly, the temptation is to increase the flow rate. This group of babies, however, may do better with a lower flow rate to assist them with respiratory stability, and reduced expectations for total oral intake.

Intervention Strategies to Alter Flow

Once it has been determined that high or low flow rate is a factor in an infant's feeding problems, there are a variety of methods to change flow rate in order to improve feeding performance.

Increasing Flow

There are several reasons to increase flow during breastfeeding. The most frequent reason is to improve the nutrition of a baby who is not achieving adequate milk transfer. This baby may be failing to gain weight or growing at an inappropriately slow rate. It is important to determine if this is due to baby-sided factors such as inability to latch or suck effectively, or due to inadequate maternal supply.

Another reason to increase flow is to improve the sucking pattern. A chomping and biting sucking pattern may be observed when the baby has difficulty generating flow at the breast, resulting in painful nursing and/or inadequate milk transfer. Increasing flow may help this baby use a more functional and appropriate sucking pattern with greater suction. Some caution is necessary when increasing flow. If the baby is intentionally limiting flow due to breathing or swallowing problems, increasing flow may be detrimental to the baby.

Increasing Flow Without a Feeding Tube Device

When the mother has an adequate milk supply, the first step is to make sure the baby is fully awake, so he or she can actively participate in breastfeeding. Parents should be taught how to fully wake their baby for feeding, and benefit from instruction in identifying feeding cues so they are able to respond to their baby at opportune times.

Optimizing latch frequently improves flow. Techniques might include activities to improve the baby's mouth opening, strengthening the baby's suck (see Chapter 11), and finding the best position (see Chapters 5 and 12).

If the baby appears to have a good latch and suck, but milk flow still seems inadequate, techniques to stimulate milk flow can be added. If there appears to be a delayed MER, with the baby frustrated and unwilling to suck long enough to stimulate milk flow, it may be helpful for mother to prepump so milk is available more quickly. While the baby is sucking, it can be effective for mother to use deep compression with moderate to strong squeezing of the breast to increase flow, and then release the compression when the baby pauses (Newman & Pitman, 2000).

For premature infants, it is common for mom to have a good milk supply, but for the baby to transfer very little milk. The strength and coordination of suction is not fully developed in the premature infant, and may lead to inability to sustain latch and transfer milk. Use of a nipple shield has been found to aid milk transfer significantly for premature infants, because more of their energy goes into removing milk and less goes into staying attached to the breast (Meier et al., 2000; Clum & Primomo, 1996). For a nipple shield to be effective in augmenting flow for the premature infant, it should be sized to the infant's mouth. Nipple shields may also aid milk transfer in term infants who have trouble sustaining suction at the breast.

If the mother has a marginal or poor milk supply, increasing her supply should increase flow. Milk supply can be increased by frequent milk expression with a rental-grade electric breast pump, use of galactogogues (such as domperidone, metoclopramide, or fenugreek and other herbs), and by spending time with the baby at the breast or in skin-to-skin contact.

Feeding Tube Devices

When the methods described in the previous section do not result in a sufficient increase in flow, or if it is clear that the mother has a low milk supply, a feeding tube device can be considered. These devices add milk flow from an external source. When recommending these devices to a mother, the lactation specialist should be sensitive to the mother's verbal and nonverbal communication, to determine her acceptance of the device. Providing adequate, hands-on instruction in the use of the device is crucial to ensuring success. Commonly used devices are the Supplemental Nursing System (SNS; Medela), the Lact-aid Nursing Trainer, and a feeding tube (such as a 5 French gavage tube) attached to a syringe or placed into a bottle of milk.

Adding flow at the breast using a feeding tube device can be a strategy to improve sucking pattern and efficiency. Some babies suck using an excessive amount of compression and limited suction, resulting in inefficient milk transfer and/or breast pain for mother. These babies may show a normal sucking pattern during each MER, but revert to a pattern of excessive compression and limited suction as the flow of milk abates. In this situation, the lactation specialist should identify the point during nursing when the baby needs increased flow to improve the sucking pattern. Although some babies will need increased flow throughout the entire feeding, others may only need it when milk flow from the MER slows. If set up prior to starting the feed, and trained in the method, most mothers are able to start the flow of the tube feeding device to correspond with the baby's needs. For a healthy infant this should increase the flow rate so that the baby swallows after most sucks. Each suck should be a long "draw" rather than a short "chomp."

Feeding tube devices can be helpful for any baby with diminished endurance and/or weak suck, including babies with prematurity or congenital heart disease. To augment milk flow, the tube feeding device may be used throughout the entire feeding or started as the baby tires. For the baby with low endurance, the lactation specialist must take care not to overwhelm the baby's suck, swallow, and breathe abilities with a flow rate that is too high. A slower flow rate with a ratio of three or four sucks per swallow may be needed to support the baby's abilities.

The rate of milk flow can be adjusted when using any of these devices. For the SNS, tube size can be selected to give the appropriate flow rate. The Lact-aid and feeding tube/syringe can be squeezed to change the flow. For tube-in-bottle supplementers, the container can be elevated to increase flow. As the flow rate is increased with any of these devices, the lactation specialist needs to be attentive to signs of excessive flow. An appropriate flow rate occurs when the baby is able to breathe regularly while sucking, and only inhibit breathing in the moment of swallowing. If the baby is breath holding, looking distressed, or coughing and sputtering, the baby's suck/swallow/breathe capacities have been overwhelmed and flow from the supplementer should be slowed.

Decreasing Flow

The unique flow characteristics at the breast usually support excellent control and coordination of sucking, swallowing, and breathing. There can be times, however, when flow at the breast leads to discoordination regardless of the mother's actual flow rate. Feeding-induced apnea, although more prevalent during bottle feeding, can also be observed during breastfeeding, even in healthy infants. Medical diagnoses such as respiratory distress can result in an elevated respiratory rate, making it difficult to coordinate swallowing and breathing even when flow rate is typical. In these cases, methods to decrease milk flow may be considered.

At times, the quantity of the mother's milk production, or the vigor of her MER, can overwhelm even a baby who has normal skills to coordinate sucking, swallowing, and breathing.

Too often, however, difficulty with coordinating sucking, swallowing, and breathing is immediately diagnosed as an "overactive let-down." The problem is attributed to the mother, when the difficulty may lie with the baby. This results in treatment strategies that do not improve the problem, because they do not deal with the root cause. The lactation specialist should carefully evaluate the baby's respiration at baseline and during feeding, how well breathing is coordinated with sucking and swallowing, and if there are any concerns about the safety of swallowing. If problems are noted, flow may need to be reduced. In identifying methods to slow the flow, the lactation specialist needs to identify which changes might be needed on the mother's part, and which changes on the baby's part.

Mother-Sided Methods

As the mother feels her MER approaching, she can momentarily take her baby off the breast and allow the strong flow to fall on a cloth. Prepumping to reduce the initial milk flow may offer a short-term solution, but in the long term can result in more milk, which compounds the problem. Feeding the baby on only one breast at each feeding may gradually lower the mother's milk supply so her MER is not as brisk. Some mothers have one breast that makes more milk or has a more brisk MER. The mother may start each feeding on the "slower" breast so the baby is not as hungry and vigorous when they get to the "faster" breast.

An additional method for slowing milk flow during breastfeeding was suggested by Carol Chamblin, IBCLC (personal communication, March 30, 2007). Carol teaches mothers to press on the breast with a flat hand to temporarily collapse some ducts when the infant shows signs of struggling with flow.

Baby-Sided Methods

Changing the baby's position during nursing can decrease flow. In positions where the baby is below the breast (such as the standard cradle or football hold) gravity assists the flow of milk, and should be avoided. Alternate positions that eliminate gravity include mother and baby lying side by side in bed, or having the mother recline with the baby lying prone on her chest. In the latter position, milk will travel slightly uphill and potentially does the most to slow the flow.

If feeding-induced apnea is present during breastfeeding, external pacing can be used to help the baby coordinate breathing with sucking and swallowing. This is a technique that systematically imposes breathing breaks for the baby who is not spontaneously breathing at appropriate intervals. During nutritive sucking, when the baby is swallowing after most sucks, the baby is helped to take a breathing break after three to five suck/swallows. For some babies, simply touching their cheek, talking to them, and/or moving them may encourage them to stop sucking and take a few breaths. Other babies need to be "unlatched" while they take two to four breaths. The baby's mouth should continue to touch the mother's breast, so the baby knows that the feeding will resume quickly. This technique sets the "pace" of breathing for the baby who does not have appropriate internal control of breathing coordination. In many cases, pacing is only needed for the first few minutes of feeding, when the baby is sucking eagerly, mother is having her first and strongest MER, and flow is very high. Although this technique may sound disruptive to nursing, it may actually make the baby who latches easily more comfortable. Feeding-induced apnea not only is exhausting for the baby, but also can lead to oxygen desaturation, microaspiration, and general stress. External pacing allows the baby to continue breastfeeding while remaining physiologically stable.

Conclusion

Rate of milk flow is an important aspect of infant feeding, and within breastfeeding there is a dynamic relationship around flow—mother and baby both contribute to the rate of milk flow. If flow is too low, because the mother has inadequate milk supply or the baby is not able to access it, the baby will not thrive at the breast. If milk flow is too high, because of abundant supply or because normal flow is too high for a particular baby, breastfeeding will be affected. Our job is to help mothers and babies adjust flow so it is not too high, and not too low, but "just right."

References

Bu'Lock, F., Woolridge, M. W., & Baum, J. D. (1990). Development of co-ordination of sucking, swallowing and breathing: Ultrasound study of term and preterm infants. *Developmental Medicine & Child Neurology, 32*(8), 669–678.

Chetwynd, A. G., Diggle, P. J., Drewett, R. F., & Young, B. (1998). A mixture model for sucking patterns of breast-fed infants. *Statistics in Medicine, 17,* 395–405.

Clum, D., & Primomo, J. (1996). Use of a silicone nipple shield with premature infants. *Journal of Human Lactation, 12,* 287–290.

Drewett, R. F., & Woolridge, M. W. (1979). Sucking patterns of human babies on the breast. *Early Human Development, 3*(4), 315–320.

Drewett, R. F., & Woolridge, M. W. (1981). Milk taken by human babies from the first and second breast. *Physiology and Behavior, 26,* 327–329.

Gewolb, I. H., & Vice, F. L. (2006). Maturational changes in the rhythms, patterning, and coordination of respiration and swallow during feeding in preterm and term infants. *Developmental Medicine & Child Neurology, 48,* 589–594.

Gewolb, I. H., Vice, F. L., Schwietzer-Kenny, E. L., Taciak, V. L., & Bosma, J. F. (2001). Developmental patterns of rhythmic suck and swallow in preterm infants. *Developmental Medicine Child Neurology, 43,* 22–27.

Hanlon, M. B., Tripp, J. H., Ellis, R. E., Flack, F. C., Selley, W. G., & Shoesmith, H. J. (1997). Deglutition apnoea as indicator of maturation of suckle feeding in bottle-fed preterm infants. *Developmental Medicine & Child Neurology, 39*(8), 534–542.

Lau, C., Alagugurusamy, R., Schanler, R. J., Smith, E. O., & Shulman, R. J. (2000). Characterization of the developmental stages of sucking in preterm infants during bottle feeding. *Acta Paediatrica, 89*(7), 846–852.

Mathew, O. P., & Bhatia, J. (1989). Sucking and breathing patterns during breast- and bottle-feeding in term neonates. *American Journal of Disease in Children, 143,* 588–592.

Mathew, O. P., Clark, M. L., Pronske, M. L., Luna-Solarzano, H. G., & Peterson, M. D. (1985). Breathing pattern and ventilation during oral feeding in term newborn infants. *Journal of Pediatrics, 106,* 810–813.

Meier, P. P., Brown, L. P., Hurst, N. M., Spatz, D. L., Engstrom, J. L., Borucki, L. C., & Krouse, A. M. (2000). Nipple shields for preterm infants: Effect on milk transfer and duration of breastfeeding. *Journal of Human Lactation, 16*(2), 106–114; quiz 129–131.

Meier, P. P., Lysakowski, T. Y., & Engstrom, J. L. (1990). The accuracy of test-weighing for preterm infants. *Journal of Pediatric Gastroenterology & Nutrition, 10,* 62–65.

Mortola, J. P., & Fischer, J. T. (1988). Upper airway reflexes in newborns. In O. P. Mathew & G. Sant'Ambrogio (Eds.), *Respiratory function of the upper airway* (Vol. 35, pp. 303–357). New York: Marcell Dekker.

Newman, J., & Pitman, T. (2000). *The ultimate breastfeeding book of answers.* Roseville, CA: Prima.

Ramsay, D. T., & Hartmann, P. (2005). Milk removal from the breast. *Breastfeeding Review, 13*(1), 5–7.

Sameroff, A. J. (1968). The components of sucking in the human newborn. *Journal of Experimental Child Psychology, 6*(4), 607–623.

Selley, W. G., Ellis, R. E., Flack, F. C., & Brooks, W. A. (1990). Coordination of sucking, swallowing and breathing in the newborn: Its relationship to infant feeding and normal development. *British Journal of Disorders of Communication, 25*(3), 311–327.

Tuchman, D. N. (1993). Physiology of the swallowing apparatus. In D. N. Tuchman & R. S. Walter (Eds.), *Disorders of feeding and swallowing in infants and children* (pp. 1–26). San Diego, CA: Singular Publishing Group.

Vice, F. L., Heinz, J. M., Giuriati, G., Hood, M., & Bosma, J. (1990). Cervical auscultation of suckle feeding in newborn infants. *Developmental Medicine & Child Neurology, 32,* 760–768.

Weber, R., Woolridge, M. W., & Baum, J. D. (1986). An ultrasonographic study of the organisation of sucking and swallowing by newborn infants. *Developmental Medicine & Child Neurology, 28,* 19–24.

Wolf, L. S., & Glass, R. P. (1992). *Feeding and swallowing disorders in infancy: Assessment and management.* Austin, TX: Pro-Ed.

Wolff, P. H. (1968). The serial organization of sucking in the young infant. *Pediatrics, 42*(6), 943–955.

Chapter 7

Breastfeeding Preterm Infants

Kerstin Hedberg Nyqvist

Breastfeeding Rates in Preterm Infants

In spite of the particular importance of breast milk feeding for children born preterm (a gestation of less than 37 weeks) or with low birth weight (LBW, < 2,500 g) (Feldman & Eidelman, 2003; Schanler, 2001; Smith et al., 2003), breastfeeding rates for these infants in industrialized countries are lower than rates observed in term infants, and show considerable variation. Differences in rates can be attributed to several factors. One major explanation is probably the general attitude to breastfeeding in society at large. Other contributing factors are mothers' right to maternity leave from work and maternal allowance during the infant's hospitalization and after discharge.

> In settings where breastfeeding is considered the norm for infant and young child feeding, mothers and personnel in neonatal units strive for "normalcy."
>
> When breastfeeding is regarded as a matter of personal choice and bottle feeding is considered normal, this attitude is reflected in lower breastfeeding incidence.

Special Characteristics and Needs of Preterm Infants

- *External characteristics:* Typical features of a preterm infant are thin arms and legs and low muscle tone when the infant is resting. The mouth is small, and the infant lacks fat pads in the cheeks, which help to stabilize movements of the tongue and jaws during oral feeding. Preterm infants' immature appearance may impart the false impression that they lack the prerequisites for oral feeding.

- *Physiological immaturity:* Cardiorespiratory immaturity with bradycardia, irregular respiration, apnea (pause in respiration of more than 20 seconds), and difficulty maintaining adequate oxygen saturation are the main concerns during feeding. Decisions about the choice of feeding method are primarily based on protecting the infant's physiological stability.

- *Metabolic immaturity:* Metabolic immaturity, with lack of sufficient subcutaneous fat, brown fat, and glycogen, contributes to increased risk of hypothermia and hypoglycemia. This necessitates protection from cold stress during breastfeeding by skin-to-skin contact or adequate clothing, and frequent feeding.

- *Neurologic immaturity:* An immature motor system and low muscle tone make it difficult for the preterm infant to attain and maintain a position with flexed hips, knees, and feet; flexed arms with the hands joined in the midline near the face; and head control. Without adequate support, the infant is unable to stay fixed at the breast, with a straight trunk and neck, without curling into a slumped posture. Low muscle tone results in poor latch, less efficient sucking, and difficulties in staying fixed at the breast.

The preterm infant spends more time in a diffuse, drowsy state, and has frequent shifts in states (e.g., between diffuse sleep and active awake). Signs of waking up are subtle (slightly more irregular respiration, gasps, grimaces, movements in lips and tongue, raised eyebrows, diffuse movements). Direct light is an obstacle to eye opening. Periods of focused alertness are short. Instead, a glassy-eyed look and a surprised look with wide-open eyes are common, indicating limited ability to handle visual stimuli.

The infant is easily overloaded by stimuli (touch, sounds, visual input, light), especially when they occur simultaneously. Habituation, the capacity to shut out common environmental stimuli, does not mature until term age. Voices in a normal conversational tone and activity in the visual field cause stress, displayed as irregular respiration and movements, and reduce the time available for activities directed at the breast.

Considering all these differences, the common assumption that breastfeeding is inappropriate until a certain maturational level is not surprising. However, research has shown that this is not the case.

Assessment of Readiness or Facilitation of Competence

Criteria for Initiation of Oral Feeding

Decisions about initiation of breastfeeding in preterm infants are often based on an assessment of readiness. A certain maturational level has been the most common criterion, such as a postmenstrual age (PMA, gestational weeks from the first day of the last menstrual period) of 34 weeks (Comrie & Helm, 1997) or 32 weeks (Cousins, 1999; Lemons, 2001; Wheeler et al., 1999). It has been suggested that infants at a gestational age (GA) of less than 32 weeks should only be allowed to suck at their mother's emptied breast, whereas mothers of infants at 32–33 weeks can be allowed to breastfeed without restriction (Meier, 2001). A minimum weight is also a common criterion. Another approach for testing readiness to feed is evaluation of sucking vigor during pacifier or finger sucking (Comrie & Helm). Several screening methods and guidelines have been elaborated for assessment of feeding skills and for introduction of oral feedings (McCain, 2003; Thoyre, Shaker, & Pridham, 2005; White-Traut, Berbaum, Lessen, McFarlin, & Cardenas, 2005). But these methods were based on bottle feeding. As I will explain later in this chapter, initiation of breastfeeding should be based on facilitation of competence instead of assessment of readiness.

Physiological Stability During Breastfeeding

Coordination of sucking, swallowing, and breathing is considered a requirement for commencing oral feeding. Because of fear of physiological compromise, preterm infants' physiological response to oral feeding has been explored extensively. However, in the absence of breastfeeding research, conclusions drawn from infants' reactions to nipple (bottle) feeding have been incorrectly applied to breastfeeding. A study of bottle feeding, which noted apnea, bradycardia, and oxygen desaturation during sucking, was that "in most preterm infants respiratory control during feeding is still immature at 35–36 weeks" (Mathew, 1988, p. 220).

> Comparisons of preterm infants' physiological responses to breast- and bottle feeding have clearly demonstrated differences in favor of breastfeeding.

Common observations during bottle feeding were uncoordinated sucking and swallowing; reduced breathing; higher incidence of bradycardia, apnea, and desaturation; lower levels of oxygen saturation; progressive postfeed decline of transcutaneous oxygen saturation; and lower temperature, whereas the same infants—also very preterm infants—remained stable during breastfeeding (Bier et al., 1997; Chen et al., 2000; Dowling, 1999). Apnea during swallowing (deglutition apnea) is more frequent in bottle-fed preterm infants than in term infants (Hanlon et al., 1997).

These differences are easily explained; at the breast the infant is in control of sucking, swallowing, and breathing in a pattern that permits physiological stability. A breastfed infant with an immature sucking pattern holds his or her breath during suckling and breathes during pauses, reflected in brief desaturations that resolve shortly after the termination of a sucking burst. After a period of rapid breathing, the respiration slows down and the infant spontaneously begins to suck again. This is no cause for concern, provided that the infant is allowed to decide the pace. Higher body temperature during breastfeeding is explained by the skin-to-skin contact and higher chest temperature in breastfeeding women, due to the effects of oxytocin (Uvnäs-Moberg & Eriksson, 1996).

Obstacles to infant self-regulation during bottle feeding are the size of the hole in the nipple, the force of gravity that makes milk flow, and manipulation by the caregiver who tries to coax the infant to continue sucking, leading to oxygen desaturation and a postfeed period with low saturation (or if the percentage of supplemental oxygen was increased during the feed, until this can be decreased to the prefeed level).

Risk of aspiration has also been considered a possible hazard. However, even very preterm infants respond with an upper airway chemo reflex to fluid in the larynx (Davies, Koenig, & Thatch, 1989). In addition, observational studies of breastfeeding in preterm infants have not found aspiration to occur in an immature sucking pattern.

> Preterm infants maintain physiologic stability during breastfeeding, provided that the mother is sensitive to the infant's behavioral and physiological cues.

Facilitation of Breastfeeding by Developmentally Supportive Care

Infant motor development is enhanced by modification of care and the caregiving environment that supports the infant's own activities for self-regulation, according to the infant's current maturational stage of central nervous system development (Nyqvist, Ewald, & Sjodén, 1996). During the intense process of brain development during the second half of the pregnancy, the organization of cortex is influenced by the infant's exposure to touch, hearing, vision, taste, odor, and proprioceptive and vestibular experience.

The Newborn Individual Developmental Care and Assessment Program (NIDCAP) is a clinical model for structured infant assessment and provision of care in harmony with infants' current developmental stage and medical status (Als et al., 1994). The infant is perceived as an active individual who responds to sensory input by signs of strength or sensitivity and activities for self-regulation. The infant's responses are observed in autonomic signs, motor behavior, behavioral states, and activities related to interaction with the social and physical environment (**Table 7-1**). Decisions on timing and progression of oral feeding are based on the infant's current threshold of tolerance (Ross & Browne, 2002). Lower age at the first oral feeding and last tube feeding were observed in preterm infants after modification of the physical environment in the nursery to make it less stressful (Becker et al., 1991). Very preterm infants who received care structured according to regular NIDCAP observations attained full bottle/breastfeeding earlier than infants with conventional care (Als et al., 1994).

The interaction between the infant and a parent or other caregiver is a dialogue, in which both participants exert a mutual influence on each other. A sensitive caregiver modifies his or her behavior and the environment according to the infant's ongoing responses. When the caregiver acts according to his or her own agenda, the infant responds by increasing the incidence and severity of signs of sensitivity (**Table 7-2**). The NIDCAP program emphasizes parents' unique role in their infant's life. All steps are taken to enable parents to be present in the unit, participate in decisions regarding infant feeding on equal terms with professionals, and take over the responsibility for their infant's feeding and care as soon as they are willing to do so.

Protecting Milk Supply

Initiation and Frequency of Breast Milk Expression

A variation in markers of the onset of copious milk secretion after birth (milk citrate, lactose, sodium, and total protein) indicates that some mothers of preterm infants may take longer to establish their milk production (Cregan, De Mello, Kershaw, McDougall, & Hartmann, 2002). This finding underscores the importance of initiation of regular, frequent milk expression as soon as possible, for example, beginning before 6 hours postdelivery (Furman, Minich, & Hack, 2002). Expressing milk at least six to seven times per 24 hours has been

TABLE 7-1   Infant Cues of Approach and Avoidance During Breastfeeding
According to NIDCAP

Cues of Approach	Cues of Avoidance
Autonomic System	
Regular heart rate and respiration	Fast or slow heart rate
	Irregular fast or slow respiration
Adequate oxygen saturation	Respiratory pauses, apnea, hypoxia
Stable skin color: pink or red	Pale, mottled, dusky, cyanotic, flushed, color shifts
Stable digestive functions	Spits up, gags
	Bowel movement grunting
	Sighs, gasps
Occasional startles and twitches	Hiccough
	Startles, twitches, tremor
Motor System	
Maintains muscle tone	Low muscle tone in hands, arms, legs, trunk, and face
	Achieves and maintains flexed arms, legs, trunk, and gaping mouth
	Shows tongue
Tucks him- or herself closer to the breast	High muscle tone: extended posture, tense
Braces hands/feet against mother's body	Active extension of arms/legs
Brings/holds hands to face or mouth	Arches head and/or trunk backwards, turns away
Smiles	Fans or splays (spreads out) fingers
Mouthing, licking	
Laps milk	
Rooting, sucking	Clenches fists
Grasping	Grimaces
Holds onto finger, breast, etc.	Stretches out tense tongue
Molds to mother's trunk	Exaggerated flexion
	Does not mold to mother's trunk
Smooth coordinated movements	Diffuse squirming
	Jerky uncoordinated movements
Behavioral States	
Stable periods of sleep or alertness	Light/diffuse sleep
Deep sleep	Low/diffuse states (drowsy, diffuse movements with closed eyes)
States are easy to distinguish	Short periods of alertness

(continues)

TABLE 7-1 Infant Cues of Approach and Avoidance During Breastfeeding According to NIDCAP (continued)

Cues of Approach	Cues of Avoidance
Behavioral States (continued)	
Looks at mother, orients, with focused look	Swift state transitions Open eyes with glassy-eyed look or stares with a tense, surprised, frightened look
Smooth state transitions: calm waking up, falls asleep easily	Difficult to calm down Irritable Frenetic activity
Shuts out stimuli easily	Crying Limited ability to shut out disturbing stimuli
Attention, Interaction	
Orients towards mother's face, voice, other objects or events	Looks away Stares in another direction
Raises eyebrows Frowns	Eyes "float" from side to side or roll around
Purses lips as if saying "oh"	Fusses, cries, turns drowsy, closes eyes
Speech movements, imitates facial expression	Yawns, sneezes
Cooing sounds	Cues of avoidance in autonomic/motor/behavioral system

associated with subsequent sufficient milk production (Hill, Brown, & Harker, 1995). Simultaneous pumping increases the chances of a higher milk yield; gentle breast massage may further increase milk production (Jones, Dimmock, & Spencer, 2001). Mothers who prefer sequential pumping can be advised to repeatedly alternate between the breasts because this may result in higher volumes.

The volume of milk produced depends on pumping strategy:

Simultaneous pumping + breast massage > simultaneous pumping without breast massage > sequential pumping + breast massage > sequential pumping without breast massage.

In industrialized countries, manual expression is mainly used as a complement to breast pumps. Because it is easier to collect colostrum by manual expression directly into a small cup, mothers should be offered instruction soon after delivery to stimulate their milk

TABLE 7-2   Maternal Behavior During Breastfeeding Preterm Infants

Sensitivity	Lack of Sensitivity
Positions the infant at the breast at signs of waking, when the infant is awake, and at subtle signs of interest in sucking.	Positions the infant at the breast when asleep and shows no signs of interest in sucking.
Selects a quiet place where the infant is shielded from direct light, noise, activity, and visual input.	Selects a place with direct light, noise, a high level of activity, and visual input for the infant.
Sits in an upright position (or lies down). Places the infant on a cushion or the like for positioning.	Sits in a reclining position.
Supports an infant position with straight trunk, head directed forwards, mouth in front of nipple.	Holds the infant with inadequate support for head and trunk, the infant's trunk is not straight, the head is turned sideways, the mouth is not in front of the nipple.
Places the infant with arms and legs flexed, using her clothes or KMC binder or the like for support and protection from cold stress. Gives consistent support for a correct position with still hands.	Holds the infant in a position with extended arms/legs. No clothes/other support for the infant's position. Does not cover the infant.
If the infant shows extension movements: Gently helps the infant to regain a flexed position. Offers the infant the breast by gently touching his lips with nipple/finger to elicit rooting.	Moves her hands often. Does not respond to extension movements. Changes the infant's position often. Does not adjust the position when needed.
When the infant does not respond: Lets him rest, waits for signs of interest in sucking/waking up. At signs of rooting, pulls the infant closer to her body, with the nose touching the breast and the chin pressed into the breast.	Opens the infant's mouth. Inserts the nipple into the infant's mouth. Continues her efforts to make the infant latch on in spite of no response. Holds the infant loosely, at some distance from her body. Nose and chin do not touch the breast, or the nose is "pressed into" the breast.
Is attentive to the infant's position at the breast	Does not notice incorrect position.
Makes appropriate adjustments when needed.	Does not make any adjustments.

(continues)

TABLE 7-2 Maternal Behavior During Breastfeeding Preterm Infants (*continued*)

Sensitivity	Lack of Sensitivity
Focuses her attention mainly at the infant; does not pay much interest in the environment.	Focuses her attention at the environment; looks at the infant occasionally.
Has a relaxed face.	Looks worried, stressed, uncomfortable, or bored.
When the infant makes long pauses during sucking: Encourages sucking by talking or gently depressing breast tissue in front of the infant's nose to elicit the sucking reflex by tactile stimulation of the hard palate. Is mainly quiet, may talk sometimes in a soft voice with the infant's father, staff, or other parents.	Does not stimulate sucking, or stimulates the infant repeatedly by tickling face and body, patting, rocking, talking, moving the breast, or repositioning. Does not notice lack of response. Talks in a loud voice with infant's father, staff, or other parents.
Lets the infant suck until he stops and lets go of the breast.	Interrupts or terminates breastfeeding while the infant is still sucking.

production. This practice also gives mothers proof of their ability to produce milk in spite of preterm birth. Ideally, these mothers who provide their infants' nutrition can borrow an electric breast pump, free of charge, for use at home during their infant's hospitalization. A hand pump may work for some mothers, but these are best for casual use, when the mother is outside the home or the hospital.

Early attainment of milk production that exceeds the infant's current needs should be encouraged (Hill, Aldag, & Chatterton, 1999). All of the mothers who attained a weekly production of more than 3,500 ml at the end of the second week were able to maintain sufficient milk production at weeks 4 and 5, whereas this was only achieved by 54% of mothers who produced 1,700 ml, and by none of the mothers with a weekly production of less than 1,700 ml.

Facilitation of Breast Milk Production

The mother can express her milk in a special pumping room. Some mothers like to express their milk at the infant's bedside, where they can look at or touch the infant during pumping—provided there are adequate arrangements for privacy. At home, the mother can arrange a cozy place for pumping where she has everything she needs within reach. Stress is an obstacle to the milk ejection reflex (MER), so the mother should be informed about what women in her situation have found helpful: sit in a comfortable chair, have something to drink, have something to read, listen to music or radio, watch TV. The MER can be triggered by gentle massage of the nipples before pumping, looking at the baby's photo, imagining the baby, and holding or smelling clothes worn by the baby.

After some time, mothers may experience reduced milk production in spite of frequent and regular pumping. Counseling about the impact of stress, pain, anxiety, exhaustion, grief, and the like on the MER and milk production is important so the mother does not believe that her milk will disappear completely. Telling her about relactation may inspire belief in her own capacity and help her to persevere in pumping or increase pumping frequency.

> The mother's milk production reflects her state of mind. In cases of decreasing milk volumes, continued frequent pumping often—but not always—results in increased milk production after some time.

Observing Breastfeeding in Preterm Infants

Breastfeeding policies for preterm infants are based on health professionals' perception of what can be expected from these infants. Meier and Anderson (1987) described a burst-pause pattern in infants at 32–36 weeks, initially with sucking bursts of 3–7 sucks or isolated sucks. A few days later, some infants managed bursts of 10–15 consecutive sucks.

The author developed the Preterm Infant Breastfeeding Behavior Scale (PIBBS) and performed the first prospective descriptive study ever of the development of preterm infants' breastfeeding behavior (**Table 7-3**; Nyqvist, Rubertsson et al., 1996). This is a method for direct observation by professionals and mothers of levels of oral motor competence (see **Figures 7-1** and **7-2**). The aim is to obtain a basis for practical suggestions to the mother about enhancement of the infant's breastfeeding competence. The method can also be applied to term infants (Radzyminski, 2003).

Early Breastfeeding Competence in Preterm Infants

Seventy-one mothers of 71 singletons, born at a GA between 26 and 35 weeks, without serious illness, used the PIBBS as a breastfeeding diary, providing more than 4,000 PIBBS records (Nyqvist, Ewald, & Sjodén, 1999). Breastfeeding was initiated as soon as the infant was able to breathe without ventilator or continuous positive airway pressure (CPAP), irrespective of current PMA, age, or weight. The mother received weekly breastfeeding counseling based on the PIBBS (**Table 7-4**). As soon as there were signs of milk intake, test-weighing was introduced before and after each breastfeed.

The first breastfeed occurred at 27 weeks PMA. Breastfeeding milestones are presented in **Table 7-5**. Irrespective of PMA on the first day with breastfeeding, all infants rooted (the majority showed obvious rooting) and latched on, half of them efficiently. Most infants stayed fixed for short periods, 5 minutes or less. Nearly all infants engaged in single sucks or short sucking bursts. Obvious rooting, efficient areolar grasp, and staying fixed at the

TABLE 7-3 Breastfeeding Observation According to the PIBBS

Mark/record data in the box for the description that agrees with the infant's best performance.

Date									
Time									

Rooting (lip movements, mouth opening, tongue extension, hand to mouth/face movements, head turning, squirming)

No rooting									
Some rooting									
Obvious rooting (simultaneous mouth opening + head turning)									

How much of the breast was inside the infant's mouth?

None, the mouth merely touched the nipple									
Part of the nipple									
Whole nipple									
Nipple and part of the areola									

Latched on and stayed fixed

Did not stay fixed									
Stayed fixed for less than 1 minute									
For how many minutes did the infant stay fixed before she/he let go of the breast (including pauses for resting or sleep, with part of the breast inside the mouth)?									

Minutes 1–≥ 10

Sucking (sucking burst = number of consecutive sucks)

No activity directed at the breast									
Did not suck, only licked/tasted milk									
Single sucks, occasional short sucking bursts (2–9 sucks)									
2 or more short sucking bursts, occasional long bursts (> 10 sucks)									
2 or more consecutive long sucking bursts									

(continues)

Longest sucking burst										
Maximum number of consecutive sucks before a pause										

Swallowing										
No swallowing was noticed										
Occasional swallowing										
Repeated swallowing										

breast for long periods were observed as early as 28 weeks. Some infants sucked in long sucking bursts, even bursts of ≥ 30 sucks, at 32 weeks. The longest sucking burst data showed large variation. Mothers perceived repeated audible swallowing at 31 weeks at the earliest.

Ninety-four percent of the infants were breastfed at discharge from hospital, 80% fully and 14% partially. Some infants reached full breastfeeding with an immature sucking pattern (mainly short sucking bursts and respiration occurring during pauses). On the day of attainment of full breastfeeding, several infants were able to ingest large volumes, whereas others mainly took small volumes, with 40 ml as maximum (Nyqvist, 2001). Infants with apnea treatment and a longer period of separation from their mothers (number of days when the mother was not living in a parent room in the unit) established breastfeeding at

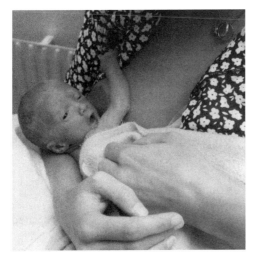

Figure 7-1 Rooting.

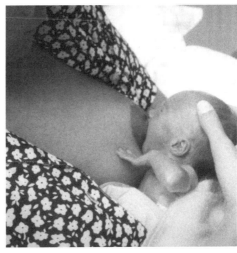

Figure 7-2 Latch.

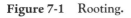

TABLE 7-4 Practical Advice Based on Breastfeeding Observation According to the Preterm Infant Breastfeeding Behavior Scale (PIBBS)

Rooting: The infant does not root.
Support and advice: Give the mother suggestions about touching the infant's lips with the nipple or a finger to elicit rooting. Inform her that (a) touching the infant's cheek or corner of the mouth may cause restless movements, but elicits the rooting reflex in a term infant, and (b) that crying is a late hunger cue.

How much of the breast is inside the infant's mouth: Nothing, part of the nipple, or the whole nipple but no areola.
Support and advice: Give the mother suggestions for how she can stimulate rooting, and pull the infant closer when she or he has a wide open mouth and the tongue down. Touching the infant's palm may stimulate mouth opening (the palmomental reflex) when she or he approaches term age. Inform her that signs of a good latch are: the tip of the infant's nose touches the breast, the chin is burrowed into the breast, and infant is able to stay fixed.

Latching on and staying fixed: The infant does not stay fixed at all or only for short periods.
Support and advice: Suggest to the mother that she pull the infant closer. If the infant's nose is pressed into the breast, she should pull the buttocks closer. Ask her to avoid pressing down breast tissue and avoid using the "scissors hold."

Sucking: The infant does not commence sucking, or takes very long pauses with calm breathing while being awake, without sucking.
Support and advice: Suggest to the mother that she talk to the infant, and depress breast tissue gently in front of the infant's nose (makes the nipple touch the hard palate, which elicits the sucking reflex). She could also touch the infant's palm.

Swallowing: No sound of swallowing is perceived (a silent sound when the airways close, or the sound of gulping in case of a rapid milk flow).
Support and advice: Inform the mother that it is difficult to hear this sound. Also tell her that it is impossible to estimate milk intake from an observation of sucking pattern, sucking duration, and sounds of swallowing.

Lack of improvement in spite of application of suggested advice.
Support and advice: If no improvement occurs in spite of application of the above-mentioned advice repeated times (the infant does not latch on, lets go of the breast repeatedly, sucks minimally in spite of being awake, ingests minimal volumes of milk or the milk consumption does not increase, in spite of sucking), suggest the use of a nipple shield and assess the effects.

a higher PMA and postnatal age (Nyqvist & Ewald, 1999). Low GA at birth was associated with early efficient breastfeeding behavior and a high incidence of full breastfeeding. This supports the theory that infant motor development occurs with experience (Thelen & Vogel, 1989). Oral motor competence is triggered when the nipple touches the infant's lips, the nipple touches the hard palate, and milk flows into the infant's mouth.

TABLE 7-5 **Developmental Milestones in Preterm Infants' Progress in Breastfeeding**

Events	n	Postmenstrual Age Median (range)	Postnatal Age Median (range)
Initiation of breastfeeding	71	33.7 (27.9–35.9)	1 (0–20)
First nutritive sucking (>5 ml)*	71	34.3 (30.6–37.7)	8 (1–46)
Exclusive breastfeeding	57	36.0 (33.4–40.0)	19 (2–68)

*Verified by test-weighing (the electronic scales in the level II nursery gave infants' weight to the nearest 5 g).

Initiation of breastfeeding in preterm infants should be based merely on cardiorespiratory stability (with severe apnea, bradycardia, and desaturation in connection with handling functioning as exclusion criteria), irrespective of current postmenstrual age, postnatal age, or weight. Initiation is possible from a postmenstrual age of 27 weeks.

Individual Sucking Patterns

Considerable variability in sucking patterns, sucking intensity and frequency, and duration of pauses were found in a study of 26 infants at 32–37 weeks PMA, using surface electromyography, or EMG (Nyqvist, Farnstrand, Edebol, Eeg-Olofsson, & Ewald, 2001; see **Figure 7-3**). The proportion of time spent sucking ranged between 10% and 60% of a breastfeeding episode. Corresponding data for mouthing (movements in lips, tongue, and jaw other than sucking) were 2–35%, and for pauses 12–67%. The longest sucking burst ranged from 5 to 96 sucks; this long sucking burst was noted at 34 weeks.

Common restrictions in the duration of breastfeeds, for example permitting a mother-infant pair a maximum time of 15 or 30 minutes, are unwarranted. The infant is not exhausted by a long time at the breast, because he or she is in control of his or her pattern of sucking, swallowing, breathing, and resting.

Mental Checklist for Practical Breastfeeding Support

Information Before the Delivery

When there is enough time, a mother admitted for impending preterm delivery (and the father) should be informed about how the infant will be fed, the lactation process and benefits of breast milk, and the value of initiating breast milk expression as early as possible. She is also told about skin-to-skin (STS) holding—the kangaroo mother care method—and when she can commence breastfeeding.

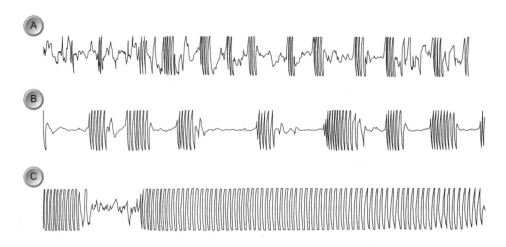

Figure 7-3 **Sucking patterns in preterm infants obtained by electromyography.**
A. PMA 33 weeks, age 25 days. Repeated short sucking bursts with mainly high sucking intensity. Pauses with considerable mouthing. **B.** PMA 33 weeks, age 17 days. Repeated short sucking bursts and occasional long bursts (3rd from the right), mainly high sucking intensity. Occasional mouthing after and between bursts. **C.** PMA 34 weeks + 6 days, age 18 days. Very long sucking bursts with high intensity. Some mouthing.

Skin-to-Skin Contact

Encouragement of early, prolonged mother-infant STS contact, without unfounded restrictions, is a fundamental strategy for support of lactation and breastfeeding. The mother immediately notices when the infant is waking up: She feels movements and changes in the respiratory pattern, hears subtle sounds, and can see eye opening and early signs of interest in sucking. This helps her to utilize her baby's short periods of alertness in an optimal way.

Prevention of Stressful Events

Plan the infant's care in order to avoid stressful events before breastfeeding. For preterm infants, diaper changes, washing, and bathing constitute stressful experience and deplete the infant's reserve of energy; they should not be performed immediately before breastfeeding (Morelius, Hellstrom-Westas, Carlen, Norman, & Nelson, 2006). On the other hand, a moderately preterm infant may wake up more easily during diaper changes.

Physiological Monitoring

For infants with tendencies for apnea, bradycardia, and desaturation, physiological monitoring of heart rate, respiration, and oxygen saturation at the mother's breast is advisable. Once the infant has shown adequate stability during breastfeeding, monitoring can be discontinued and replaced by the mother's assessment of her baby's breathing pattern and skin color.

Armchair, Footstool, and Pillow

Provide the mother with an armchair of the right height. Assist her in finding a comfortable, upright position, with adequate support for her back and arms. Offer her a pillow as a positioning aid, and a footstool to rest her feet and to facilitate the infant's position close to her body, with the head at the same height as the breast.

Breastfeeding Positions

Encourage the mother to hold her preterm baby STS under her clothes, covered by a blanket and—if the infant is very small—wearing a cap, in order to prevent heat loss. Suggest that she try different breastfeeding positions. The over-hand (transitional) hold is the most practical position for small infants (**Figure 7-4**), followed by the football hold (**Figure 7-5**), but there are alternative ways of achieving a functional position. Describe how to hold the infant close to her trunk, with the infant's head extended, neck and trunk aligned, and flexed arms and legs (with the lower arm tucked around the mother's body, under the breast). Explain why a preterm infant needs adequate head support in order to stay at the breast.

A Supportive Physical Environment

If possible, breastfeeding should take place in privacy in a parent room or a separate breastfeeding room. In the nursery, the mother can be offered privacy by a curtain, screen, or partitioning wall, or by placing the armchair with her back turned against the room. It is essential that the environment is as calm as possible, with conversations taking place in a low voice and disturbing sounds removed. The infant's eyes should be protected from direct light and activity in the visual field.

A Professional's Presence

Offer your presence in connection with the first few breastfeeding sessions, sitting down by the mother, in order to guide her interaction with the infant and to answer questions.

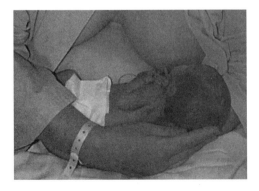

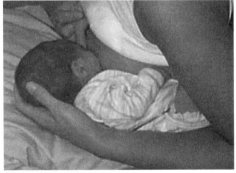

Figure 7-4 Overhand position.   **Figure 7-5** Football hold.

No Unfounded Restrictions

The infant's time at the breast should not be restricted unless there are definite reasons, such as a medical procedure that must take place at a certain time. Instead, the mother should be encouraged to allow the infant plenty of time to suck and rest between periods of activity.

Realistic Expectations

GA at birth, past and present medical problems, normal variations in development, and individuality contribute to infants' progress. Maturational level alone cannot be applied as a criterion for expectation on incidence and duration of periods of alertness, feeding frequency, sucking behavior, or milk intake.

Guidance of Mother-Infant Interaction

By interpreting infant behavior according to the NIDCAP model, optimal opportunities are created for the infant's activities directed at the breast: Point out the infant's signs of alertness and robustness, which signal availability for stimulation at the breast, and signs that the infant is tired and needs to rest, when stimulation should be withheld.

Tell the mother about preterm infants' response to touch; advise her to hold the infant with still hands once a comfortable position has been achieved. Caressing, patting, tickling, and rocking usually result in movements that obstruct successful breastfeeding (squirming, extension of arms and legs, arching head and trunk, pulling away from the breast, and irregular respiration with pauses).

Use of Alternative Feeding Methods Related to Breastfeeding

Aims of a Breastfeeding-Supportive Feeding Policy

To support optimal infant growth, satisfy infants' need for sucking, and achieve a feeding situation that is as normal as possible with respect to parent-infant contact and physical environment, entrust parents with the normal parental task of feeding as soon as possible, enable mothers to breastfeed, terminate a regulated feeding schedule with fixed times and volumes as soon as possible, and support breastfeeding (ideally exclusive breastfeeding).

Cup Feeding

Cup-fed infants soon learn how to take milk from the cup, and the method is not time-consuming, provided that it is performed correctly (Gupta, Khanna, & Chattree, 1999; Malhotra et al., 1999). Before a parent cup feeds the first time, a nurse should demonstrate how to hold the baby in an upright position and how to hold the cup; spillage is measured in order to ensure prescribed milk intake (Dowling, Meier, DiFiore, Blatz, & Martin, 2002; Nyqvist & Strandell, 1999). Compared to bottle feeding, preterm infants are more stable during cup feedings with lower heart rates, higher oxygen saturations, and lower incidence of oxygen desaturation (Marinelli, Burke, & Dodd, 2001; Rocha, Martinez, & Jorge, 2002), because the infant controls the pace and volume of milk intake (Lang, 1994).

> Cup feeding is the first choice of an alternative oral feeding method, when full oral feeding cannot be achieved wholly by breastfeeding, and can be introduced from a PMA of 29 weeks. A cup is used (a) when the infant is awake for a feed in the mother's absence, and (b) after a breastfeed when the infant has not taken enough milk, does not want to suck, and is awake.

Tube Feeding

Compared to bottle supplements, preterm infants who received supplementation by tube were more likely to be breastfeeding at discharge (Kliethermes, Cross, Lanese, Johnson, & Simon, 1999). The use of a permanent indwelling naso- or orogastric feeding tube is common during the period of transition from full enteral to full oral feeding, but may negatively influence sucking. Shiao et al. (1995) observed lower minute ventilation and tidal volume, lower pulse rate, and lower oxygen saturation when the infant sucked with a nasogastric tube than without the tube. Infants sucked more forcefully and took more milk without the tube. Pacifier sucking during tube feeding has been associated with decreased intestinal transit time and more rapid weight gain (Bernbaum, Pereira, Watkins, & Peckham, 1983) and a decrease in restless states (DiPietro, Cusson, Caughy, & Fox, 1994).

One approach is to regard tube feeding as an invasive practice and limit tube feeding to situations when an infant cannot be fed by cup because of prematurity, medical problems, or exhaustion. This policy is supported by evidence of risks for poor sucking ability and feeding problems in infancy in infants with prolonged exposure to tube feeding (Bier, Ferguson, Cho, & Vohr, 1993; Hawdon, Beauregard, Slattery, & Kennedy, 2000). On the other hand, the use of an indwelling tube is justified when the infant cannot be fed orally because of serious illness or because he or she needs frequent tube feeding. An infant with an occasional requirement of tube feeding can have a new tube inserted and removed in connection with each feed. Staff can offer to teach parents how to tube feed as soon as the infant shows sufficient physiologic stability during feeding. Parents can also be offered the opportunity to perform tube insertion, especially in case of early discharge for home care.

Bottle Feeding: An Exception When the Mother Intends to Breastfeed

In addition to the negative physiological effects it causes, bottle feeding constitutes an obstacle to breastfeeding, because facial muscles are activated in a way that differs from the oral motor pattern used during breastfeeding. Bottle feeding promotes the view of feeding as the provision of fixed volumes at fixed intervals, by anybody—it does not require the

> **A breastfeeding-friendly tube-feeding policy should include the following components:**
>
> - Preferably, the infant is held by a parent while he or she is fed.
> - An infant who has commenced breastfeeding is tube fed at the mother's breast.
> - An infant who cannot be positioned at the mother's breast during tube feeding, including infants with ventilator or CPAP treatment, is offered either
>   - The opportunity to suck a pacifier during each tube feed
>   - A small portion of breast milk, 0.5–1 ml, in the beginning of each tube feed by gentle administration via a syringe on one side of the tongue, combined with pacifier sucking.

mother's presence. Furthermore, it is mainly a feeding method, in contrast with breastfeeding which is also the newborn infant's main strategy for self-regulation during the process of adaptation to the extra-uterine environment.

In a feeding policy based on prioritizing breastfeeding, bottle feeding is considered appropriate when the mother:

- Is unable to breastfeed for medical reasons
- Is unable to attain a milk production that satisfies her infant's needs in spite of efforts
- Does not intend to breastfeed, which should be the result of an informed decision, and can have psychological explanations
- Explicitly demands to use a bottle after being provided information about the advantages of cup feeding and reasons for a restrictive attitude toward bottle feeding

Nipple Shield

For term infants, caution is recommended by some authors regarding the use of nipple shields because of a possible risk of reduced milk transfer. In contrast, mothers' use of a nipple shield while breastfeeding their preterm babies was associated with higher milk consumption (Meier et al., 2000). Indications for nipple shield use mentioned by these authors were that the infant had difficulties in latching onto or staying fixed at the breast. The shield also helped to remind infants about sucking when they kept falling asleep at the breast: It resulted in longer sucking bursts and longer periods of wakefulness.

Transition from Full or Partial Enteral Feeding to Full Breastfeeding

The following guidelines are based on evidence and clinical experience in the unit where the author is working. Since their introduction, the PMA when infants reach full breastfeeding has decreased gradually. Healthy preterm infants are often discharged with full breastfeeding around one month before the expected date of birth, many at 34 weeks, and several at 33 weeks. A few infants reach full breastfeeding at 32 weeks (**Table 7-6**).

Initiation of Breastfeeding

Breastfeeding is initiated as soon as the infant has been weaned off the ventilator and CPAP and does not show severe physiologic instability, irrespective of current PMA, age, or weight.

TABLE 7-6   Breastfeeding Progress in a Very Preterm Girl

Infant: GA at birth: 30 weeks + 5 days, birth weight 1,525 g, length 41 cm, ventilator treatment 8 hours, CPAP 12 hours.

Mother: Multipara, age 39 years, nonsmoker

Day	PMA	Weight, g	Events Related to Feeding/Breastfeeding
0	30 + 5	1,525	Tube feeding, every 3 hours donor milk and colostrum.
1	30 + 6	1,525	Tube feeding, donor milk, and mother's own milk.
2	31 + 0	1,495	Commenced breastfeeding. Nurses' report: "Sucks very well, hungry." Cup fed in mother's absence.
3	31 + 0	1,425	Lowest weight (−7%)
4	31 + 2		Mother transfers to parent room in the NICU.
5	31 + 3	1,445	Milk intake 9 times: 1–25 ml. Tube fed 4 times.
9	32 + 0	1,530	Regained birth weight.
10	32 + 1	1,555	Semi-demand feeding introduced. Tube fed once.
			Transferred from incubator to water bed in open crib.
11	32 + 2	1,555	Reached exclusive breastfeeding: 20–50 ml. "Spent the night in the mother's bed."
12	32 + 3	1,595	Test-weighing is terminated.
14	32 + 5	1,645	Water bed removed from open crib.
15	32 + 6	1,650	Home care by parents.
18	33 + 2	1,749	Discharged from hospital. Follow-up at neonatal follow-up clinic in hospital and local child health center.

(Exceptions can be made for moderately preterm infants with CPAP who are sufficiently stable and dissatisfied with just pacifier sucking.) Additional oxygen via nasal prongs (nasal cannula) is no obstacle. The first time a mother positions her infant at the breast suggestions should be given about alternative breastfeeding positions and a breastfeeding observation should be made. Breastfeeding sessions should not be restricted in frequency or duration. The timing and volume of supplementary feeds need to be planned on an individual basis, to ensure attainment of a sufficient daily milk volume. The assessment of the infant's need for supplementation, timing, volume, and feeding method is made jointly by the mother and nurse in charge.

Breastfeeding mothers in the maternity unit also are encouraged to come for breast-feeding during the night, and—upon agreement—the nurse telephones the mother when her infant wakes. When a mother leaves the neonatal unit, she informs the nurse regarding how long she will be absent and how she can be reached (telephone, cell phone).

Transition from Scheduled Interval Feeding, to Semi-demand Feeding, to Demand Feeding

Internationally, feeding regimens based on feeds every 2, 3, or 4 hours are common in infants who are not breastfed fully. However, small infants tolerate frequent feeding intervals of 2 hours, with small volumes, more easily. The advantage of an initial feeding schedule every 2 hours is the message conveyed to the mother that a frequent feeding pattern, resembling breastfeeding, is natural. For very small preterm infants, hourly feeds may be even more appropriate.

Test-weighing is introduced when there are signs of milk intake at the breast: audible swallowing or appearance of fresh milk when feeding tube location is assessed by aspiration of gastric contents with a syringe. The goal is to reduce the number of tube feeds and the duration of the infant's exposure to a tube, and to facilitate early attainment of exclusive breastfeeding. Mothers who find test-weighing stressful are offered alternative strategies for reduction of supplementation (see next section).

As soon as the infant ingests about half of the volume of milk prescribed for a feed (once is enough), the scheduled interval feeding regimen is terminated, and a total daily milk volume is prescribed. The mother is reminded that a variable intake pattern is normal in breastfed children. The mother is encouraged to offer the infant the breast (a) whenever he or she shows any sign of interest, and (b) when a maximum of about 3 hours have passed since the last breastfeed, in order to encourage state transition; the sensation of the nipple touching the mouth and the taste of milk may elicit awakening.

The volumes of milk taken at the breast are recorded and added up. The mother and the nurse should decide jointly when the infant needs supplementation by tube or cup in order to reach the daily volume. The nurse responsible for each shift has the ultimate responsibility for ensuring consumption of the target daily volume. When the infant reaches full breast-feeding (or partial, when mixed feeding is required), test-weighing is discontinued. The infant is weighed once a day or every 2–3 days initially, to ensure adequate weight gain.

Definitions

Semi-demand feeding (or ad libitum feeding): Constant assessment of the infant's feeding cues for facilitation of frequent breastfeeding, combined with active encouragement of breastfeeding after long periods of rest, with supplemental feeds given whenever needed, in order to reach the daily prescribed milk volume.

Demand feeding: The infant's neurological development has reached a stage when the brain is able to co-regulate behavioral states with hunger and satiety, and feeding can be based entirely on the infant's hunger cues.

When the infant reaches term age, the immature sucking pattern is replaced by a mature sucking pattern with long bursts and rhythmical sucking interspersed with breathing, and the infant can safely be fed on demand. Many infants are discharged home from hospital fully breastfeeding when they are still premature. Their mothers usually need to keep up the semi-demand regimen for some time. They may have to awaken the infant, day and night, in order to avoid overly long inter-feed intervals and reach a sufficient number of feeds per day. This is crucial for avoiding "breastfeeding malnutrition": an infant who does not consume enough milk does not grow or may even lose weight, present with late hyperbilirubinemia, and become dehydrated with high levels of sodium and chloride (hypernatremic dehydration), a serious condition that is prevented by adequate breastfeeding/feeding (Cooper, Atherton, Kahana, & Kotagal, 1995).

The infant's feeding plan is established jointly by the mother/parents and the nursing staff. A graph like the one shown in **Figure 7-6** can be used to identify the infant's current phase in the establishment of breastfeeding together with the mother, and to prepare her for the following phases.

Strategies for the Transition from Enteral Feeding to Breastfeeding

Test-Weighing

When the infant shows progress in milk intake, test-weighing boosts mothers' confidence. It proves their infant's actual intake, is helpful for planning supplementation, and may reduce the time required to reach full breastfeeding. No difference in breastfeeding confidence was found between mothers of preterm infants who used test-weighing during hospitalization and those who did not (Hall, Shearer, Mogan, & Berkowitz, 2002). Mothers of preterm infants who are discharged early in the process of establishing breastfeeding may find test-weighing particularly valuable (Kavanaugh et al., 1995), because the primary concern of these mothers is adequacy of their milk production and milk transfer to their infants (Hill, Hanson, & Mefford, 1994).

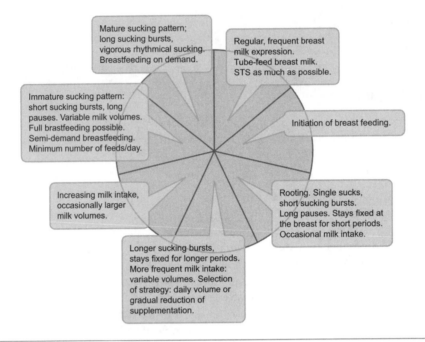

Figure 7-6 Phases in the mother and infant's progress in breast milk feeding and breastfeeding.

Gradual Reduction of Supplementation or Reduction According to Clinical Indices

Another alternative for transitioning is to reduce supplementation gradually according to a schedule. A third approach is to base decisions on the assessment of the infant's sucking vigor and pattern and sounds of audible swallowing, so called "clinical indices" of milk intake. However, this method is not reliable for evaluation of milk intake when used by mothers and nurses, not even in healthy children born at term (Meier et al., 1996).

Individual Strategies

A middle course between these strategies is to ask mothers what they perceive as helpful. When the infant's progress is slow, the test-weighing procedure may become an additional source of stress and disappointment for the mother. Instead of opportunities for enjoyable interaction, breastfeeding may be perceived as merely a way of providing nutrition, a duty to be fulfilled. In that case, gradual reduction of milk volumes is preferred. If the mother wishes, test-weighing can be performed for a 24-hour period once or twice a week for assessment of the pace of supplement reduction.

Early Discharge and Home Care

Usual criteria for transfer of the infant to home care in Sweden are medical stability, absence of apneic episodes, ability to maintain normal body temperature in an open crib (with clothes, cap, and adequate bedding) or by STS, and some oral intake at the breast. Parental criteria are readiness to take their infant home, ability to feed by tube and/or cup, and reported confidence in taking over the infant's care. Basic requirements are a safe home environment, access to a telephone, and means for transportation to the hospital. Scales should be provided free of charge as long as the infant is test-weighed. A minimum period of one or a couple of days at home before the infant's formal discharge from hospital, with telephone support, is required as a trial period. Daily rounds and communication about the infant's growth and planning of the infant's feeding occur over the telephone. The parents have access to telephone counseling by a nurse and neonatologist around the clock and can return to the hospital whenever they wish. Before formal discharge from the neonatal unit, relevant information about the infant, including breastfeeding status, is communicated to the local child health center. (Child health services are provided free of charge in Sweden.) The infant's health and growth are monitored carefully at the neonatal follow-up clinic and the child health center.

The Kangaroo Mother Care Method

At the same time as practices evolved in industrialized countries stipulating assessment of preterm infants' readiness to feed and advocating caution in introduction of oral feeding, the Kangaroo Mother Care (KMC) method was launched in Colombia (Gomez, Sanabria, & Marquette, 1993). KMC is based on kangaroo position, kangaroo feeding policy, and early discharge in kangaroo position. Alternative articles of clothing used for holding an infant in the kangaroo position are shown in **Figures 7-7** and **7-8**. Cup or spoon feeding is used to supplement breastfeeding. Outcomes of improved lactation and breastfeeding have been noted (Hurst, Valentine, Renfro, Burns, & Ferlic, 1997). In a multi-center study of KMC, the breastfeeding/breast milk feeding rates at discharge were 83%, 98%, and 80%, in the three hospital studies (Cattaneo, Davanzo, Worky et al., 1998).

In the Western world, STS periods of about one hour per day are common, not necessarily occurring every day. But as evidence of benefits of the method kept appearing, the International Network on Kangaroo Mother Care recommended that in settings with ample health and medical care resources "KMC can be applied to LBW infants of any postconceptional age from 28 weeks and onward, of any gestational age, of any weight (as low as 600 g), ... as tolerated by the mother-infant dyad, by the family and by the health care system" (Cattaneo, Davanzo, Uxa et al., 1998, p. 442). In 2003, the World Health Organization (WHO) included KMC among methods recommended for high quality neonatal care and published guidelines for practical implementation (WHO, 2003).

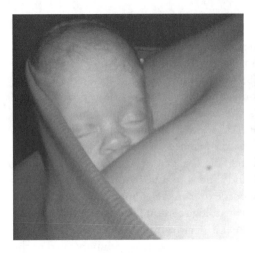

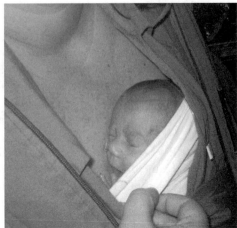

Figure 7-7   Kangaroo care blouse.   **Figure 7-8**   Kangaroo care top.

Table 7-7 describes a moderately preterm infant who had nearly uninterrupted STS contact with his mother (father acting as substitute) during his hospital stay. He was placed on his mother's chest immediately after birth and transported in this position to the NICU, where his parents roomed-in with him in a parent room. The mother breastfed at any subtle cue of interest from her baby, initially twice per hour. During nights the mother co-slept with him in the kangaroo position. As his mother breastfed him frequently and he sucked well, no supplementation was introduced. Regular blood glucose tests were made and his weight was followed closely. The reader is reminded that most preterm infants require variable periods of supplementation by tube and/or cup before they are breastfed fully. This case report is presented to highlight the need for re-evaluation of current common feeding policies and practices with a view to modifying them so they agree with infants' actual abilities. In an industrialized country such as Sweden, continuous KMC (including uninterrupted KMC from birth)—when possible—may be accepted by most parents, have a favorable impact on breastfeeding, and reduce the duration of infants' hospital stay.

Conclusion

By learning from evidence and experience from different parts of the world, lactation consultants can improve policies and practices, which will help mothers and preterm infants to attain their personal goals for breastfeeding in the best possible way.

TABLE 7-7   Continuous Kangaroo Mother Care from Birth

Infant: GA 34 weeks + 4 days, birth weight 2,835 g, vaginal birth, Apgar 9-9-10

Mother: multipara, age 30 years, nonsmoker

Day	PMA	Weight, g	Events Related to Feeding/Breastfeeding
0	34 + 4	2,835	Uninterrupted skin-to-skin contact with mother from birth. Very frequent breastfeeding (initially twice/hour). No supplementation. Regular B-Glucose tests.
3	35 + 0	2,578	Lowest weight (−9%).
4	35 + 1	2,635	STS interrupted for photo-therapy on water bed in an open crib one day because of hyperbilirubinemia.
5	35 + 2	2,670	Bilirubin levels do not require treatment. B-Glucose tests never showed any hypoglycemia. Home care program.
8	35 + 5	2,734	Discharge from hospital with exclusive breastfeeding. Never required any supplementation. Follow-up at neonatal follow-up program in hospital and local child health center.

References

Als, H., Lawhon, G., Duffy, F. H., et al. (1994). Individualized developmental care for the very low-birth-weight preterm infant. *Journal of the American Medical Association, 272,* 853–858.

Becker, P. T., Grunwald, P. C., Moorman, J., & Stuhr, S.. (1991). Outcomes of developmentally supportive nursing care for very-low-birth-weight infants. *Nursing Research, 140*(3), 150–155.

Bernbaum, J. C., Pereira, G. R., Watkins, J. B., & Peckham, G. J. (1983). Nonnutritive sucking during gavage feeding enhances growth and maturation in premature infants. *Pediatrics, 71*(1), 41–45.

Bier, J. A., Ferguson, A., Cho, C., Oh, W., & Vohr, B. (1993). The oral motor development of low-birth-weight infants who underwent orotracheal intubation during the neonatal period. *American Journal of Diseases in Children, 147*(8), 858–862.

Bier, J. A., Ferguson, A. E., Morales, Y., Liebling, J., Oh, W., & Vohr, B. (1997). Breastfeeding infants who were extremely low birth weight. *Pediatrics, 100,* e3.

Cattaneo, A., Davanzo, R., Worky, B., Surjono, A., Echeverria, M., Bedri, A., et al. (1998). Kangaroo mother care for low birthweight infants. A randomized controlled trial in different settings. *Acta Paediatrica, 87*(9), 976–985.

Cattaneo, A., Davanzo, R., Uxa, F., & Tamburlini, G. for the International Network on Kangaroo Mother Care. (1998). Recommendations for the implementation of Kangaroo Mother Care for low birthweight infants. *Acta Paediatrica, 87*(4), 440–445.

Chen, C.-H., Wang, T.-M., Chang, H.-M., et al. (2000). The effect of breast- and bottle-feeding on oxygen saturation and body temperature in preterm infants. *Journal of Human Lactation, 16,* 21–27.

Comrie, J. D., & Helm, J. M. (1997). Common feeding problems in the intensive care nursery: Maturation, organization, evaluation and management strategies. *Seminars of Speech and Language, 18,* 239–261.

Cooper, W. O., Atherton, H. D., Kahana, M., & Kotagal, U. R. (1995). Increased incidence of severe breastfeeding malnutrition and hypernatremia in a metropolitan area. *Pediatrics, 96*(5 Pt 1), 957–960.

Cousins, R. (1999). Breast feeding the preterm infant in the special care baby unit: The first feed. *Journal of Neonatal Nursing, 5,* 10–14.

Cregan, M. D., De Mello, T. R., Kershaw, D., McDougall, K., & Hartmann, P. E. (2002). Initiation of lactation in women after preterm delivery. *Acta Obstetrica Gynecologica Scandinavica, 81,* 870–877.

Davies, A. M., Koenig, J. S., & Thatch, B. T. (1988). Upper airway chemoreflex responses to saline and water in preterm infants. *Journal of Applied Physiology, 64*(4), 1412–1420.

DiPietro, J. A., Cusson, R. M., Caughy, M. O., & Fox, N. A. (1994). Behavioral and physiologic effects of nonnutritive sucking during gavage feeding in preterm infants. *Pediatric Research, 36*(2), 207–214.

Dowling, D. A. (1999). Physiological responses of preterm infants to breast-feeding and bottle-feeding with the orthodontic nipple. *Nursing Research, 48,* 78–85.

Dowling, D. A., Meier, P. P., DiFiore, J. M., Blatz, M., & Martin, R. J. (2002). Cup-feeding for preterm infants: Mechanics and safety. *Journal of Human Lactation, 18,* 13–20.

Feldman, R., & Eidelman, A. I. (2003). Direct and indirect effects of breast milk on the neurobehavioral and cognitive development of premature infants. *Developmental Psychobiology, 43,* 109–119.

Furman, L., Minich, N., & Hack, M. (2002). Correlates of lactation in mothers of very low birth weight infants. *Pediatrics, 109*(4), e57:1–7.

Gomez, H. M., Sanabria, E. R., & Marquette, C. M. (1992). The mother kangaroo programme. *International Journal of Child Health, 3*(1), 55–67.

Gupta, A., Khanna, K., & Chattree, S. (1999). Cup feeding: An alternative to bottle feeding in a neonatal intensive care unit. *Journal of Tropical Pediatrics, 45,* 108–110.

Hall, W. A., Shearer, K., Mogan, J., & Berkowitz, J. (2002). Weighing preterm infants before & after breastfeeding: Does it increase maternal confidence and competence? *MCN American Journal of Maternal and Child Nursing, 27*(6), 318–326.

Hanlon, M. B., Tripp, J. H., Ellis, R. E., Flack, F. C., Selley, W. G., & Shoesmith, H. J. (1997). Deglutition apnea as indicator of maturation of suckle feeding in bottle-fed preterm infants. *Developmental Medicine and Child Neurology, 39,* 534–542.

Hawdon, J. M., Beauregard, M., Slattery, J., & Kennedy, G. (2000). Identification of neonates at risk of developing feeding problems in infancy. *Developmental Medicine and Child Neurology, 42*(4), 235–239.

Hill, P. D., Aldag, J. C., & Chatterton, R. T. (1999). Effects of pumping style on milk production in mothers of non-nursing preterm infants. *Journal of Human Lactation, 15,* 209–215.

Hill, P. D., Brown, L. P., & Harker, T. L. (1995). Initiation and frequency of breast expression in breastfeeding mothers of LBW and VLBW infants. *Nursing Research, 44,* 352–355.

Hill, P. D., Hanson, K. S., & Mefford, A. L. (1994). Mothers of low birthweight infants: Breastfeeding patterns and problems. *Journal of Human Lactation, 10,* 169–176.

Hurst, N., Valentine, C. J., Renfro, L., Burns, P., & Ferlic, L. (1997). Skin-to-skin holding in the neonatal intensive care unit influences maternal milk volume. *Journal of Perinatology, 17*(3), 213-217.

Jones, E., Dimmock, P. W., & Spencer, S. A. (2001). A randomised controlled trial to compare methods of milk expression after preterm delivery. *Archives of Disease in Childhood, Fetal Neonatal Edition, 85,* F91-F95.

Kavanaugh, K., Mead, L., Meier, P., et al. (1995). Getting enough: Mothers' concern about breastfeeding a preterm infant after discharge. *Journal of Obstetric, Gynecologic and Neonatal Nursing, 24,* 23-32.

Kliethermes, P. A., Cross, M. L., Lanese, M. G., Johnson, K. M., & Simon, S. D. (1999). Transitioning preterm infants with nasogastric tube supplementation: Increased likelihood of breastfeeding. *Journal of Obstetric, Gynaecologic and Neonatal Nursing, 28,* 264-273.

Lang, S. (1994). Cup-feeding. An alternative method. *Midwives Chronicle & Nursing Notes, 107,* 171-176.

Lemons, P. K. (2001). Breast milk and the hospitalized infant: Guidelines for practice. *Neonatal Network, 20,* 47-52.

Malhotra, N., Vishwambaran, L., Sundaram, K. R., et al. (1999). A controlled trial of alternative methods of oral feeding in neonates. *Early Human Development, 54,* 29-38.

Marinelli, K. A., Burke, G. S., & Dodd, V. L. (2001). A comparison of the safety of cupfeedings and bottlefeedings in premature infants whose mothers intend to breastfeed. *Journal of Perinatology, 21,* 350-355.

Mathew, O. P. (1988). Respiratory control during nipple feeding in preterm infants. *Pediatric Pulmunology, 5,* 220-224.

McCain, G. C. (2003). Evidence-based guidelines for introducing oral feeding to healthy preterm infants. *Neonatal Network, 22*(5), 45-50.

Meier, P., & Anderson, G. C. (1987). Responses of small preterm infants to bottle- and breastfeeding. *MCN American Journal of Maternal and Child Nursing, 12*(2), 97-110.

Meier, P. M., Brown, L. P., Hurst, N. M., Spatz, D. L., Engstrom, J. L., Borucki, L. C., et al. (2000). Nipple shields for preterm infants: Effect on milk transfer and duration of breastfeeding. *Journal of Human Lactation, 16*(2), 106-114.

Meier, P. P., Engstrom, J. L., Fleming, B. A., et al. (1996). Estimating milk intake of hospitalized preterm infants who breastfeed. *Journal of Human Lactation, 12,* 21-26.

Meier, P. P. M. (2001). Breastfeeding in the special care nursery. Prematures and infants with medical problems. *Pediatric Clinics of North America, 48,* 425-442.

Morelius, E., Hellstrom-Westas, L., Carlen, C., Norman, E., & Nelson, N. (2006). Is a nappy change stressful to neonates? *Early Human Development, 82*(10), 669-676.

Nyqvist, K. H. (2001). The development of preterm infants' milk intake during breast feeding. *Journal of Neonatal Nursing. 7,* 48-52.

Nyqvist, K. H., & Ewald, U. (1999). Infant and maternal factors in the development of breastfeeding behavior and breastfeeding outcome in preterm infants. *Acta Paediatrica, 88,* 1194-1203.

Nyqvist, K. H., Ewald, U., & Sjodén, P.-O. (1996). Supporting a preterm infant's behavior during breastfeeding: A case report. *Journal of Human Lactation, 12*(3), 221-228.

Nyqvist, K. H., Ewald, U., & Sjodén, P.-O. (1999). Development of preterm infants' breastfeeding behavior. *Early Human Development, 55,* 247-264.

Nyqvist, K. H., Farnstrand, C., Eeg-Olofsson, K., & Ewald, U. (2001). Early oral behaviour in preterm infants during breastfeeding: An EMG study. *Acta Pediatrica, 90,* 658-663.

Nyqvist, K. H., Rubertsson, C., Ewald, U., et al. (1996). Development of the preterm infant breastfeeding behavior scale (PIBBS), a study of nurse-mother agreement. *Journal of Human Lactation, 12*(3), 207-219.

Nyqvist, K. H., & Strandell, E. (1999). Evaluation of a cup feeding protocol in a neonatal intensive care unit. *Journal of Neonatal Nursing, 2,* 31–36.

Radzyminski, S. (2003). The effect of ultra low dose epidural analgesia on newborn breastfeeding behaviors. *Journal of Obstetric Gynecologic and Neonatal Nursing, 32*(3), 322–331.

Rocha, N. M. N., Martinez, M. E., & Jorge, S. M. (2002). Cup or bottle for preterm infants: Effects on oxygen saturation, weight gain, and breastfeeding. *Journal of Human Lactation, 18,* 132–138.

Ross, E. S., & Browne, J. V. (2002). Developmental progression of feeding skills: An approach to supporting feeding in preterm infants. *Seminars in Neonatology, 7,* 469–475.

Schanler, R. (2001). The use of human milk for premature infants. *Pediatric Clinics of North America, 48,* 207–219.

Shiao, S. Y. P. K., Youngblut, J. A. M., Anderson, G. C., et al. (1995). Nasogastric tube placement: Effects on breathing and sucking in very-low-birth-weight infants. *Nursing Research, 44*(2), 82–88.

Smith, M. M., Durkin, M., Hinton, V. J., et al. (2003). Influence of breastfeeding on cognitive outcomes and age 6–8 years: Follow-up of very low birth weight infants. *American Journal of Epidemiology, 158,* 1075–1082.

Thelen, E., & Vogel, A. (1989). Toward an action-based theory of infant development. In J. Lockman & N. Hazen (Eds.), *Action in social context* (pp. 123–164). New York: Plenum.

Thoyre, S. M., Shaker, C. S., & Pridham, K. F. (2005). The early feeding skills assessment for preterm infants. *Neonatal Network, 24*(3), 7–16.

Uvnäs-Moberg, K., & Eriksson, M. (1996). Breastfeeding: physiological, endocrine, and behavioural adaptations caused by oxytocin and local neurogenic activity in the nipple and mammary gland. *Acta Paediatrica, 85,* 525–530.

Wheeler, J. L., Johnson, M., Collie, L., et al. (1999). Promoting breastfeeding in the neonatal intensive care unit. *Breastfeeding Review, 7,* 15–18.

White-Traut, R. C., Berbaum, M. L., Lessen, B., McFarlin, B., & Cardenas, L. (2005). Feeding readiness in preterm infants. *MCN American Journal of Maternal and Child Nursing, 30*(1), 52–59.

World Health Organization, Department of Reproductive Health and Research. (2003). *Kangaroo mother care. A practical guide.* Geneva, Switzerland: WHO.

Chapter 8

The Influence of Anatomic and Structural Issues on Sucking Skills

Catherine Watson Genna

Ankyloglossia (Tongue-Tie)

Ankyloglossia or tongue-tie is considered a minor anomaly. It may be isolated or may occur with other midline defects. Ankyloglossia is caused by insufficient apoptosis during prenatal differentiation of the tongue from the floor of the mouth. The cells that attach the tongue to the floor of the mouth normally regress from anterior to posterior, leaving a small remnant of attachment called the lingual frenulum. The lingual frenulum is an extension of the oral mucosa to the tongue, and is poorly vascularized and poorly innervated at birth. If the lingual frenulum is too inelastic, too short, failed to regress and extends along the underside of the tongue, or is placed too close to the gum ridge, tongue function will be restricted. Many combinations of length, placement, and elasticity are possible, affording a wide range of potential effects on feeding skills.

Tongue Mobility

Tongue mobility is often assessed by the infant's ability to extend the tongue tip over the gum ridge. Tongue extension in a tongue-tied infant generally decreases as the infant opens the mouth wider (tongue retraction increases with gape). Because a wide gape is vital to a deep latch, and the tongue contacting the breast is the stimulus for latch, tongue retraction interferes with attachment. Retraction (pulling back) with gape may cause the infant who can keep the tongue over the gum ridge while sucking an adult finger to be unable to do so during breastfeeding, where a wider gape is required (see **Figure 8-1**). The presence of the tongue tip over the lower gum during sucking is important to prevent the bite reflex from being stimulated. Normally, the tongue tip extends over the lower lip with the mouth wide open. Tongue extension can be elicited by a touch to the front (not the tooth-bearing surface) of the lower gum in infants (see **Figure 8-2**). Infants with slightly more posterior tongue attachments may be able to extend the tongue over the gum ridge, but traction from the restrictive frenulum will cause the tongue tip to be pulled under and the posterior tongue to elevate (see **Figure 8-3**).

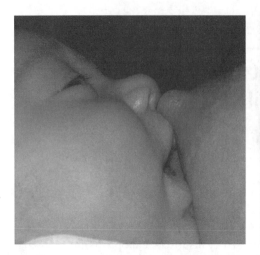

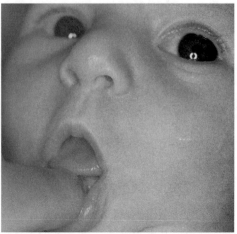

Figure 8-1 Tongue retraction with gape prevents the infant from grasping the breast.

Figure 8-2 Stimulating tongue extension by touch to the front surface of the lower gum. Note that in normal tongue extension, the tongue tip remains flat and extends well out over the lower lip.

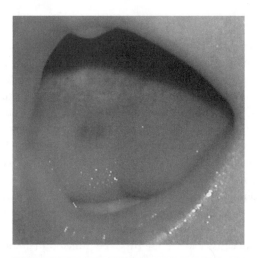

Figure 8-3 Restricted extension due to tongue tie.

Tongue elevation is more vital in suckling, because elevation of the anterior tongue stabilizes the breast in the mouth while the posterior tongue depresses to draw milk out. The sequential front to back wavelike movements of the anterior tongue may also move milk toward the nipple, and are probably important in initiating the smooth coordination of sucking and swallowing. Tongue elevation can be assessed during crying. The infant should be able to elevate the tongue blade straight to the palate with the mouth at least half open (see **Figure 8-4**). Infants who cry with the tongue flat in the mouth or with just a small portion of the anterior tongue curled back are tongue tied. If no opportunity is found to observe crying (the author certainly is not in favor of stimulating it!), holding the alert infant in an en face position and talking to him will stimulate reciprocal mouth movements and allow visualization of the upper surface (dorsum) of the tongue. A dent or pulled down area at the forward extent of the lingual frenulum may be noted as the infant "talks back." Lifting the tongue with a grooved director, tongue depressor, or finger will generally reveal a restrictive frenulum, as will palpation under the tongue with a fingertip coming from the side to midline (see **Figures 8-5** and **8-6**).

The sides of the tongue need to elevate to groove the tongue longitudinally to help form a teat from the nipple and surrounding areola, to stabilize it in the mouth, and to help form milk into a bolus for a controlled swallow. In some tongue-tied infants, the frenulum is sufficiently elastic for the grooving to occur; in others grooving is weak (see **Figure 8-7**). Grooving can be assessed by allowing the infant to suck a finger, and assessing how well the sides of the tongue hug the finger.

Lateralization (the ability to move the tongue tip to the sides of the mouth) is more important in eating solids than during suckling, when lateralization moves food repeatedly to the chewing surfaces of the teeth and after the meal allows the tongue tip to remove food trapped between teeth (see **Figure 8-8**). Nevertheless, inability to lateralize the tongue tip to at least the corners of the mouth without twisting the body of the tongue is a good sign of ankyloglossia that requires treatment (see **Figure 8-9**). Twisting of the tongue is a normal movement that is useful for pushing solids to the teeth during chewing (Hiiemae & Palmer, 2003), but does not substitute for lateralization (see **Figure 8-10**). Lateralization is uncommonly observed spontaneously in young infants, but can be stimulated by running a finger along the outside of the lower gum ridge from one side to the other. The tongue tip should be able to follow the finger at least to the corners of the lips with the body of the tongue held stationary in midline.

Examination of the hard palate may help to identify tongue-tied infants who require treatment. The palate forms from three plates, a small anterior midline primary palate, and larger lateral palatine shelves. The shelves grow over the tongue and meet each other in midline, and merge with the primary palate. Normal tongue movements in utero spread the forming palate into a broad "U" shape (see **Figure 8-11**). Ankyloglossia prevents palatal spreading, and will leave tongue-tied infants with a high arched and narrow palate (see **Figures 8-12** and **8-13**). The severity of the palatal distortion is proportional to the degree of tongue restriction. Reduced tongue strength, tone, and range of motion due to neurological disorders can also lead to abnormal palate shape (see Chapter 11).

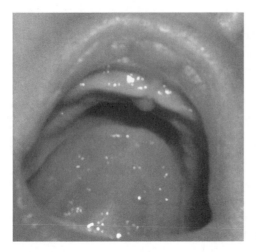

Figure 8-4 Normal tongue elevation.

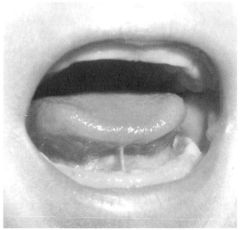

Figure 8-5 Restricted tongue elevation due to ankyloglossia (tongue-tie).

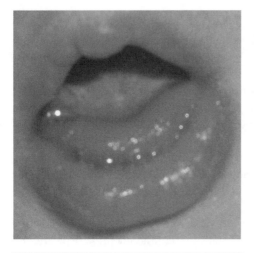

Figure 8-6 Posterior tongue-tie from above. Note how the tongue is pulled down strongly by the frenulum well behind the tongue tip.

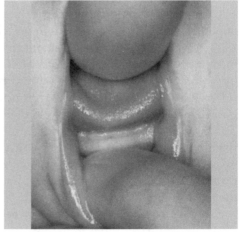

Figure 8-7 Weak grooving due to ankyloglossia.

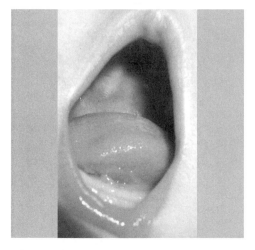

Figure 8-8 Normal lateralization.

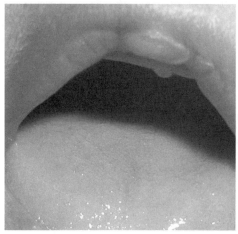

Figure 8-9 Restricted lateralization in complete tongue-tie. Note the large sucking blister on the upper lip.

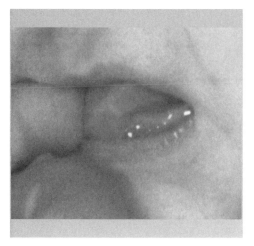

Figure 8-10 Twisting on lateralization in posterior (partial) tongue-tie.

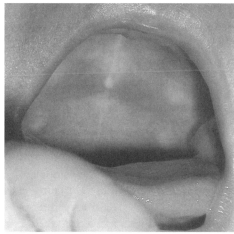

Figure 8-11 Normal palate.

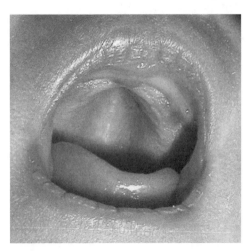

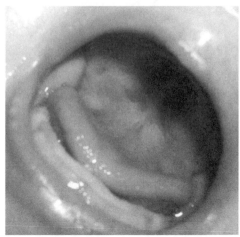

Figure 8-12 High, narrow, "V"-shaped palate in an infant with type 3 tongue-tie.

Figure 8-13 High, narrow palate in an infant with type 1 tongue-tie. Note the flat, retracted tongue.

Finally, allowing the infant to suck on a (suitably clean and covered) finger can be particularly helpful in assessing tongue mobility. Most infants will suck differently with and without fluid flow, so use of an eyedropper or syringe of milk is important to get the true picture. Curved-tip syringes are particularly useful for this purpose, because they are inexpensive and the tip can be inserted against the finger without disrupting the infant's lip seal. An infant with normal tongue mobility will use a biphasic pattern during sucking—a rapid backward wavelike movement along the anterior tongue, and then a slower downward movement of the posterior tongue associated with a slight opening of the jaw while the anterior tongue and lips remain sealed on the finger. Graduation of pressure is normal; most infants will use progressively more positive and negative pressure until milk is delivered. Tongue retraction so that the lower gum ridge is felt, excessive positive pressure such that the sucking is uncomfortable, and sliding, thrusting, excessive humping, or bumping movements of the tongue are all abnormal. In some tongue-tied infants, tongue elevation is so restricted that the finger can be withdrawn from the mouth without any resistance. Infants who make no negative pressure in the mouth should also be examined for the presence of a submucosal or overt cleft of the hard or soft palate (which are discussed later in this chapter).

Alison Hazelbaker advocated the examination of multiple tongue movements in her Assessment Tool for Lingual Frenulum Function (ATLFF; Hazelbaker, 1993). The ATLFF identifies the most severe ankyloglossia and has been used to identify infants requiring treatment in newborn nursery and lactation clinic settings (Ballard, Auer, & Khoury, 2002). Substantial inter-rater reliability was found in the function section for the characteristics of lift (elevation), extension, and lateralization (Amir, James, & Donath, 2006), with excellent agreement that frenotomy is indicated if the score on these three items is 4 or lower. Other authors, however, have found that sole reliance on this tool yields a high rate of false negatives (Ricke, Baker, Madlon-Kay, & DeFor, 2005). This is not surprising in light of the explosion of knowledge about breastfeeding mechanics since the ATLFF was designed. Still, the approach of scrutinizing both the appearance *and* function of the tongue remains helpful.

Effect on Breastfeeding

Tongue-tie often has a negative effect on latch, breastfeeding efficiency, and maternal comfort (Ballard, Auer, & Khoury, 2002; Dollberg, Botzer, Grunis, & Mimouni, 2006; Griffiths, 2004; Livingstone, Willis, Abdel-Wareth, Thiessen, & Lockitch, 2000). Some tongue-tied infants are able to latch and transfer milk, though most are less efficient than their peers with unrestricted tongue motion (Ramsay et al., 2004a). Others are unable to attach to breast at all. Some attach but fail to transfer enough milk to sustain growth and stimulate maternal supply; or cause maternal nipple or breast damage. The presence of tongue-tie triples the risk of weaning in the first week of life (Ricke et al., 2005).

Some of the variability in breastfeeding effectiveness can be attributed to maternal breast characteristics. Elasticity, nipple protractility, and maternal motor skills are all important in allowing the tongue-tied infant to perform at his best. The more elastic the breast, the easier it is for the infant to grasp a good portion of the areolar tissue for good milk transfer. Nipples that retract when grasped make it more difficult for any infant to attach to breast, but may make it impossible for tongue-tied infants. Good maternal motor planning skills or previous breastfeeding experience improve the support and assistance she is able to give to her infant to help him obtain an optimal latch. Optimal latch is vital to filling the mouth and stabilizing the tongue so it can function as well as possible during sucking.

Think of yourself with a rocket-shaped lollipop that has a narrow tip and widens toward the base. If you put only the slender tip of the rocket pop into your mouth, you need to lift your tongue tip to your upper gum ridge to press the pop there, and purse your lips to hold it in. If you put the slender tip way back nearly to your soft palate, you have the much wider base at your lips, so you can hold onto it without pursing, and your tongue can gently groove against the wide base of the lollipop without straining. Even if your tongue attachment is slightly tight, you should have enough "give" to press the lollipop further up to your palate with your tongue. If your tongue is very tight and unable to lift off the floor of your mouth, your lips and jaws will have to do all the work of keeping the pop in your mouth.

Classification of Ankyloglossia

Ankyloglossia or tongue-tie can be classified according to the sites of attachment of the lingual frenulum on the tongue and the floor of the mouth (see **Table 8-1**). Much of the disagreement in the literature on this subject is due to differing definitions of tongue-tie. It is generally more helpful to describe both the sites of attachment and the relative elasticity of the frenulum, as well as which specific tongue movements are restricted or altered. Griffiths (2004) classified tongue-tie by the proportion of the length of the tongue that was attached by the lingual frenulum. He found that even a thick, inelastic frenulum against the base of the tongue (0% tongue-tie) restricted tongue mobility, and that treatment of these very posterior frenula had positive outcomes in at least 50% of infants (personal communication, 2004).

Tongue range of motion is the most important factor in infant ability to breastfeed with ankyloglossia. A thin, elastic frenulum will generally impact tongue movement less than a thick, fibrous one (see **Figures 8-14** and **8-15**). Seventy-five percent of thick frenula were associated with breastfeeding difficulties in one case-control study (Messner, Lalakea, Aby, McMahon, & Bair, 2000). The elasticity of the floor of the mouth is another important component in tongue mobility. A very elastic mucosal floor may partially compensate for a restrictive lingual frenulum. If the floor of the mouth is tight and the frenulum is short and inelastic, the infant is at risk for very poor tongue function. The extent of the lingual frenulum along the underside of the tongue is another important determinant of function, with a longer attachment generally (but not always) restricting tongue elevation and extension more than a shorter one.

Often the most severe cases of ankyloglossia are not recognized because the infant has such limited ability to elevate the tongue that there is no telltale notching on the tongue tip, nor is there a heart-shaped anterior tongue. An infant with a severely restrictive lingual frenulum will usually keep the tongue behind the gum line, especially as the mouth opens (see

TABLE 8-1   Classification of Ankyloglossia

Type	Superior Attachment	Inferior Attachment	Characteristics of Frenulum
1	Tip of tongue	Alveolar ridge	Often thin, may be elastic
2	2–4 mm behind tongue tip	On or just behind alveolar ridge	Often thin, may be elastic
3	Mid-tongue	Middle of floor of mouth	Usually thicker, more fibrous, inelastic
4	Submucosal	Floor of mouth at base of tongue	Usually thick, fibrous, shiny, and inelastic

Source: Courtesy of Elizabeth V. Coryllos, MD, FAAP, FACS, IBCLC.

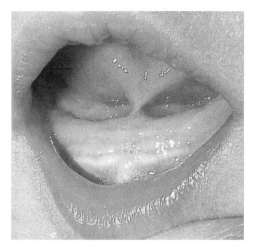

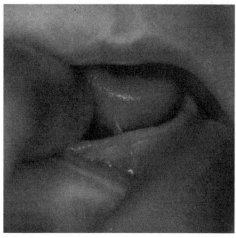

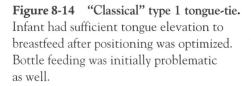

Figure 8-14 "Classical" type 1 tongue-tie. Infant had sufficient tongue elevation to breastfeed after positioning was optimized. Bottle feeding was initially problematic as well.

Figure 8-15 Severe type 1 tongue-tie. This lingual frenulum is thick and inelastic, and required treatment.

Figure 8-16). The tongue will appear flat, or bunched into an unusual configuration. Touch to the future tooth-bearing surface of the exposed lower gum ridge triggers reflexive biting, which is normally inhibited by the presence of the tongue tip there. If the infant retracts the tongue during sucking, the lower gum is exposed to the breast, and a normal phasic bite (bite-release-bite) takes place. The upper gum may also damage the breast if the infant keeps the mouth tight in order to help maintain attachment or move milk when the tongue is not sufficiently mobile. The combination of inability to elevate the tongue for wavelike movements (see **Figures 8-17** and **8-18**) and the triggering of the normal phasic bite reflex causes these infants to chew at the breast. Ultrasound studies are not capable of imaging the very front of the mouth, because the sound waves bounce off the bone of the jaw, leaving a black shadow. The consistency of maternal reports and the bruising or skin injury seen on the areola from the infant's gums leave little doubt that biting is occurring, however.

Normal feeding requires the anterior tongue to cup (curve gently upward) to grasp the breast while the body of the tongue flattens and pulls the breast into the mouth. Once the breast is in place, the anterior tongue presses against the breast in an anterior to posterior wave while the jaw assists by closing. This is believed to push milk toward the nipple (Ardran, Kemp, & Lind, 1958). As the wave passes to the posterior tongue, the jaw opens and the posterior tongue depresses and grooves, to enlarge the volume of the oral cavity, creating negative pressure. This negative pressure opens the nipple pores and pulls milk from the breast. Recent

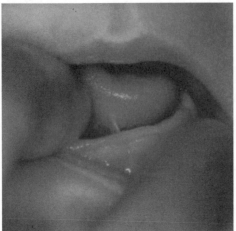

Figure 8-16   Type 2 tongue-tie.

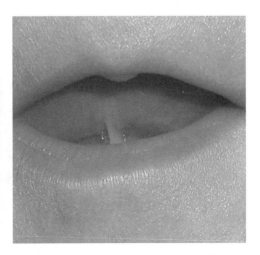

Figure 8-17   Type 3 tongue-tie.
Tongue tip can elevate when mouth is not
open widely.

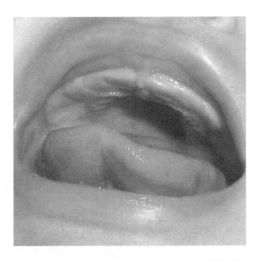

Figure 8-18   Type 3 tongue-tie.
When the mouth is open, only the edges of
the tongue are able to elevate.

ultrasound studies have revealed that the degree of depression of the posterior tongue is extremely important to the quantity of milk transferred per suck (Ramsay et al., 2004b). The grooved tongue collects the milk into a bolus and allows the infant to hold it there until enough milk builds up to trigger a swallow. The grooving of the posterior tongue is essential to controlled coordination of swallowing and breathing. Without grooving of the posterior tongue, milk may flow into the pharynx before the child is ready to swallow. Gulping that is poorly coordinated with breathing, aerophagia (swallowing excessive air), and even aspiration can result, making feeding uncomfortable, stressful, or scary for the infant. Poor ability to handle milk flow is a common cause of fussiness during feeding or even feeding refusal.

The tongue is a bundle of muscle that is anchored to the floor of the mouth by the root of the genioglossus muscle at the posterior floor of the mouth. When it is anchored along much of its length by the midline frenulum, normal range of motion is not available and the tongue is mainly able to redistribute its muscle mass backward or laterally. This results in a thick, bunched appearance of the tongue (see **Figure 8-19**) that progresses into an elevation of the muscle mass of the tongue posteriorly, creating an unusually large "hump" in the posterior tongue (see **Figure 8-20**). The repetitive stress of this pistoning movement against the breast or nipple can cause considerable trauma (see **Figure 8-21**).

Another compensation for restrictive tongue attachment is the use of a sliding motion of the tongue from anterior to posterior. This was seen in the author's ultrasound studies when the geniohyoid and mylohyoid muscles over-contract to assist tongue elevation. As the tongue retracts, the posterior tongue elevates and rubs against the maternal nipple. Mothers describe the sensation as feeling like sandpaper on their nipples. The infant can usually be observed to pull the breast in and out of the mouth when using this sucking pattern.

Infants with poor tongue function or a shallow latch may use a sweeping movement of the upper lip in an attempt to move milk from the breast with positive pressure, or in an attempt to hold onto the breast while the tongue slides or slips. This strategy generally causes severe sucking blisters on the infant's lips (see **Figures 8-22** through **8-24**). Ultrasound studies confirm that tongue-tied infants latch more shallowly than infants without a restrictive lingual frenulum (Ramsay et al., 2004a). Lip sweeping is not specific to tongue-tie, and is sometimes seen in infants with short mandibles as well.

Excessive jaw excursions are also seen in tongue-tied infants. The anterior tongue normally stays applied to the breast while the posterior tongue and mandible drop to make a small pocket of negative pressure in the mouth, which expands the nipple and pulls milk from the nipple pores. If the front of the tongue is not capable of elevating or remaining cupped and grooved around the breast as the back of the tongue drops, it is pulled by the frenulum to the floor of the mouth. Then the mandible must drop more in order to create negative pressure in the entire mouth, rather than in the small pocket behind the nipple. This increases the workload of the lips and cheeks; the cheeks may collapse or dimple (see **Figure 8-25**), and the baby may fall off the breast if the lips are not sufficiently strong to maintain the latch. Some infants compensate by fixing the lips and overusing the orbicularis oris muscle (see **Plate 3**). Tightening this circular sling of muscle around the lips often

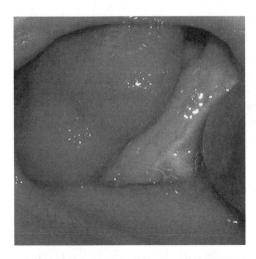

Figure 8-19 Attempts to mobilize the restricted tongue cause the thick, bunched configuration.

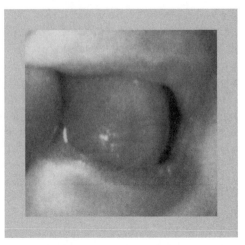

Figure 8-20 Posterior tongue elevation in type 3 tongue-tie.

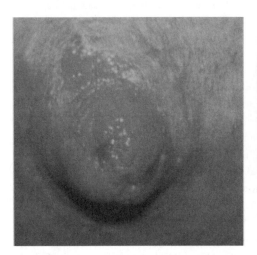

Figure 8-21 Nipple damage from posterior tongue elevation and pistoning after one week of healing.

Note the deep fissure at the nipple shaft just posterior to the face, and a compression fissure across the face of the nipple, leading to mastitis and candidiasis. Mother reported feeling the infant's tongue forcefully bumping into her nipple with each suck. Finger feeding with counterpressure on the posterior tongue helped the infant change her tongue movements so that feeding was then comfortable and more effective (see Figure 11-41 in Chapter 11).

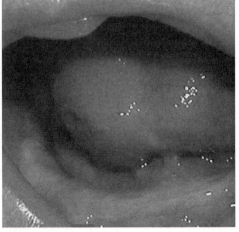

Figure 8-22 Infant with type 2 tongue-tie and large friction blister on upper lip. Compare the position of the blister in this photo and in Figure 8-24. This infant has a tight superior labial frenulum as well, so the blister is on the inner vermillion.

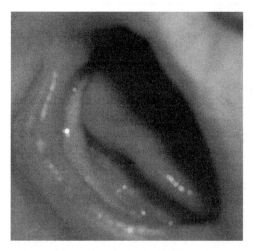

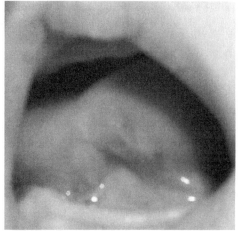

Figure 8-23 Type 4 tongue-tie is recognized by poor tongue mobility in a neurologically healthy infant with no visible frenulum.

Figure 8-24 Infant with type 4 tongue-tie pulls up the floor of the mouth to elevate the tongue. Note the huge friction blister in the typical position in midline on the upper lip.

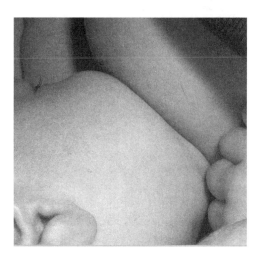

Figure 8-25 Excessive jaw excursion—note the flattened, dimpled cheek.

causes the baby to slide toward the nipple as the feed progresses, especially if the anterior tongue is not doing its part to help maintain attachment.

Treatment for Ankyloglossia

The obvious solution to symptomatic ankyloglossia is to divide the lingual frenulum against the underside of the tongue, releasing the restriction of tongue movements. Frenotomy was once routinely performed, until bottle feeding became the norm in Western culture. Now that breastfeeding initiation is increasing, articles advocating frenotomy for breastfeeding problems in infants with ankyloglossia are again appearing in the medical literature. Several randomized controlled trials have been conducted, indicating that 96% of infants who did not improve with intensive lactation consultant assistance substantially improved their feeding skills after frenotomy (Hogan, Westcott, & Griffiths, 2005), and that maternal pain and latch improve after frenotomy but not after a sham procedure (Dollberg et al., 2006).

Frenotomy in young infants is generally an outpatient or office procedure. Some practitioners use flavored benzocaine gel as a topical anesthetic; others use no anesthesia. The infant is immobilized by an assistant, and the tongue is lifted either with gloved fingers or a grooved director, a tool designed for performing frenotomy. Surgical scissors or a surgical laser is used to cut the frenulum either in midline or at the underside of the tongue. Care is taken to avoid the orifices of the submandibular glands on the floor of the mouth. The frenulum is usually avascular. If there is a blood vessel, it can be sutured above and below the frenotomy site and then the division made between the two sutures. Pressure to the incision site with gauze square is sufficient to prevent or stop bleeding in most cases. (See Chapter 9 for a detailed explanation of frenotomy procedures.)

After frenotomy, the majority of infants spontaneously correct their tongue movements during sucking. If improvement is not marked after 3–4 days, the infant should be re-examined to see if the tongue-tie was reduced but not eliminated. Further treatment is usually helpful in these cases. It is possible to perform simple frenotomy on infants with type 3 and 4 ankyloglossia. When the fibrous, posterior frenulum is snipped it opens up into a diamond shape, allowing more tongue movement in each direction. A more complex procedure such as transverse-vertical frenuloplasty is an option, though general anesthesia is then required. For infants with very poor tongue motion, the lifelong benefits of improved tongue function can outweigh the risks of anesthesia.

Management of Ankyloglossia Without Frenotomy

Infants who do not self-correct their suck within 4 days, and those who are not treated, may benefit from exercises to help improve tongue extension and elevation to the extent possible. In the author's practice, a subset of infants with severe restriction of tongue movement were able to breastfeed by about 6–9 weeks of age without frenotomy. In these cases, infants were fed expressed milk by bottle or Hazelbaker FingerFeeder, and breastfeeding was attempted periodically until gradually the infant was able to transition to exclusive breastfeeding. If frenotomy is unacceptable or unavailable to the parents, they can be encouraged to:

- Maintain a full milk supply by pumping at least eight times each day with a rental-grade breast pump or efficient manual expression

- Maintain practice at breast by putting baby to breast after a partial alternate feeding ("breast for dessert")

- Focus on obtaining the deepest asymmetrical latch possible

- Reduce posterior tongue elevation and retraction with oral exercises

Anticipatory guidance is important. Parents should be counseled to expect feedings to be less efficient, and to be patient if their infant needs to feed more often or for longer periods of time.

Even in tongue-tied infants who are able to breastfeed without maternal pain, feeding is less efficient. The infant may fatigue before being satiated, and milk supply will calibrate downward if mom fails to pump or express. Tremors of the tongue and/or mandible are common in tongue-tied infants, due to the fatigue involved in using less ergonomic compensatory tongue, jaw, and lip movements. This enhanced physiologic tremor is a reliable sign that the infant is working too hard. If tremor is seen in a neurologically healthy infant, oral anatomy and oral motor function should be assessed, and the infant's growth followed closely. If growth is suboptimal, supplementation with expressed milk fed in a way that supports breastfeeding (see Chapter 11) is important.

Latch Alterations

Attachment to the breast requires the tongue tip be down in the mouth and in contact with the breast. This is more difficult for infants with tongue-tie, who generally gape less well and may retract the tongue more as they open wider (see **Figure 8-3** earlier in the chapter). Several management alterations can help improve a tongue-tied infant's ability to latch. Giving good positional stability and shaping the breast to help the infant get a larger mouthful are covered in Chapter 5. Several additional strategies are helpful for tongue-tied infants.

Healthy, neurotypical infants with ankyloglossia may attach better if simply given optimal positioning and allowed to self-attach. This gives more time for them to organize their tongue movements to drop the tongue and grasp the breast. Optimal positioning includes holding baby diagonally against mom, with the baby's belly snuggled to mom's ribcage, hips flexed around mom's side, chest brought to mom's breast, chin on the areola, and philtrum to the nipple (see **Figure 8-26**). Mom should be encouraged to support baby's shoulders and back and keep her fingers off the head and neck, to allow the head to extend as the baby gapes widely and lunges for the breast (see **Figure 8-27**). Mom supports baby's movements by snuggling the baby straight toward her as the baby grasps the breast (see **Figure 8-28**).

If the baby is unable to bring the tongue down sufficiently and fails to grasp the breast repeatedly, the baby's entire body can be slid slightly toward the other breast, exposing a larger and easier to grasp circle of breast to the infant's tongue tip. The shoulders can be pressed in as well during this maneuver, to bring the chin and tongue tip closer to the breast.

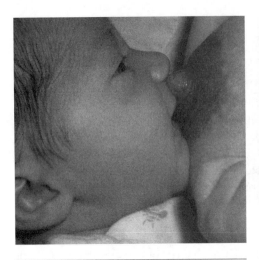

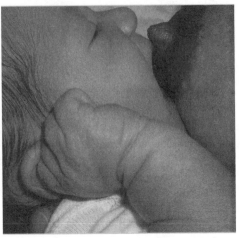

Figures 8-26   Asymmetrical attachment: chin on breast, philtrum to nipple.

Figure 8-27   Asymmetrical attachment: allows baby to gape.

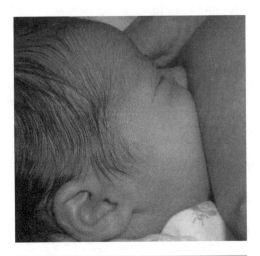

Figure 8-28   Asymmetrical attachment: baby snuggled in for a deep latch.

Another strategy that is particularly useful if the baby slides the lower lip and tongue tip toward the nipple during latch is to "dent" the breast at or just beyond the margin of the areola with one finger to form a firmed, billowed out area of breast for baby to grasp. The baby's chin is snuggled in the hollow created by the denting finger, which helps prevent the lower lip from sliding toward the nipple as the baby latches.

Finger Feeding Tongue-Tied Infants

The most important consideration for a tongue-tied infant who will not be treated is to help reduce some of the negative effects of sucking compensations. For infants who retract the tongue tip and/or use forceful posterior elevation, modified finger feeding can be helpful in reducing the excessive shifting of the tongue mass toward the back of the mouth. The finger and tube are held across both of the infant's lips with the well-filed fingernail on the philtrum, to simulate the feeling of the breast on the lower lip and the nipple touching the philtrum (see **Figure 8-29**). When the infant gapes widely, the fingertip is slid against the palate to reduce the chance of stimulating the gag reflex. Ideally, the infant will grasp the finger with the tongue and suck it deeply into the mouth, until the finger pad rests on the back of the hard palate, and the nail side of the finger is against the tongue in midline. Good contact with tongue and palate and alignment of the finger in midline is important as modeling for the position of the teat in breastfeeding, and helps to stimulate central grooving of the tongue that is so important in both stabilizing the teat and bolus control for safe swallowing (see **Figure 8-30** and **Figure 8-31**).

When the infant begins to suck, milk is delivered either by the infant's efforts (Hazelbaker FingerFeeder, or feeding tube in a bottle) or by the feeder (curved tip syringe or syringe and feeding tube). Feeder-controlled methods are particularly effective for operant conditioning. Milk delivery is stopped when the tongue retracts or the posterior tongue is pistoned against the finger, and resumed when the tongue tip is brought back over the gum ridge and the posterior tongue drops slightly. A slight reduction of the excessive posterior elevation may be enough to keep mom comfortable. The goal is not to completely flatten the tongue, but to help the infant maintain the tongue tip over the gum ridge to inhibit the bite reflex. It is important to remember that posterior tongue elevation is an important part of normal sucking; it is the *degree* to which the mass of the tongue is distributed backward and the force of the elevation that are abnormal in ankyloglossia.

Counter-pressure from the feeder's finger can also be used to discourage *excessive* posterior tongue elevation or tongue retraction. If there is posterior elevation but the tongue tip stays over the lower gum ridge, the feeder can simply angle the fingertip down against the over-elevated tongue until it drops slightly. Usually, the tongue is retracted as well, and a slight traction toward the front of the mouth is helpful. The finger is angled downward against the humped tongue and the humped area is pushed slightly toward the front of the mouth. The corrective force is provided with minimal finger movement, to avoid disrupting the infant's attachment to the finger.

Tongue Exercises

No oral exercise is capable of curing ankyloglossia, but specific targeted interventions may help reduce maladaptive or "limiting" compensations. With knowledge of tongue movements during normal suckling and infant sensory reflexes, exercises can be easily constructed to address each infant's needs. It is vital to respect the infant's autonomy and body integrity, and to make the exercise a game that the infant enjoys and actively participates in. Therefore,

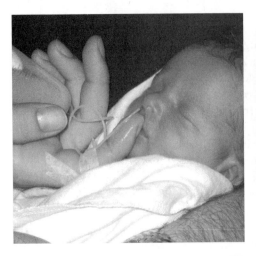

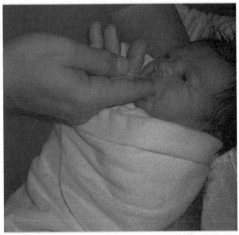

Figure 8-29 Presenting finger for finger feeding.

Figure 8-30 Finger feeding with head extended over arm in infant with respiratory disorder.

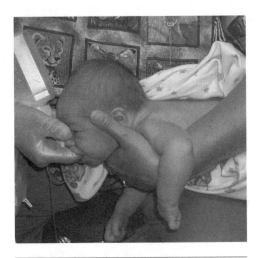

Figure 8-31 Finger feeding in prone position for infant with severe laryngomalacia.

the infant should be in a receptive (quiet alert or early active alert) state. The more predictable the sequence of stimuli and movements elicited, the more the infant is likely to tolerate and even enjoy the exercise.

Any exercise should show some signs of effectiveness in early trials. If the infant rejects it or it is ineffective in changing tongue movements even slightly, a different exercise or strategy should be used. Ideally, an infant with oral motor issues will be working with both a lactation consultant and a speech or occupational therapist with expertise in feeding.

Press-Down Exercise

This exercise was designed for an infant with a short mandible who was still using excessive posterior tongue elevation after frenotomy, but did not like having a finger in her mouth. Touch stimulation was given to chin, nose, and philtrum, and when the baby opened in response to touch on the philtrum, brief fingertip pressure was applied to the humped area of the tongue and the finger quickly withdrawn. A different sound was made with each touch, but the sound and tone for each specific touch was kept consistent, further adding to the predictability (and tolerability) of the stimulation. The sounds were silly (beep, bip, bop, boop) to help make it fun for the infant, and to provoke cross-modal processing to reinforce the effectiveness of the sequence. The adult performing the sequence smiled and made eye contact with the baby to reinforce the playfulness of the interaction. As soon as the baby failed to "play along" and open her mouth, the exercise was terminated for that session. After a few repeats, the baby was starting to drop her posterior tongue slightly when she opened her mouth. Her mother was encouraged to try this game very briefly before feedings, or between breasts if baby was too hungry to tolerate delaying the feeding a few seconds (see **Figure 8-32a–e**).

Tongue Massage

Infants with severe tongue retraction may respond to a small amplitude circular massage on the anterior tongue. The baby is stimulated to open the mouth by touch to the philtrum, and the finger pad is placed on the surface of the tongue just behind the tongue tip. The fingertip is rotated in a small circle without losing contact with the tongue (see **Figure 8-33**). The infant should improve the shape and extension of the tongue at least slightly during this massage. The infant will generally attempt to suck the finger; the finger can then be upended in the mouth so the finger pad is on the palate, and massage can continue with the (well trimmed and filed) nail side of the finger on the posterior tongue. Forward traction can be added to the massage by accentuating the portion of the circular movement that is moving anteriorly. Massage can precede finger feeding in an infant who is unable to latch onto the breast due to the severity of the tongue-tie. Sometimes just one brief session of tongue massage with or without finger feeding is sufficient to improve tongue extension enough for the baby to be able to attach to breast, though it might take many weeks before the infant is able to latch consistently and suckling is painless for the mother and efficient for the infant.

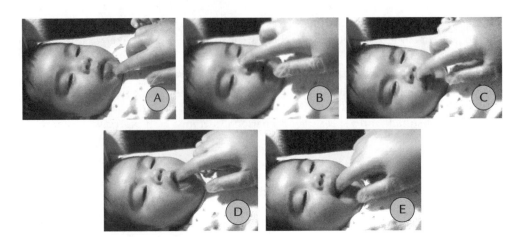

Figure 8-32 Press-down exercise.

Increasing Tongue Lateralization

After frenotomy, the infant may need some assistance to extend and lateralize the tongue. This exercise helps to stimulate the transverse tongue reflex, where the tongue tip follows a fingertip around the gum from center to side. The baby is stimulated to open the mouth by touching the philtrum or lips. When the infant opens, the fingertip is placed on the center of the lateral surface (outside) of the lower gum ridge and, maintaining contact with the gum ridge, moved around to the side, then lifted off and returned to center (see **Figure 8-34**). This is repeated three times in the same quadrant, and then repeated in the other quadrants of the mouth, lower gums first, and then upper. The immediate repetition in each quadrant gives the infant time to anticipate and follow the finger.

Desensitizing the Palate

Infants with high palatal arches occasionally resist a deep latch because stimulation to the relatively naïve apex of the palate stimulates their gag reflex. Many tongue-tied infants have strong and more anteriorly provoked than usual gag reflexes. The sensory characteristics of the soft breast and the provision of milk allow many infants to inhibit the gag. For infants with a gag that is difficult to inhibit, systematic desensitization can be helpful.

The infant is stimulated to open with touch to the philtrum or upper lip, and the fingertip touches the anterior hard palate in midline. The finger is gently slid back along the hard palate, stopping just before the spot at which the gag was stimulated previously (see **Figure 8-35**). (If the infant begins to gag as soon as the finger presses the anterior palate, firm pressure from the finger may help inhibit it.) Over several sessions or days, the infant generally learns to tolerate normal touch pressure to the palate. Desensitization

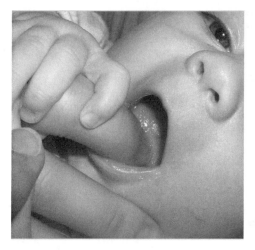

Figure 8-33 Tongue massage.

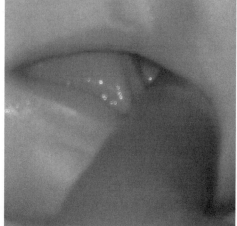

Figure 8-34 Stimulating tongue lateralization.

requires finesse to find the right balance of gentle challenge to help the infant tolerate touch yet avoiding pushing the infant too far and reinforcing their discomfort.

For the rare infant whose gag reflex is so hypersensitive that they cannot breastfeed, use of a mini-Haberman feeder until that is tolerated and then switching to the longer teat of the regular-size Haberman after a few days has been helpful as a transition to the breast in the author's practice.

Oral motor exercises designed for neurologically impaired infants can sometimes be useful for improving sucking in tongue-tied infants. These are found in Chapter 11. In choosing or designing exercises, it is important to identify the normal movements that are not being produced and encourage those, while discouraging the compensatory movements that are inefficient for the infant or painful for the mother.

Using a Nipple Shield

A thin silicone nipple shield used to preform the breast may assist infants with significant tongue retraction who are otherwise unable to latch. For tongue-tied infants, the widest diameter nipple shield teat that will fit completely in the mouth is optimal, because their restricted tongue grooving makes a narrow teat difficult to grasp. It is important to draw the entire nipple and significant areola into the shield teat. A particularly effective method of applying a nipple shield was innovated by professional engineer and IBCLC Linda Pohl (personal communication). The nipple shield is held on the fingers of both hands, with the thumbs on either side of the teat. The teat is partially inverted by bringing the thumbs toward the fingers and rotating the hands slightly away from each other. The shortened

Figure 8-35
Pressure on the anterior palate
helps desensitize a hypersensitive
gag response.

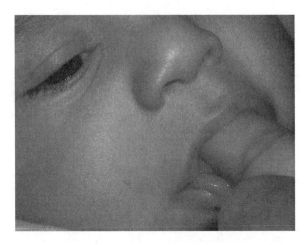

teat is placed over the nipple, and two fingers from each hand press into the folded area of the teat, first back toward the chest wall, and then outward toward the sides of the breast. The nipple and much of the surrounding tissue is drawn into the teat as it everts.

The breast should be presented as much as if the nipple shield were not there as possible, to preserve oral searching and gaping behaviors for eventual direct breastfeeding. Presenting the tip of the teat to the infant's philtrum helps create an asymmetrical latch and assists the infant in taking some of the area surrounding the teat, at least in the lower part of the mouth. (See **Figures 10-12** through **10-16** in Chapter 10.)

There are potential pitfalls of using a nipple shield in this population. For infants with significant tongue retraction, the shield becomes a stimulus for the bite reflex, and may actually increase maternal pain. Tongue-tied infants with high palates generally have an accentuated gag response, which may be stimulated by the shield. Expressing a few drops of milk into or onto the shield may help the infant inhibit the gag. Tongue-tied infants are less effective feeders, and the nipple shield may not allow good milk transfer. Whenever possible, test-weights should be performed when trying a nipple shield, and the shield abandoned if milk transfer is problematic. If milk transfer is substantial, but still suboptimal, brief breastfeeding for practice combined with pumping and alternate feeding may be the best use of the mother's time until baby's sucking improves.

Restricted tongue movements due to an anteriorly placed, short, or inelastic lingual frenulum can cause infants to use alternate, and less efficient, movements during feeding. Common movement patterns include posterior tongue elevation (humping) and pistoning, excessive compression and chewing, upper lip sweeping, and anterior-posterior sliding of the tongue. Each of these patterns has specific disadvantages to both mother and infant during feeding, and can usually be eliminated by frenotomy.

Superior Labial Frenulum

The lips are attached to the gum ridge in midline by frenula as well. If the superior (upper) labial frenulum is very tight, it might interfere with the infant's ability to maintain attachment to the breast. Generally, increasing head extension will allow the infant to grasp the breast sufficiently. If the labial frenulum is inserted into the upper gum ridge, it will cause a gap between the central incisors. Treatment in infancy can improve breastfeeding (Wiessinger, 1995), and can cause the frenulum to regress by interrupting its blood supply. Treatment in adulthood is much more difficult, and involves dissecting the labial frenulum from the gum ridge.

Hemangioma

Hemangiomas are the most common tumor in infancy. They are benign, and may be present at birth or appear during the early weeks of life. Hemangiomas grow rapidly, and then regress by about age nine (Smolinski & Yan, 2005). However, hemangiomas of the face may cause distortion of form and function, and those on mucosal areas such as the lip may ulcerate and cause pain, bleeding, and feeding difficulties (Band, 2000). The use of a topical anesthetic before feeding along with pain-relieving medication can help infants with an ulcerated hemangioma to breastfeed. Asymmetrical latch with head extension will help reduce upper lip stress, and make feeding as comfortable as possible. If breastfeeding is temporarily impossible, the infant may be more comfortable with cup or syringe feeding, to avoid contact with the ulcerated lip (see **Plate 2**).

Micrognathia and Mandibular Hypoplasia

There is no standard definition of what constitutes micrognathia (unusually short lower jaw). Clinically, if the infant's lower lip and jaw are completely subsumed by the maxillary (upper) gum ridge, the difference in jaw lengths is relevant. Newborns normally have recessed mandibles, partially due to in utero positioning with their head flexed into the chest. Breastfeeding provides normal muscular stresses on the jaws and may improve mandible growth (Page, 2001, 2003). However, Luz et al. (2006) failed to find a difference in the persistence of a short mandible in 5- to 11-year-old children breastfed for greater than versus less than 6 months.

Infants with shorter than usual lower jaws are likely to have feeding difficulties related to displacement of the tongue, reduced mechanical advantage, and restricted tongue movements. When the mandible is short, the tongue attachment is generally closer to the gum ridge, restricting elevation of the mid to posterior tongue. The habitual position of the tongue tip is often elevated and held to the palate, perhaps due to lack of space for the normal resting posture of the tongue tip over the lower lip. Micrognathia is associated with a narrower upper airway (Gunn, Tonkin, Hadden, Davis, & Gunn, 2000). A recent study found shorter mandibles as measured by a higher mandibular index in infants who had suffered an apparent life-threatening event vs. controls (Horn, 2006). Infants with short or retroplaced mandibles generally extend their heads and fix their tongues to the palate to help stabilize and enlarge the airway. (Compare **Plates 6** and **7** of tongue tip elevation and tongue fixing; the excessive muscle activity of fixing is obvious.) If the tongue is particularly long, it may be curled or humped in the mouth. These abnormal positions can be a poor basis for normal muscle strength and activation during sucking. Some infants with relatively long tongues have difficulty with coordination, and may use a tongue thrust pattern that pushes the breast out of the mouth. The use of a thin silicone nipple shield may help the infant maintain a deep attachment while tongue movements improve. If the infant cannot feed even with the shield, finger feeding can help strengthen the tongue and improve anticipatory tongue positioning for feeding.

Asymmetrical attachment to the breast is essential for infants with short jaws. Positioning the infant with the head well extended and the body snuggled under the mother's contralateral breast is often sufficient to improve feeding efficiency (see **Figures 8-36a–b** and **Figure 8-37a–b**). Sidelying may allow better head extension, depending on mother and baby's geometry (see **Figure 8-38**). Concerns about hyperextension of the neck in infants may be overstated; for at least the first 3 months of life the epiglottis and soft palate are in contact, and swallowing is not stressed by extension (Takagi & Bosma, 1960). Of course the effect of every intervention needs to be observed and evaluated to avoid destabilizing the infant.

The combination of a short tongue and lower jaw may cause the infant to use excessive positive pressure during suckling. Consistent unrelieved pressure may interfere with nipple perfusion and stimulate nipple vasospasm. Vasospasm (blanching of the nipple due to vaso-

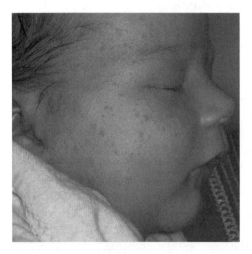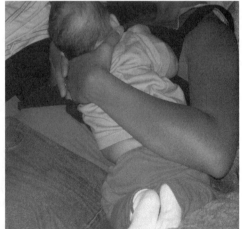

Figure 8-36 A modified kneeling prone position brought this baby's short jaw forward and improved baby's ability to manage milk flow.

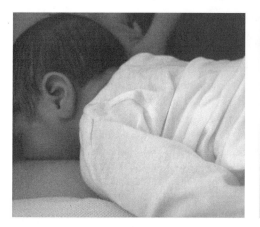
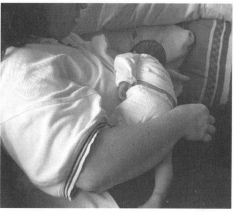

Figure 8-37 Prone positioning improves ability to manage milk flow in micrognathic infants with respiratory instability.

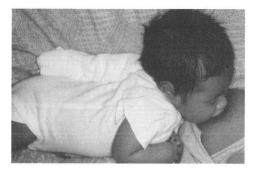

Figure 8-38 Sidelying allows greater head extension. This much head extension was required for painless feeding in the early weeks in this dyad.

constriction) is usually accompanied by stabbing, shooting, or stinging pain. Chilling of the nipple or evaporative cooling may increase the severity of reflex vasospasm, and may even trigger it in women with Reynaud's phenomenon. Wool nursing pads in the bra have helped reduce spontaneous nipple vasospasm in women with a previous diagnosis of Raynaud's. For feeding-related vasospasm, drying the nipple immediately after the baby releases it and providing a dry heat source (a hot water bottle or a rice sock—raw rice microwave heated in a cotton sock) may relieve pain and stimulate the constricted arterioles to dilate. Vitamin B_6 or calcium-magnesium supplements help some women. Pharmacologic treatment with calcium channel blockers can help reduce the incidence and pain of vasospasm in mothers with significant difficulty. Visible blanching of the nipple may continue for some months after the pain resolves.

Impeccable attention to attachment along with infant growth usually improves the situation. If extreme asymmetrical latch with head extension does not markedly improve maternal comfort, tongue mobility should be assessed, because tongue-tie can and does co-occur with micrognathia. If pain remains problematic, milk expression and alternate feeding may need to be used for several feedings per day to preserve the mother's ability to continue breastfeeding. In the author's clinical practice, most infants with shorter than average mandibles were breastfeeding without maternal discomfort by 12 weeks of age.

Macroglossia

Macroglossia (large tongue) can occur in isolation or as part of a genetic overgrowth disorder such as Beckwith-Wiedemann syndrome (see **Figures 8-39** and **8-40**). There is no standard definition of macroglossia, which is usually diagnosed clinically when the infant has difficulty keeping the tongue in the mouth, function is affected, or the jaw is distorted by pressure from the large tongue.

Infants with macroglossia may be inefficient feeders, perhaps due to insufficient room in the mouth for normal posterior tongue depression during suckling, even with wide jaw excursions. Pre- and postfeeding test weights can be used to determine whether maternal accommodations such as increasing frequency and duration of feeds are likely to be sufficient. Maintaining generous milk production by brief postfeed pumping may increase the speed of maternal milk flow and will provide human milk for alternative feedings. Surgical reduction of the tongue may improve feeding ability in infants with severe macroglossia (Kveim, Fischer, Jones, & Gruer, 1985; Maturo & Mair, 2006) (see **Figure 8-41**). Maintenance of milk production and allowing the baby to breastfeed "for dessert" even if little milk is transferred helps protect feeding skills until tongue reduction can be attempted. If bottle feeding is used, it is important to use the widest based teat possible, to allow use of the entire tongue.

> Anatomical variations of the tongue and jaw reduce feeding efficiency and predispose to reduced milk transfer. Careful monitoring of the infant for sufficient milk intake, and encouraging milk expression and alternative feeding when needed, can help maintain breastfeeding until growth or treatment improve feeding abilities.

Breastfeeding and Oral Clefts

Although clefts of the lip are obvious, lactation consultants may be the first professional to identify a cleft of the palate. A recent study conducted in the United Kingdom (Habel, Elhadi, Sommerlad, & Powell, 2006) identified a 28% incidence of delayed detection of overt

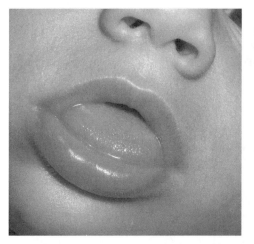

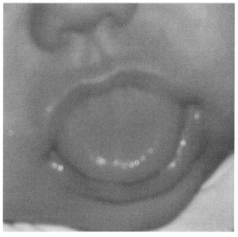

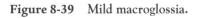

Figure 8-39 Mild macroglossia.

Figure 8-40 Macroglossia associated with Beckwith-Wiedemann Syndrome (BWS).

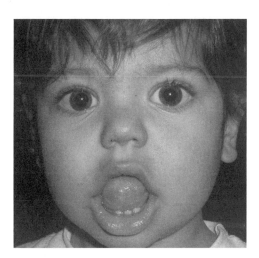

Figure 8-41 Child with BWS after tongue reduction surgery.
Breastfeeding ability improved markedly after tongue reduction surgery.

clefts. Even relatively large clefts of the hard palate were not identified, several for years after birth, especially if the physician examining the infant after birth performed only digital examination and was not specifically instructed in cleft detection. The authors recommend visual inspection with a light and a tongue depressor in addition to a digital exam.

Overt Clefts

Infants with hard palate clefts tend to rest their tongue tip in the defect, which can influence the development of tongue movements (see **Figure 8-42**). Another major issue in breastfeeding an infant with a cleft is the inability to produce negative pressure in the mouth unless the cleft can be occluded. Mild negative pressure helps to hold the breast in the mouth during sucking. More importantly, negative pressure is necessary for normal milk removal from the breast. Previously, wavelike tongue movements were thought to "strip" or press milk from the breast. Recent ultrasound studies have suggested that the negative pressure generated by depression of the posterior tongue and mandible at the end of the peristaltic wave is most important to the amount of milk transferred (Ramsay & Hartmann, 2005). If the hard palate is not intact, and the soft palate is not able to seal with the back of the tongue, no negative pressure can be created in the mouth.

Infants move milk from the breast by compartmentalizing the oropharynx (mouth) from the nasopharynx (nasal air space) and the hypopharynx (the area above the esophagus). The soft palate behaves like a hinged flap attached to the posterior hard palate. It flips

Figure 8-42
Infants with unilateral clefts frequently press the tongue tip into the cleft, distorting normal tongue movement patterns.

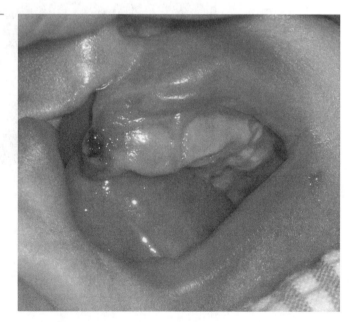

downward to lie against the back of the tongue, isolating the oropharynx. The anterior tongue cups and compresses the breast; the posterior tongue then depresses while the mandible drops slightly. This enlarges the space in the mouth. As long as the anterior tongue stays sealed on the breast and the cheeks are able to resist collapsing inward, the pressure in the mouth is reduced and milk flows from the breast along the pressure gradient onto the depressed grooved tongue until a sufficient bolus size is reached for swallowing. Then the soft palate elevates to seal off the nasopharynx, the vocal folds adduct (pull together), the epiglottis depresses to direct milk around the vocal folds adding another layer of protection for the airway, and the swallow is initiated.

Feeding difficulties contribute to a higher risk of growth deficiencies in cleft-affected infants (Montagnoli, Barbieri, Bettiol, Marques, & de Souza, 2005). Clefts provide an alternate route for air to enter the oropharynx, potentially preventing the isolation necessary for the production of negative pressure (see **Figure 8-43**). If the cleft is confined to the lip and the tongue incompletely seals the breast, breast tissue or the mother's finger can occlude the cleft sufficiently to prevent air from rushing into the mouth. If there are small clefts in the anterior hard palate, breast tissue or a thin silicone nipple shield may provide sufficient surface to occlude the cleft and allow near normal suction levels. If the cleft extends farther than the breast tissue can reach, an obturator (an acrylic prosthesis that covers the palate) may be made. Kogo et al. (1997) reported successful partial breastfeeding with a Hotz type plate, modified to include a posterior ridge to seal with the tongue and replace the function of the soft palate. If an obturator is used, it should be smoothed on the oral side to avoid irritating the breast.

Figure 8-43
Cleft of the soft palate.

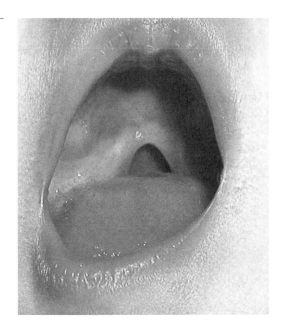

If the nares are occluded, negative pressure can be created throughout the nasopharynx, oropharynx, and hypopharynx together. Because this creates so large a volume of airspace, it would take a greater deflection of the tongue and mandible to pull milk from the breast. It is unknown if anatomic limits allow enough range of movement to provide appropriate negative pressure in so large a volume. There is evidence that some cleft-affected infants are able to transfer some milk from the breast, but the mechanisms have not been studied.

Some infants with clefts are able to maintain attachment to the breast if they are held snugly by the shoulders, and the mother uses one hand to hold the breast in the mouth. This hand can be used to compress the breast or to manually express milk into the infant's mouth. If the cleft is small and the infant's major issue is maintaining attachment, firming the anterior breast with two adjacent fingers ("scissors hold") may help. The mother needs to be cautious to keep the fingers sufficiently far back on the breast to avoid blocking the infant's access to the areola and creating a shallow latch.

Pierre Robin Sequence

Pierre Robin sequence (PRS) consists of micrognathia, retroplaced tongue, and a high or "U"-shaped cleft palate (see **Figure 8-44**). It is called a malformation sequence because the extremely small mandible causes the other features. The small jaw causes the tongue to be placed more posteriorly and hump up more in the mouth, preventing the palatal shelves from closing or causing a very high palate. The major difficulty in PRS is the infant's inability to maintain an airway, particularly during feeding. Some researchers believe that the anatomical changes are insufficient to cause the airway obstruction, and postulate a brainstem abnormality (Abadie, 2002), but a large prospective study showed four different anatomical mechanisms of obstruction (Marques et al., 2001), as well as poor function of the genioglossus muscle. Marques et al. found that feeding difficulties were proportional to

Figure 8-44
Complete "U"-shaped cleft palate in an infant with Pierre Robin sequence.

Note the short mandible and retroplaced tongue.

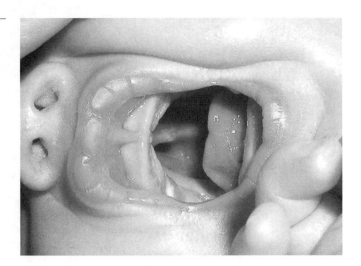

airway instability: infants with the most difficulty breathing were the poorest feeders. Abnormalities of the facial nerve have been found in the majority of autopsies of infants with PRS (Gruen, Carranza, Karmody, & Bachor, 2005, p. 606). Because the facial nerve innervates many of the facial muscles used during feeding, this compounds the feeding problems.

Feeding in a prone or semi-prone position with head extension can be helpful for infants with PRS (Takagi & Bosma, 1960). Infants with PRS without a cleft may be able to breastfeed, but will likely be inefficient, and growth may be poor. Infants with clefts will usually need alternative feeding, along with the use of special positioning strategies.

Breastfeeding Cleft-Affected Infants

Active supplementation at breast can also be used to give cleft palate infants the experience of breastfeeding even if they are unable to transfer milk. This can help to normalize tongue movements and provide traction on the palate for normal spreading. Commercial or homemade supplementer devices that rely on negative pressure (Medela SNS, Lact-Aid, or a feeding tube in a bottle of milk) may not work for cleft palate infants, unless the tube end can be placed between the tongue and the breast, and the breast occludes the cleft sufficiently. A feeding tube (5 French or finer) or a butterfly catheter with the needle cut off on a syringe full of milk can supply milk during suckling (see **Figure 8-45**). The tube is best taped or held to the breast with the end of the tube at the tip of the nipple, and the tube running along the breast where the center of the infant's lower lip will contact it during latch and direct it into the mouth, between the tongue and breast. Alternatively, a periodontal syringe (a syringe with a curved, tapered tip) can be used, but care must be taken to direct the milk where it will not enter the cleft. The Lactation Institute sells flexible tip covers for curved tip syringes used in infants' mouths if the rigid tip is a concern. Most lactation consultants who use them rest the tip of the periodontal syringe against the breast rather than the infant's oral mucosa.

Figure 8-45
Active supplementation at breast with syringe and feeding tube.

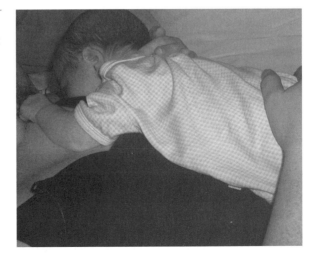

During active supplementation, the mother synchronizes the delivery of milk from the syringe with the infant's suckling. When the infant lowers the mandible and posterior tongue, the feeder presses the plunger of the syringe to deliver a small bolus (approximately 0.5 ml, or as much as the infant can safely swallow) into the infant's mouth. The goal is to achieve a normal sucking pattern if possible: a 1:1 suck:swallow ratio for bursts of 10–20 sucks, followed by a 5- to 6-second respiratory pause, for at least the initial 5–10 minutes of the feeding. Thereafter, pauses will likely increase in length as the infant fatigues. Lack of swallowing is a sign that boluses are too small, and loss of milk from the lips or unco-ordinated swallowing sounds are signs that the bolus is too large. Finger splaying, eye widening, or avoidance responses are signs that pacing is too rapid. The mother is super-vised until she correctly synchronizes milk delivery with the infant's sucking and stops delivering milk during respiratory pauses. This process can be particularly tricky with cleft-affected infants who have been using alternate swallowing movements in utero.

Positioning may prevent loss of milk into the nasopharynx during sucking and swal-lowing. Use a reclining maternal position so the infant is prone on the mother's chest and the throat is "uphill" from the breast or a straddle position where the infant's legs straddle the mother's thigh and the infant rests upright along the mother's trunk to reach the breast.

Alternate Feeding for Cleft-Affected Infants

If active supplementation during breastfeeding is insufficient to provide for optimal growth, alternate feeding will be necessary. The goal of any alternate feeding method is to provide as close to the normal sensory motor experience of feeding as possible, particularly to promote normal tongue movements, including normal coordination of swallowing and breathing.

The Haberman Feeder (Special Needs Feeder)

The Haberman Feeder (marketed in the United States as the Special Needs Feeder by Medela) was designed by the mother of an infant with Stickler syndrome. The teat is isolated from the bottle by a one-way valve, which allows the infant to use compression alone to move milk. The feeder can squeeze the teat to assist the infant's efforts. In addition, the nipple has a slit design that allows the feeder to control the bolus size by the orientation of the nipple in the baby's mouth. If the slit is parallel to the plane of the tongue, the flow is slowest, if perpendicular, the flow is fastest. The teat is molded with three raised lines to indicate the flow. The relative length of the line that points to the nose indicates the flow setting. The teat comes in a long (regular) version intended to promote central grooving of the tongue, and a shorter (mini) version that is useful for infants with strong gag reflexes or tiny preterm infants. The Haberman teat has a narrow base, and promotes a tighter lip seal than breast-feeding does, but no wide-based teat exists for cleft-affected infants at this time.

Using the Haberman Feeder. The feeder should help the infant preserve the gape response (a wide open mouth) by presenting the teat to the upper lip or philtrum, or crossing the teat across both lips, so the tip rests on the philtrum. When the infant opens wide, the feeder can touch the base of the feeder nipple to the tongue and then tip the feeder into the mouth, allowing the baby to assist with the tongue (see **Figure 8-46**). These two nuances help simulate drawing the breast into the mouth to preserve normal feeding behaviors. It can be helpful to begin with the slowest flow (shortest line on the teat pointing to the infant's nose), and to rotate the feeder in the infant's mouth until a 1:1:1 suck:swallow:breathe ratio with good coordination of swallowing and breathing is achieved. If the infant is not able to handle that rapid a flow, the flow is reduced until the infant feeds without signs of stress (splayed fingers, widened eyes, furrowed forehead, worried expression, color changes) or dysphagia (coughing, congestion that increases as the feeding progresses, gulping or other poorly coordinated swallowing sounds).

If the teat is squeezed to assist the infant's tongue movements, care should be taken to coordinate the pressure with the infant's feeding efforts to avoid overwhelming the capacity to coordinate swallowing and breathing.

The Pigeon Feeder. The Pigeon feeder is a pliable plastic bottle with a valved teat. The teat looks like a normal latex bottle nipple, but has a softer and a firmer side. The softer side is placed against the tongue, and milk streams from the nipple in response to compression of the teat by the tongue. The teat is narrow based, which uses a mouth position unlike breastfeeding, and necessitates more activation of the orbicularis oris than breastfeeding does. The flow is rather high from the Pigeon feeder, and not all infants can handle the flow safely. For infants that can handle the flow rate, the Pigeon feeder can allow the infant more autonomy than using a squeeze feeder.

Figure 8-46
Using a Haberman feeder in a semi-prone position with head extension to feed an infant with PRS and airway instability.

Note splayed fingers and toes.

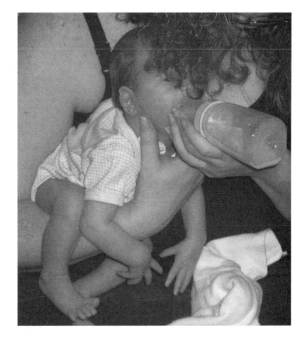

The Mead Johnson Feeder. This feeder consists of a soft, squeezable bottle with a tip shaped like a short plastic straw. The feeder squeezes the container to direct milk into the infant's mouth. If skillfully used in synchrony with the infant's feeding efforts, milk can be delivered without causing respiratory stress, but this is rarely the case in practice. The feeder does not promote normal tongue movements, is extremely narrow, promotes feeding with an open mouth, and does not allow the infant much participation in feeding other than swallowing milk that is delivered into the mouth. The outlet tends to migrate toward the front of the mouth in use, making it more difficult for the infant to keep milk from leaking into the nasopharynx through the cleft. In general, this device provides nutrition but little normal feeding development.

Finger Feeding. Finger feeding is sometimes useful for cleft-affected infants, particularly those with Pierre Robin sequence, who may have difficulty maintaining airway patency with other feeding devices even when fed in a semi-prone position. An active flow device such as a syringe and feeding tube is needed for these infants, who cannot create negative intraoral pressure. The infant can be held sitting or prone, with the head extended to improve airway patency (Takagi & Bosma, 1960; see **Figure 8-47**). The feeder should stimulate the gape response, and slide the clean (parent) or gloved (therapist) finger along the palate when the infant opens wide. The infant will soon learn to use the tongue to draw the finger deep into the mouth, to where the junction of the hard and soft palate would be if there were no cleft. The infant's sucking efforts determine the pace of feeding. The feeder delivers small boluses of milk when the infant sucks, and stops when the infant pauses.

Figure 8-47
Finger feeding a prone infant with mild head extension can provide slow pacing and encourage improved tongue movements.

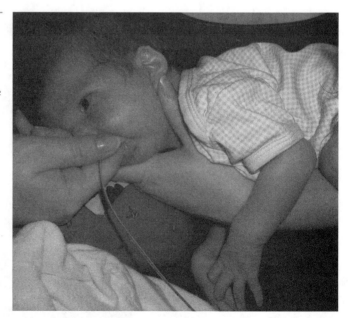

Submucous Clefts and Velopharyngeal Inadequacy

Submucous clefts of the junction of the hard and soft palate (velum) can disrupt the normal arrangement of the muscles of the soft palate, causing prolonged feeding (> 40 minutes) and nasal regurgitation (loss of milk through the nose during quiet feeding) (Moss, Jones, & Pigott, 1990). Submucous clefts are uncommon in the general population, but occur in 36% of children with cleft lip (Gosain, Conley, Santoro, & Denny, 1999). One result of submucous clefting is velopharyngeal inadequacy (inability of the soft palate and pharyngeal muscles to close off the nasopharynx). Neurological mechanisms (poor strength, timing, or coordination of muscular contractions) can also cause velopharyngeal incompetence, as can other anatomical issues such as hypoplasia (undergrowth) of the velum.

Infants with velopharyngeal inadequacy can usually breastfeed, but may become irritated by milk loss from the nose (see **Figure 8-48**). Some suffer nasal regurgitation after or between feedings, or seem inexplicably unable to breastfeed well (see **Figure 8-49**). Suspicion of velopharyngeal inadequacy is raised when the infant displays short sucking bursts, has harsh sounding respiration during feeding without cyanosis, and at least occasional nasal regurgitation. Positional changes (straddle, sidelying, or prone) can reduce milk loss through the nose. Exercises to improve bolus handling by stimulating better tongue grooving are recommended by feeding therapists (Morris & Klein, 2000).

Physical signs of submucous cleft palate include bifid uvula, notching at the junction of the hard and soft palate, absence of the posterior nasal spine at the posterior hard palate, a prominent midline palatal suture, and paranasal bulging (Stal & Hicks, 1998). Occult

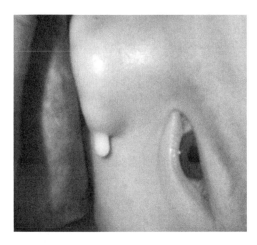

Figure 8-48   Nasal regurgitation due to velopharyngeal inadequacy.

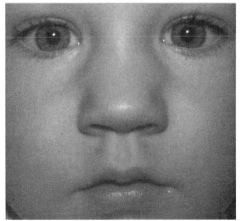

Figure 8-49   Child with velopharyngeal insufficiency and subtle signs of submucous cleft, including paranasal bulges and mild "gull wing" upper lip.

submucous cleft occurs without a bifid uvula, and can be difficult to detect without MRI. Velopharyngeal inadequacy can be diagnosed by nasal endoscopy. The physician may discourage the mother from breastfeeding, but infants in the author's practice with this condition were better able to breastfeed than bottle feed, even with the use of a Haberman feeder and careful pacing (see **Figure 8-50a–b**). The Haberman feeder can be used in addition to breastfeeding until the infant is able to meet all his needs at breast. Feeding resistance may occur at about the third month of life due to discomfort or stress of having milk penetrate the nasopharynx. Gentle encouragement and distraction of the infant during feeding is usually helpful. Some infants respond well to having a toy to hold during feeding, others to the mother walking around while feeding in a sling.

Infants with overt or submucous clefts may feed less efficiently than necessary, and maternal milk supply may decline over time if pumping or expression is not maintained. Infant growth should be monitored frequently, and expression and supplementation with mother's milk by alternate feeding methods instituted if necessary. Alternate feeding should have the dual goal of providing nutrition and normalizing oral motor skills. It is important that the infant participate as fully as possible in feeding, that milk is not simply squeezed into the infant's mouth. Normal tongue movements should be encouraged and required by the feeding method, to provide a good basis for future tongue functions.

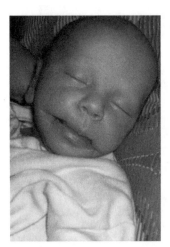 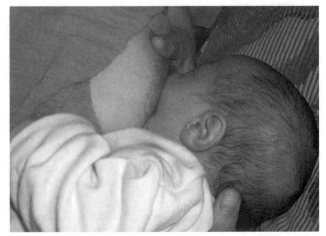

Figure 8-50 Bilateral transverse facial clefts (macrostomia). This condition can be isolated, or can occur with hemifacial microsomia, or undergrowth of the mandible and midface. This infant breastfed well by taking a large mouthful of breast, but was unable to seal on the bottle.

Congenital Abnormalities of the Airway

The work of feeding requires an increase in oxygen intake, while the intermittent presence of food in the shared areas of the pharynx requires intricate coordination of swallowing and breathing. Healthy infants given a normal flow of milk are up to the challenge. Infants who are working harder to breathe at rest due to instability or malformation of their respiratory tract have less reserve of energy and oxygen to devote to feeding, and may require more calories to support the increased work of breathing (Goberman & Robb, 2005). When baseline respiratory rate is high, there are less spaces available between breaths for safe swallowing. Feeding refusal or failure to thrive result when the infant is forced to choose between inhibiting breathing in order to swallow or going hungry. (See Chapter 6.) The increased intrathoracic pressures generated by the respiratory efforts predispose infants with airway anomalies to gastroesophageal reflux (GER; Bibi et al., 2001). In addition to the loss of milk that the infant obtained at high cost, GER causes pain and increased risk of aspiration (Suskind et al., 2006) that may lead to increased feeding resistance. Management of feeding for infants with respiratory issues involves modifying flow, improving the infant's ability to handle flow, maintaining airway patency by positioning the infant with head extension, and treating reflux if present (see **Figure 8-51**).

Figure 8-51
Worried expression and preferred posture of head extension in an infant with a respiratory issue.

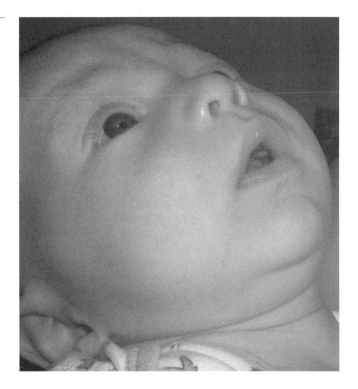

Laryngomalacia

Laryngomalacia is the most common cause of neonatal stridor, a high-pitched squeaky sound during breathing that indicates a narrowed airway. Three variants have been identified (Kay & Goldsmith, 2006), but all cause narrowing of the airway due to collapse of the epiglottis and/or related structures (Daniel, 2006). Severe cases can lead to failure to thrive, usually between 2 and 4 months of age (Manning, Inglis, Mouzakes, Carron, & Perkins, 2005). Lactation consultants can generally reduce the risk for growth failure by providing compensatory strategies for feeding that can allow the infant to get sufficient calories despite increased difficulty coordinating swallowing and breathing (Glass & Wolf, 1994).

Symptoms of laryngomalacia include inspiratory stridor (stridor when the infant breathes in) that appears or worsens during supine positioning, feeding, or crying, and suprasternal retractions (sucking in of the suprasternal notch immediately above the breastbone). During feeding, sucking bursts are likely to be very short (3–5 sucks per burst) and respiratory pauses significantly longer than the average 3–5 seconds. The child may have a worried expression and pallor or cyanosis (blueness) of the hands and feet or around the mouth and orbits. Holding the infant in a sidelying or prone position with the head extended can help reduce respiratory distress.

Head extension during feeding helps to elevate the larynx and reduce airway resistance, and may ease coordination of swallowing and breathing. Head extension can be increased in response to stridor by snuggling the infant's shoulders and sliding slightly toward the infant's feet. The mother can recline while feeding to allow the infant to be in a prone position during feeding to help increase head extension and ease coordination of swallowing and breathing. Brief, frequent feedings are generally helpful, but some infants prefer to take longer, more leisurely feedings with long respiratory pauses. If milk flow is rapid, the infant should be free to release the breast and rest. Holding the baby by the shoulders rather than the head and neck allows both head extension and self-pacing.

Milk expression may be necessary if the infant is an inefficient feeder. Expressed milk can be fed to the infant with a Haberman feeder used at the lowest setting, or by finger feeding. Infants with severe respiratory instability may finger feed best in a prone position with the head extended. Laryngomalacia generally begins to improve by 4–6 months of age, and resolves by 18 months in most infants. Supplemental feedings can be gradually phased out as respiratory capacity and coordination of sucking, swallowing, and breathing improve. Infants who are unable to grow well with feeding compensations should be referred to a specialist (ENT/ear, nose, and throat, or otorhinolaryngologist) to rule out vascular malformations, webs, or masses that can cause the same symptoms, and to assess the need for surgery.

Tracheomalacia

Although far less common than laryngomalacia, tracheomalacia is the most common malformation of the lower airway. In this condition, the cartilage rings that maintain the stiffness of the trachea during air flow are abnormally shaped and/or weak. Bernoulli discovered that rapid air movement decreases surrounding air pressure. The strength of this pressure differential allows airplanes to fly, and partially collapses the trachea as the infant breathes. Air flow through the narrowed trachea causes stridor. Adults with tracheomalacia exhibit expiratory stridor, because exhalation is usually more rapid than inhalation in adults, causing a greater pressure differential on breathing out. Infants with tracheomalacia generally have inspiratory stridor. Use of accessory muscles for breathing (Altman, Wetmore, & Marsh, 1999) pulls the sternum or abdomen in, resulting in a retracted appearance (see **Figure 8-52**).

Feeding concerns are similar to those with laryngomalacia, as are interventions. Head extension, prone positioning for feeding, allowing the infant to self-pace, and offering frequent feedings to compensate for reduced efficiency are all helpful (see **Figure 8-53**). Infants with sternal retractions and biphasic stridor (stridor with both inhalation and exhalation) should receive a medical workup, because they are more likely to have compression of the trachea from a tumor or vascular ring (Spencer, Yeoh, Van Asperen, & Fitzgerald, 2004).

Vocal Fold (Cord) Paralysis

Stridor and hoarse cry are signs of vocal fold paralysis (VFP) in infants (Daniel, 2006). Paralysis can be either unilateral or bilateral. The etiology (cause) can be neurological, structural, or due to birth trauma. Most infants recover from VFP within 24–36 months. Bilateral VFP in the adducted (closed) position can be life-threatening and requires intubation (Kaushal,

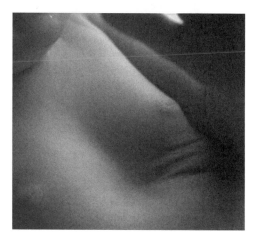

Figure 8-52   Sternal retraction in an infant with tracheomalacia.

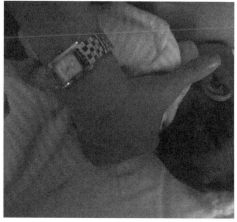

Figure 8-53   Strong head extension can help infants with respiratory malformations by reducing airway resistance to airflow.

Upadhyay, Aggarwal, & Deorari, 2005). In the past, tracheostomy was performed to open the airway for adducted vocal folds. Partial removal of the arytenoid cartilage with a surgical laser restores the airway and often allows the tracheotomy tube to be removed (Bower, Choi, & Cotton, 1994; Brigger & Hartnick, 2002; Hartnick, Brigger, Willging, Cotton, & Myer, 2003). When the VFP is in the abducted position (open) bilaterally, the airway is unprotected during swallowing and the infant is at risk for aspiration. Many different surgical techniques are possible for abducted VFP. Infants with unilateral abducted VFP feed best with the undamaged cord downward (dependent) for best airway protection (Tunkel, 1994, p. 37).

Subglottic Stenosis

Subglottic stenosis, or narrowing of the lumen of the cricoid cartilage, causes excessive work of respiration and biphasic stridor (stridor during both inhalation and exhalation; Daniel, 2006). This condition is usually self-limiting, and resolves as the child grows, but during early infancy feeding can be difficult. Breastfeeding can be particularly important both in providing optimal pacing of feeding and to help prevent airway inflammation that would exacerbate the condition.

Nasal Blockages

Choanal atresia (blockage of the posterior nasal opening in the skull) can be unilateral or bilateral. When bilateral, it can cause severe breathing difficulties and cyanosis that are relieved by crying (Daniel, 2006). An infant with reduced nasal airway patency from any cause will release the breast repeatedly during a feeding to breathe through the mouth. Short, frequent feedings and referral for medical evaluation are warranted. Other causes of nasal obstruction include small nares and nasopharyngeal tumors. One case of mouth breathing and breastfeeding difficulties in a young infant resolved when a salivary gland tumor in the nasopharynx was identified and removed (Cohen, Yoder, Thomas, Salerno, & Isaacson, 2003).

Congenital Heart Disease (CHD)

Although there are many types of malformations of the heart, they are currently classified as those that reduce pulmonary blood flow, those that increase it, and those that obstruct it. Infants with CHD have reduced energy and endurance, increased hypoxia with effort, and breathlessness. There is generally a higher metabolic need for calories, at the same time that fluids may need to be restricted in order to prevent congestive heart failure. The appropriate renal solute load of human milk is particularly advantageous for infants with CHD. Children with CHD are particularly prone to infections, and need the anti-infective properties of human milk even more than their well peers.

In the past, breastfeeding was thought to be too much effort for infants with CHD, but studies have shown better growth and shorter hospitalization (Combs & Marino, 1993) and better oxygen saturation during feeding (Marino, O'Brien, & LoRe, 1995) for breastfed vs. bottle-fed infants with heart defects. Support, staff education, and accessibility of breast pumps and lactation consultants increased the rate of breastfeeding among infants with CHD in one institution (Barbas & Kelleher, 2004). Feeding compensations recommended for infants with CHD include short, very frequent feeding and supplementation at breast with *hindmilk,* high fat milk expressed at the end of feedings if additional calories are needed to support growth (Lambert & Watters, 1998). Minimal mother-baby separation may reduce infant stress and increase the percentage of calories that can go towards growth.

Feeding is aerobic exercise, and requires normal cardiorespiratory function. Infants with airway anomalies or cardiac issues are vulnerable to failure to thrive if their need to feed frequently for short durations is not accommodated. Depending on the severity of the condition, feeding compensations may be insufficient to allow the infant to meet caloric needs, and alternative feeding may be necessary. Careful pacing of the feeding will help avoid hypoxia and reduce the risk of aspiration. Infants who are unable to feed without substantial accommodations should be referred for medical evaluation, because delayed identification of cardiorespiratory malformations is not uncommon.

Other Structural Issues

Congenital Muscular Torticollis

The etiology of torticollis is still debated, but is thought to result from either restricted intrauterine positioning or vascular injury to one sternocleidomastoid (SCM) muscle before or during birth (Do, 2006). A contracted SCM causes the head to be rotated to the contralateral (opposite) side and tilted to the ipsilateral (same) side. There are associated facial asymmetries, including changes in eye height and size, unequal mandible opening (Wall & Glass, 2006), and lowering and posterior rotation of the ear on the same side as the muscle imbalance. The contralateral ear is usually flattened. If untreated, progressive fibrosis (replacement of muscle tissue with inelastic fibrous tissue) may occur (Hsu et al., 1999). Treatment consists of stretching exercises performed by the parents under direction of a physician or physical therapist, and is most effective if started before one year of age (Cheng et al., 2001). The neck movement deficits in persistent cases are treated surgically, or more recently, by injections of botulinum toxin (Joyce & de Chalain, 2005; Oleszek, Chang, Apkon, & Wilson, 2005).

Breastfeeding issues posed by torticollis include difficulty attaching and transferring milk due to the asymmetrical mandible and twisted neck position (see **Figure 8-54** and **Figure 8-55**). The infant should be positioned at breast in a way that maintains the preferred head position until therapy begins to yield results (see **Figure 8-56**). Milk transfer should be assessed to ensure that the infant is able to drive milk production, and pumping and alternate feeding used if necessary. Two infants in Wall and Glass's case series (2006) and several in the author's practice showed improved milk transfer and ease of attachment with a nipple shield.

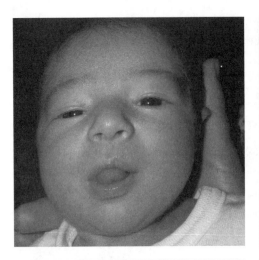

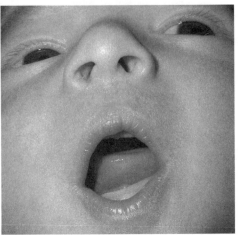

Figure 8-54 **Infant with torticollis.**
Note the rotated and tipped head, and
asymmetrical face and eyes.

Figure 8-55 **Asymmetrical mandibular opening in torticollis.**

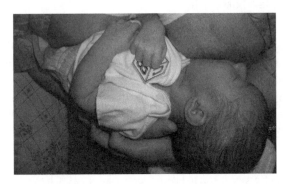

Figure 8-56 **Allowing infant to latch with head rotated to the preferred side.**

Creative positioning may be required when an infant has structural effects from a restricted uterine environment. Torticollis is frequently under-recognized, and any alteration in neck mobility and facial symmetry should be brought to the attention of the infant's health care provider.

Developmental Dysplasia of the Hip

Although hip dysplasia does not affect the mouth directly, instability of the hips reduces stability of the jaw and tongue. Treatment consists of a rigid metal frame that immobilizes the legs from pelvis to feet, which can make positioning for feeding a challenge. The mother may need protection from the brace in the form of a towel or pillow between the metal and her body. One option for feeding in a hip brace is to lay the infant's trunk and legs on a pillow placed next to the mother's thigh, and bring the infant's chin to the breast at the lateral (outer) side of the nipple.

Conclusion

Structure and function of the body are intimately intertwined. Anatomical variations and anomalies of the tongue and jaw have the most obvious effects on feeding, but alterations of other parts of the body may also be relevant due to their effect on stability. Anomalies that affect cardiorespiratory function leave less energy and oxygen for feeding. Breastfeeding is the easiest method of feeding for infants with reduced aerobic capacity, because they are in control of pacing.

References

Abadie, V., Morisseau-Durand, M. P., Beyler, C., Manach, Y., & Couly, G. (2002). Brainstem dysfunction: A possible neuroembryological pathogenesis of isolated Pierre Robin sequence. *European Journal of Pediatrics, 161*(5), 275–280.

Altman, K. W., Wetmore, R. F., & Marsh, R. R. (1999). Congenital airway abnormalities in patients requiring hospitalization. *Archives of Otolaryngology—Head and Neck Surgery, 125*(5), 525–528.

Amir, L. H., James, J. P., & Donath, S. M. (2006). Reliability of the Hazelbaker assessment tool for lingual frenulum function. *International Breastfeeding Journal, 1*(1), 3.

Ardran, G. M., Kemp, F. H., & Lind, J. (1958). A cineradiographic study of breast feeding. *British Journal of Radiology, 31*(363), 156–162.

Ballard, J. L., Auer, C. E., & Khoury, J. C. (2002). Ankyloglossia: Assessment, incidence, and effect of frenuloplasty on the breastfeeding dyad. *Pediatrics, 110*(5), 63.

Band, C. (2000). Breastfeeding an infant with an ulcerated hemangioma on the lip. *Current Issues in Clinical Lactation, 1*, 68–71.

Barbas, K. H., & Kelleher, D. K. (2004). Breastfeeding success among infants with congenital heart disease. *Pediatric Nursing, 30*(4), 285–289.

Bibi, H., Khvolis, E., Shoseyov, D., Ohaly, M., Ben Dor, D., London, D., et al. (2001). The prevalence of gastroesophageal reflux in children with tracheomalacia and laryngomalacia. *Chest, 119*(2), 409–413.

Bower, C. M., Choi, S. S., & Cotton, R. T. (1994). Arytenoidectomy in children. *The Annals of Otology, Rhinology, and Laryngology, 103*(4 Pt 1), 271–278.

Brigger, M. T., & Hartnick, C. J. (2002). Surgery for pediatric vocal cord paralysis: A meta-analysis. *Archives of Otolaryngology—Head and Neck Surgery, 126*(4), 349–355.

Cheng, J. C., Wong, M. W., Tang, S. P., Chen, T. M., Shum, S. L., & Wong, E. M. (2001). Clinical determinants of the outcome of manual stretching in the treatment of congenital muscular torticollis in infants. A prospective study of eight hundred and twenty-one cases. *Journal of Bone and Joint Surgery, American, 83-A*(5), 679–687.

Cohen, E. G., Yoder, M., Thomas, R. M., Salerno, D., & Isaacson, G. (2003). Congenital salivary gland anlage tumor of the nasopharynx. *Pediatrics, 112*(1 Pt. 1), 66–69.

Combs, V. L., & Marino, B. L. (1993). A comparison of growth patterns in breast and bottle-fed infants with congenital heart disease. *Pediatric Nursing, 19*(2), 175–179.

Daniel, S. J. (2006). The upper airway: Congenital malformations. *Paediatric Respiratory Review, 7*(Suppl. 1), 260–263.

Do, T. T. (2006). Congenital muscular torticollis: Current concepts and review of treatment. *Current Opinions in Pediatrics, 18*(1), 26–29.

Dollberg, S., Botzer, E., Grunis, E., & Mimouni, F. B. (2006). Immediate nipple pain relief after freno-tomy in breast-fed infants with ankyloglossia: A randomized, prospective study. *Journal of Pediatric Surgery, 41*(9), 1598–1600.

Glass, R. P., & Wolf, L. S. (1994). Incoordination of sucking, swallowing, and breathing as an etiology for breastfeeding difficulty. *Journal of Human Lactation, 10*(3), 185–189.

Goberman, A. M., & Robb, M. P. (2005). Acoustic characteristics of crying in infantile laryngomala-cia. *Logopedics Phoniatrics Vocology, 30*(2), 79–84.

Gosain, A. K., Conley, S. F., Santoro, T. D., & Denny, A. D. (1999). A prospective evaluation of the prevalence of submucous cleft palate in patients with isolated cleft lip versus controls. *Plastic and Reconstructive Surgery, 103*(7), 1857–1863.

Griffiths, D. M. (2004). Do tongue ties affect breastfeeding? *Journal of Human Lactation, 20*(4), 409–414.

Gruen, P. M., Carranza, A., Karmody, C. S., & Bachor, E. (2005). Anomalies of the ear in the Pierre Robin triad. *Annals of Otology, Rhinology, and Laryngology, 114*(8), 605–613.

Gunn, T. R., Tonkin, S. L., Hadden, W., Davis, S. L., & Gunn, A. J. (2000). Neonatal micrognathia is associated with small upper airways on radiographic measurement. *Acta Paediatrica, 89*(1), 82–87.

Habel, A., Elhadi, N., Sommerlad, B., & Powell, J. (2006). Delayed detection of cleft palate: An audit of newborn examination. *Archives of Disease in Childhood, 91*(3), 238–240.

Hartnick, C. J., Brigger, M. T., Willging, J. P., Cotton, R. T., & Myer, C. M. III. (2003). Surgery for pe-diatric vocal cord paralysis: A retrospective review. *Annals of Otology, Rhinology, and Laryngology, 112*(1), 1–6.

Hazelbaker, A. K. (1993). *The assessment tool for lingual frenulum function (ATLFF): Use in a lactation con-sultant private practice.* Unpublished master's thesis, Pacific Oaks College, Pasadena, CA.

Hiiemae, K. M., & Palmer, J. B. (2003). Tongue movements in feeding and speech. *Critical Reviews in Oral Biology and Medicine, 14*(6), 413–429.

Hogan, M., Westcott, C., & Griffiths, M. (2005). Randomized, controlled trial of division of tongue-tie in infants with feeding problems. *Journal of Paediatrics and Child Health, 41*(5–6), 246–250.

Horn, M. H. (2006). Smaller mandibular size in infants with a history of an apparent life-threatening event. *Journal of Pediatrics, 149*(4), 499–504.

Hsu, T. C., Wang, C. L., Wong, M. K., Hsu, K. H., Tang, F. T., & Chen, H. T. (1999). Correlation of clin-ical and ultrasonographic features in congenital muscular torticollis. *Archives of Physical Medicine and Rehabilitation, 80*(6), 637–641.

Joyce, M. B., & de Chalain, T. M. (2005). Treatment of recalcitrant idiopathic muscular torticollis in infants with botulinum toxin type a. *Journal of Craniofacial Surgery, 16*(2), 321–327.

Kaushal, M., Upadhyay, A., Aggarwal, R., & Deorari, A. K. (2005). Congenital stridor due to bilateral vocal cord palsy. *Indian Journal of Pediatrics, 72*(5), 443–444.

Kay, D. J., & Goldsmith, A. J. (2006). Laryngomalacia: A classification system and surgical treatment strategy. *Ear, Nose and Throat Journal, 85*(5), 328–331.

Kogo, M., Okada, G., Ishii, S., Shikata, M., Iida, S., & Matsuya, T. (1997). Breast feeding for cleft lip and palate patients, using the Hotz-type plate. *Cleft Palate-Craniofacial Journal, 34*(4), 351–353.

Kveim, M., Fischer, J. C., Jones, K. L., & Gruer, B. (1985). Early tongue resection for Beckwith-Wiedemann macroglossia. *Annals of Plastic Surgery, 14*(2), 142–144.

Lambert, J. M., & Watters, N. E. (1998). Breastfeeding the infant/child with a cardiac defect: An informal survey. *Journal of Human Lactation, 14*(2), 151–155.

Livingstone, V. H., Willis, C. E., Abdel-Wareth, L. O., Thiessen, P., & Lockitch, G. (2000). Neonatal hypernatremic dehydration associated with breast-feeding malnutrition: A retrospective survey. *Canadian Medical Association Journal, 162*(5), 647–652.

Luz, C. L., Garib, D. G., & Arouca, R. (2006). Association between breastfeeding duration and mandibular retrusion: A cross-sectional study of children in the mixed dentition. *American Journal of Orthodontics and Dentofacial Orthopedics, 130*(4), 531–534.

Manning, S. C., Inglis, A. F., Mouzakes, J., Carron, J., & Perkins, J. A. (2005). Laryngeal anatomic differences in pediatric patients with severe laryngomalacia. *Archives of Otolaryngology—Head and Neck Surgery, 131*(4), 340–343.

Marino, B. L., O'Brien, P., & LoRe, H. (1995). Oxygen saturations during breast and bottle feedings in infants with congenital heart disease. *Journal of Pediatric Nursing, 10*(6), 360–364.

Marques, I. L., de Sousa, T. V., Carniero, A. F., Barbieri, M. A., Bettiol, H., & Gutierrez, M. R. (2001). Clinical experience with infants with Robin sequence: A prospective study. *Cleft Palate and Craniofacial Journal, 38*(2), 171–178.

Maturo, S. C., & Mair, E. A. (2006). Submucosal minimally invasive lingual excision: An effective, novel surgery for pediatric tongue base reduction. *Annals of Otology, Rhinology, and Laryngology, 115*(8), 624–630.

Messner, A. H., Lalakea, M. L., Aby, J., McMahon, J., & Bair, E. (2000). Ankyloglossia: Incidence and associated feeding difficulties. *Archives of Otolaryngology—Head and Neck Surgery, 126*(1), 36–39.

Montagnoli, L. C., Barbieri, M. A., Bettiol, H., Marques, I. L., & de Souza, L. (2005). Growth impairment of children with different types of lip and palate clefts in the first 2 years of life: A cross-sectional study. *Jornal de Pediatrica, 81*(6), 461–465.

Morris, S. E., & Klein, M. D. (2000). *Pre-feeding skills*. San Antonio, TX: Therapy Skill Builders.

Moss, A. L., Jones, K., & Pigott, R. W. (1990). Submucous cleft palate in the differential diagnosis of feeding difficulties. *Archives of Disease in Childhood, 65*(2), 182–184.

Oleszek, J. L., Chang, N., Apkon, S. D., & Wilson, P. E. (2005). Botulinum toxin type a in the treatment of children with congenital muscular torticollis. *American Journal of Physical Medicine and Rehabilitation, 84*(10), 813–816.

Page, D. C. (2001). Breastfeeding in early functional jaw orthopedics (an introduction). *The Functional Orthodontist, 18*(3), 24–27.

Page, D. C. (2003). "Real" early orthodontic treatment. From birth to age 8. *The Functional Orthodontist, 20*(1–2), 48–54.

Ramsay, D. T., et al. (2004a). Ultrasound imaging of the effect of frenulotomy on breastfeeding infants with ankyloglossia. *Abstracts of the Proceedings of the 2004 International Society for Research in Human Milk and Lactation Conference.*

Ramsay, D. T., et al. (2004b). Ultrasound imaging of the sucking mechanics of the breastfeeding infant. *Abstracts of the Proceedings of the 2004 International Society for Research in Human Milk and Lactation Conference.*

Ramsay, D. T., & Hartmann, P. (2005). Milk removal from the breast. *Breastfeeding Review, 13*(1), 5–7.

Ricke, L. A., Baker, N. J., Madlon-Kay, D. J., & DeFor, T. A. (2005). Newborn tongue-tie: Prevalence and effect on breast-feeding. *Journal of the American Board of Family Practice, 18*(1), 1–7.

Smolinski, K. N., & Yan, A. C. (2005). Hemangiomas of infancy: Clinical and biological characteristics. *Clinical Pediatrics (Philadelphia), 44*(9), 747–766.

Spencer, S., Yeoh, B. H., Van Asperen, P. P., & Fitzgerald, D. A. (2004). Biphasic stridor in infancy. *Medical Journal of Australia, 180*(7), 347–349.

Stal, S., & Hicks, M. J. (1998). Classic and occult submucous cleft palates: A histopathologic analysis. *Cleft Palate and Craniofacial Journal, 35*(4), 351–358.

Suskind, D. L., Thompson, D. M., Gulati, M., Huddleston, P., Liu, D. C., & Baroody, F. M. (2006). Improved infant swallowing after gastroesophageal reflux disease treatment: A function of improved laryngeal sensation? *Laryngoscope, 116*(8), 1397–1403.

Takagi, Y., & Bosma, J. F. (1960). Disability of oral function in an infant associated with displacement of the tongue: Therapy by feeding in prone position. *Acta Paediatrica Scandinavia, 49*(Suppl), 62–69.

Tunkel, D. E. (1994). Surgical approach to diagnosis and management: Otolaryngology. In D. N. Tuchman & R. S. Walter (Eds.), *Disorders of feeding and swallowing in infants and children* (pp. 131–152). San Diego: Singular Publishing Group.

Wall, V., & Glass, R. (2006). Mandibular asymmetry and breastfeeding problems: Experience from 11 cases. *Journal of Human Lactation, 22*(3), 328–334.

Wiessinger, D. (1995). Breastfeeding difficulties as a result of tight lingual and labial frena: A case report. *Journal of Human Lactation, 11*(4), 313–316.

Chapter 9

Minimally Invasive Treatment for Posterior Tongue-Tie (The Hidden Tongue-Tie)

Elizabeth V. Coryllos

Catherine Watson Genna

Judy LeVan Fram

The need for frenotomy when infants are unable to breastfeed effectively or without causing maternal pain is increasingly well recognized (Griffiths, 2004; Kupietzky & Botzer, 2005; Messner, Lalakea, Aby, Macmahon, & Bair, 2000; Ricke, Baker, Madlon-Kay, & DeFor, 2005). Improvements in breastfeeding ability and maternal comfort after frenotomy have been confirmed in randomized controlled trials (Dollberg, Botzer, Grunis, & Mimouni, 2006; Hogan, Westcott, & Griffiths, 2005; Srinivasan, Dobrich, Mitnick, & Feldman, 2006).

Since the publication of our article for the AAP Breastfeeding Section newsletter (Coryllos, Genna, & Salloum, 2004), and our presentations on our ultrasound research on more subtle cases of ankyloglossia, we have been contacted by women throughout the world who have had difficulty obtaining treatment for their infants who are struggling to latch, maintain attachment, or transfer milk. We hope to remedy this situation by detailing the conservative management (modified frenotomy in early infancy without general anesthesia) reintroduced and expanded by the author (Coryllos).

Recognition

The first step toward treating any issue is recognition of the problem. Practitioners who merely look for a heart-shaped tongue tip are likely to miss restrictive frenula that restrict only the mid or posterior tongue. Those that extend the entire length of the tongue or are particularly tight can completely impede tongue elevation, preventing the elevation of the sides of the tongue that produce the heart shape. Frenula remnants that extend along the posterior half of the tongue, or that are buried behind the oral mucosa, reduce tongue mobility without producing an indentation in the tongue tip. Normal tongue mobility includes elevation of the tongue tip to the palate with the mouth fully open, extension of the tongue tip over the lower lip without pulling down of the tongue tip, and lateralization of the tongue tip to the corners of the mouth without twisting of the body of the tongue. (See Chapter 8.)

In addition to observing tongue movement, elevation of the tongue and palpation of the base of the tongue are necessary to avoid missing submucosal frenula.

Breastfeeding History and Assessment

Breastfeeding history can help to determine the need for a frenotomy. If positioning and management are optimal, yet the dyad is frustrated by poor milk transfer, prolonged feeding, difficulty coordinating swallowing and breathing, or maternal pain, frenotomy may be indicated. The presence of compensatory tongue movements during breastfeeding can be observed on ultrasound with a transvaginal transducer placed submentally (beneath the baby's chin). Nipple compression and distortion is readily visible, and is one mechanism by which milk flow is obstructed.

Clinical breastfeeding assessment should focus on attachment, milk transfer, ability to sustain attachment, and efficiency of bolus handling (soft, rhythmic swallowing without gulping, mistimed swallows, coughing, or milk loss from the lips, and without stress signs). An entire feeding should be observed, because some infants with posterior ankyloglossia are able to feed well for short periods of time and then fatigue and display tremors of the tongue and jaw or push off the breast and cry or fall asleep without getting sufficient calories. Subtle signs of sucking difficulties related to tongue-tie include dimpling of the cheeks with excessive jaw excursions, upper lip sweeping, or movement of the breast into and out of the mouth.

Family history of problems related to ankyloglossia is also explored. The need for speech therapy, orthodontia, or sleep apnea treatment in family members may expose previously unrecognized tongue-tie. Bleeding disorders and allergy to topical anesthetic agents should be ruled out before performing a frenotomy. Relative contraindications to frenotomy include Pierre Robin sequence, congenital amyotonia, or macroglossia, where it might increase the risk of upper airway obstruction.

The Frenotomy Procedure and Modifications for Posterior Tongue-Tie

The baby is observed lying down on his or her back, then swaddled, and gently but firmly restrained at the head and shoulders. It is usually best if someone other than the family performs this task so they are in the baby's line of sight and can provide verbal reassurance. Swaddling and being held still will generally elicit crying. Although troubling for parents, this enables the doctor to better visualize the tongue and nearby structures. The physician looks for the presence of a white cord of tissue or a membranous film that attaches along the midline of the underside of the tongue to the floor of the mouth. The baby then is offered a gloved finger to suck, which will provide soothing, as well as more information about tongue mobility. Starting in midline at the tip of the tongue, the finger is then slid along the underside of the tongue, until it presses against the leading edge of the tissue where the tongue base meets the floor of the mouth (see **Figure 9-1**). If there is resistance, a tongue-tie is present. A restrictive residual frenulum indicates an incomplete separation between the tongue and the floor of the mouth. If reduced tongue mobility suggests tongue-tie, but nothing is visualized, the examination is repeated with the tongue elevated with a grooved director or notched tongue depressor. The presence of a faint white line from the base of the tongue to the floor of the mouth that resists when pressed against indicates the presence of a submucosal (type 4) tongue-tie (see **Figures 9-2** through **9-5**). A residual frenulum may cause a deep crease down the middle of the tongue's underside at the base of the tongue, extending forward between the anterior fibers of the genioglossus muscle (see **Figure 9-6**). Rather than the resilient feel of the muscle fibers, the practitioner feels a resistant "string," which prevents the tongue from elevating.

The diagnosis of ankyloglossia, especially the posterior variants, is based more on lack of normal function of the tongue than appearance. The tongue's normal range of motion includes extension over the lower gum ridge and lip, lateralization to each corner of the mouth without twisting, and the ability to elevate the tongue to the hard palate *with the mouth wide open*. Infants with posterior tongue-tie may have some tongue tip elevation, but only the tip of the tongue may curl back while the bulk of the tongue remains flat (see **Figure 9-7**). The tongue may extend, even over the lip, but the tip of the tongue will be pulled down, causing the tongue to look rolled under itself. As the infant gapes, the tongue generally retracts in tongue-tied infants. A wide gape is critical for optimal attachment to the breast, as is the ability of the tongue edges to stabilize the breast in the mouth. Therefore, all functions should be tested with the mouth wide open.

A topical anesthetic (benzocaine gel) is applied to both sides of the lingual frenulum with a cotton swab, and the infant is held and comforted while the anesthetic is given time to numb the tissues. The infant is returned to the treatment table, and is firmly restrained with one adult holding the sides of the head over the ears, and another holding the shoulders with their hands, and immobilizing the body with their arms.

When performing frenotomy, it is important to get as close as possible to the tongue without cutting into the tongue itself. During the release, the tongue is lifted as high as possible, to make the tissue as taut as possible—this makes the clipping more accurate and allows the scissors to be further from the floor of the mouth. This allows the physician to avoid injury to the orifices of the submandibular glands at the floor of the mouth. The use of a grooved director stabilizes the tongue and provides a better field of view.

Posterior tongue-ties tend to bleed more than the simple, thin, more anterior restrictions because the physician is clipping through the more vascular oral mucosa or a thicker frenulum remnant. The incision is continued posteriorly until a popping sensation occurs, and the tissue opens into a diamond shape, providing the tongue a greater freedom of motion in all planes and more functional length. Linear incisions are expected to heal within 24 hours, while the diamond-shaped opening may take 3–4 days, with a white to yellow eschar persisting for a week (see **Figure 9-8**). When treating submucosal (type 4) frenula, it is sometimes necessary to clip more than once (see **Figure 9-9**). The first snip just releases the soft mucosal covering over the leading edge of the frenulum, and there may be a less noticeable "pop" during the release (see **Figure 9-10**). A white strip may still remain that may only be visible when the tongue is elevated strongly, and will require a second snip. A partial release that frees the soft tissue but not the tighter cord in midline may lead to only partial improvement in tongue function (see **Figure 9-11**). After a successful release, the tongue should elevate to the palate, and reveal the new diamond-shaped opening at the base of the tongue when the infant cries (see **Figure 9-12**).

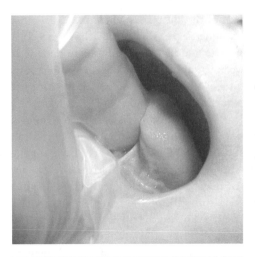

Figure 9-1 Identifying a posterior frenulum by palpation.

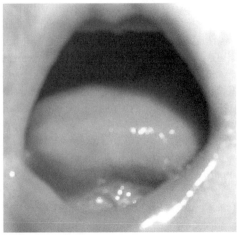

Figure 9-2 Submucosal tongue-tie makes the tongue appear short or the floor of the mouth webbed.

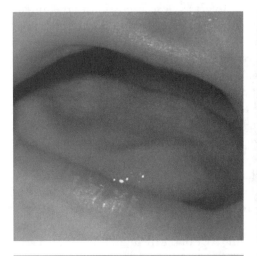

Figure 9-3 Asymmetrical, limited tongue elevation due to submucosal tongue-tie.

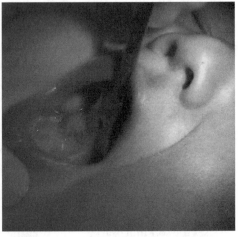

Figure 9-4 The faint white string of a submucosal tongue-tie.

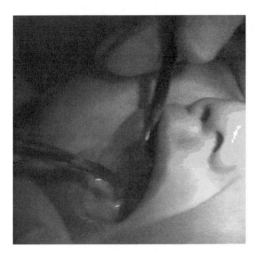

Figure 9-5 The string becomes more apparent when the tongue is stretched.

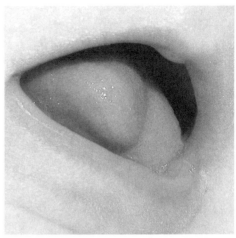

Figure 9-6 Restriction along midline by the lingual frenulum distorts tongue shape.

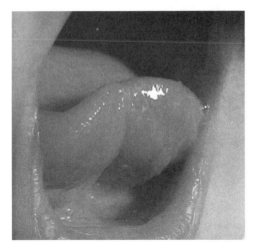

Figure 9-7 Limited elevation due to type 3 tongue-tie.

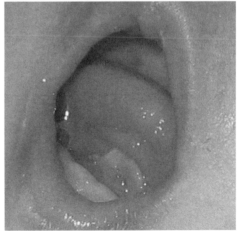

Figure 9-8 Healing eschar one week postfrenotomy.

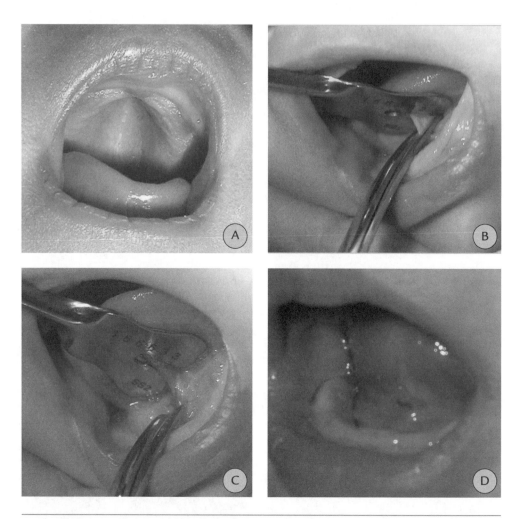

Figure 9-9 Treatment of type 3 tongue-tie requiring two snips to release the tongue sufficiently.

Bleeding is controlled with direct pressure for about 2 minutes using sterile gauze. The infant's sucking efforts usually signal the cessation of bleeding. The baby can be immediately offered the breast to ensure that sufficient release was performed to improve attachment, milk transfer, and maternal comfort. The first feeding postfrenotomy is usually a good indicator of the degree of eventual improvement. Soreness may impede feeding for 24 hours or more, and can be managed with analgesics. The newly released tongue may initially be weak. If frenotomy is delayed until the second half of the first year, rehabilitation of tongue movements may take longer than in newborns. Chapter 8 contains suggestions for postoperative oral exercises for use if feeding issues do not resolve spontaneously.

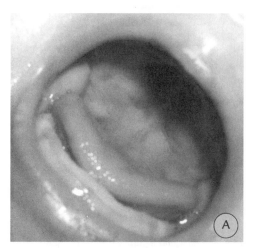

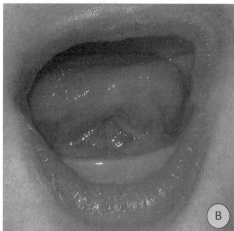

Figure 9-10 **This posterior frenulum required only one snip.** There is still some submucosal restriction, but release was sufficient for breastfeeding to become comfortable and effective.

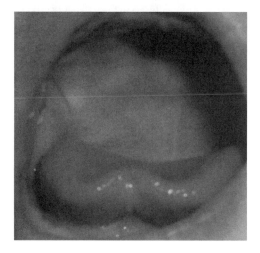

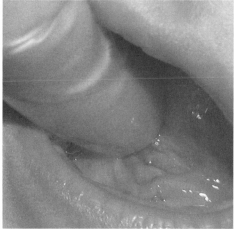

Figure 9-11 Incompletely treated tongue-tie increased maternal pain during feeding.

Figure 9-12 Postoperative appearance of infant in Figure 9-3: Note the folds of the mucosa that were attached to the tongue laterally to the midline frenulum. Treatment consisted of one snip to open the mucosa to expose the frenulum, another to divide the frenulum, and spreading of the mucosa with blunt Metzenbaum scissors.

Conclusion

Many sucking problems that make breastfeeding difficult, painful, or frustrating are due to variable degrees of restricted tongue movement due to tongue-tie. Effective, minimally invasive treatment is possible in infancy, without general anesthesia.

References

Coryllos, E., Genna, C. W., & Salloum, A. C. (Summer 2004). Congenital tongue-tie and its impact on breastfeeding. *Breastfeeding, Best for Baby and Mother.*

Dollberg, S., Botzer, E., Grunis, E., & Mimouni, F. B. (2006). Immediate nipple pain relief after frenotomy in breast-fed infants with ankyloglossia: A randomized, prospective study. *Journal of Pediatric Surgery, 41*(9), 1598–1600.

Griffiths, D. M. (2004). Do tongue ties affect breastfeeding? *Journal of Human Lactation, 20*(4), 409–414.

Hogan, M., Westcott, C., & Griffiths, M. (2005). Randomized, controlled trial of division of tongue-tie in infants with feeding problems. *Journal of Paediatrics and Child Health, 41*(5–6), 246–250.

Kupietzky, A., & Botzer, E. (2005). Ankyloglossia in the infant and young child: Clinical suggestions for diagnosis and management. *Pediatric Dentistry, 27*(1), 40–46.

Messner, A. H., Lalakea, M. L., Aby, J., Macmahon, J., & Bair, E. (2000). Ankyloglossia: Incidence and associated feeding difficulties. *Archives of Otolaryngology—Head and Neck Surgery, 126*(1), 36–39.

Ricke, L. A., Baker, N. J., Madlon-Kay, D. J., & DeFor, T. A. (2005). Newborn tongue-tie: Prevalence and effect on breast-feeding. *Journal of the American Board of Family Practice, 18*(1), 1–7.

Srinivasan, A., Dobrich, C., Mitnick, H., & Feldman, P. (2006). Ankyloglossia in breastfeeding infants: The effect of frenotomy on maternal nipple pain and latch. *Breastfeeding Medicine, 1*(4), 216–224.

Chapter 10

Sensory Integration and Breastfeeding

Catherine Watson Genna

What Is Sensory Integration?

Sensory integration (SI) is the process by which the brain coordinates all the information coming in from the senses in order to plan and execute appropriate and responsive (adaptive) behavior. This theory of brain-behavior relationships was posited by occupational therapist A. Jean Ayres (1979) from careful observation and testing of young children with learning disabilities. SI theory continues to be refined by both therapists and scientists. It is important for professionals working with infants to understand the principles of sensory integration because feeding difficulties can result from or be exacerbated by poor sensory processing.

The Process of Sensory Integration: Important Concepts

Registration is the intake and noting of sensory information. If information is not registered, it cannot be acted on. Each person has an individual threshold for sensory intake. Stimuli falling below the threshold intensity are not taken in; those above it are. A hungry infant who ignores touch from the nipple could be displaying poor registration due to an unusually high threshold, or deliberately withdrawing from too much incoming "traffic" due to a low threshold.

Next, information needs to be modulated. In the process of *modulation,* the neural signals are strengthened (facilitated) or weakened (inhibited). Useful information is normally facilitated, and extraneous, repetitive stimulation such as the feeling of clothing on the body is usually inhibited. Selection of stimuli for facilitation is a vital step in this process. If extraneous detail is focused on, the important stimuli that guide feeding are going to get lost in the static. The balance between excitatory (norepinephrine, serotonin, and dopamine) and inhibitory (GABA) neurotransmitters provides the mechanism for accommodation, the ability to stop responding to repetitive stimuli while retaining sensitivity to novelty.

Comparison is the next step in sensory processing. The cortex is arranged in layers and tracts. This arrangement allows an organized three-dimensional association of information, because it can travel both up/down and side to side through the brain. New sensory information is compared to previous experience in the associative cortex and emotional

nuances are added by the limbic system. Imagine you are preparing to cross the street. You will see the cars coming, hear the air they displace, and make a judgment based on past experience about whether or not it is safe to cross, decide how fast you need to walk, then implement that speed. This *cross-modal* processing of visual and auditory cues improves your accuracy. If you've previously had a "close call" while crossing the street, your limbic system will add some fear to encourage you to either speed up or to wait for a safer opportunity to cross. This process of association may lead infants who are frustrated with past difficulties to refuse to feed even though they are hungry. One toddler diagnosed with leukemia in the author's practice refused to breastfeed or take milk in any form during chemotherapy, though she would eat other foods. It took some detective work to reveal the association she formed between exacerbated nausea from moving into a breastfeeding position with the taste of her mother's milk. When given antiemetic medication that eliminated her nausea, she returned to breastfeeding.

The Special Senses

Children are traditionally taught that there are five senses: visual (sight), auditory (hearing), tactile (touch), olfactory (smell), and gustatory (taste). There are actually several more special senses that are important to our sense of the body and its orientation and movement in space. These include the vestibular (balance and gravity), kinesthetic (joint movement), and proprioceptive (body position) senses.

The *vestibular* apparatus is located in the inner ear. Information from the otoliths and semicircular canals is used to sense head orientation and movement and to subtract out the static effects of gravity while allowing changes in orientation to gravity (falling or tilting) to be noted. The ability to hold a steady gaze uses similar mechanisms derived from the vestibular sense (Green & Angelaki, 2003). Infants with difficulty processing vestibular information may be terrified of movement due to gravitational insecurity, and may flail and startle when moved toward the breast.

Kinesthesia and *proprioception* likewise interact with the tactile system to form the *body schema,* which maps the position of the body and its movement in space. The proprioceptive sense delivers information from stretch receptors in joint capsules and muscle spindles to be processed into a global sense of body position. The kinesthetic sense uses similar information to identify the movement of each individual joint. Neonates are dealing with unrestricted movement after having been constrained snugly in the uterus, and with gravity after having lived in a fluid, low gravity environment. These factors along with neurological immaturity and inexperience with the postbirth environment lead infants to have poorly graded (jerky) movement.

Work on tactile extinction (Vaishnavi, Calhoun, & Chatterjee, 2001) reveals that there are actually three mental representations or maps that are formed and refined by cross-modal processing between tactile-proprioceptive-kinesthetic and visual input:

- Personal space is defined from the skin in.
- Peripersonal space is from the skin surface to the surrounding space within the reach of one's limbs.
- Extrapersonal space is that which is out of reach but within visual range.

The existence of these maps explains the disorienting "closed in" feeling that a near-sighted person gets upon removing eyeglasses or contact lenses, as the extrapersonal space no longer agrees with the brain's map. It seems reasonable that children with poorly constructed maps will feel similar disorientation when their maps and reality fail to coincide perfectly.

Accurate modeling of the body is required for *praxis*. Praxis is the ability to conceive of, plan, and execute novel motor tasks. Infants and children with poor praxis are said to have dyspraxia, whereas adults who have lost this ability are diagnosed with apraxia. The difficulty in motor planning can occur in any of the three components. The child may lack the ability to think about new ways to use the body, may be unable to plan a sequence of movement, and/or may have difficulty performing the movements. Dyspraxic children are "clumsy" and require more environmental stability and practice to develop good motor skills. For breastfeeding infants with dyspraxia, keeping the environment as simple and similar as possible for each feeding will facilitate feeding.

Forward Modeling

When the motor system is activated, a neural signal called a *corollary discharge* is sent to sensory areas in the brain, forming a prediction of the sensations resulting from the action. This prediction is called a *forward model*. The refinement of movement is dependent on rapid comparison in the cerebellum of the model with actuality. The greater the difference between the predicted and actual sensation, the more the incoming sensations will be amplified (facilitated) so the conflict can be resolved. (For example, if you are walking down stairs, and a step is missing, you'd suddenly be very aware of your body and where it is in space.) If a movement produces self-touch, the forward model is likely to be quite accurate, and the tactile sensations are attenuated (muted). This explains both why we cannot tickle ourselves (Blakemore, Wolpert, & Frith, 2000) and why children with oral defensiveness can better tolerate mouthing an object voluntarily than having the same object introduced into their mouths. Letting the infant maintain control allows him to more accurately predict the sensations resulting from his action. Conversely, seeing a touch occur that is not felt actually increases tactile sensitivity. Subjects tricked with mirrors into seeing the opposite hand brushed reported feeling touch to both hands, and experienced increased sensitivity to touch in the unbrushed hand for several minutes after the experiment (Ro, Wallace, & Hagedorn, 2004). This phenomenon may be responsible for the crawling sensation one feels after brushing away a seen but unfelt insect.

It is postulated that an *efference copy* of motor commands remains in the brain for each movement. An efference copy is a complete copy of the outgoing (efferent) signals from the brain to the muscles, analogous to how outgoing email is copied to the "sent" folder. Efference copies may provide templates to guide future repetitions of the same movement, and may help explain the automatic, subconscious nature of well-practiced movements. The efference copy may be sufficient to produce correct movements, even when feedback is disrupted (Lewis, Gaymard, & Tamargo, 1998).

Putting It All Together: Sensory Integration

Constant refinement of these processes occurs with practice. The first time one picks up a heavy object, the amount of force needed may be misjudged, leading to the object not moving or moving too quickly. The brain must then adjust the instructions to the muscles after taking in the feedback received from the senses that show that the action is not occurring as intended (when compared with the forward model). The circular process of sensory integration consisting of sensory intake and registration, modulation and association, adaptive motor behavior with forward modeling, and finally sensory feedback, which provides more input, becomes more rapid and more finely tuned over time.

The process of sensory integration is important to maintaining a learning-ready state. Williamson and Anzalone (2001) explain how sensory integration maintains the four A's: arousal, attention, affect, and action (or adaptive behavior). *Arousal* is the balance of excitatory and inhibitory transmission in the brain. Too much arousal and the child is jittery or jumpy, and can't settle down to feed. Too much inhibition and the baby may not even notice a feeding opportunity exists. *Attention* requires sensory filtering: attention needs to be focused on the sensations that are relevant or changing rather than on the static ones. A baby who is paying too much attention to his clothing brushing his face may root toward his collar rather than toward the breast, whereas a baby with low attention will "filter out" the sensations of the breast and not respond to them. *Affect* is the emotional state, related to mood. A relatively positive, stable affect is best for feeding. Too low an affect is often associated with passiveness and "happy to starve" behavior in infants, and too high an affect may lead to disorganization and make it more difficult for the baby to produce feeding-directed behavior.

Cross-modal processing, or the use of several senses together, is important in correcting and refining adaptive behavior. It also allows us to have a "gestalt" (sense of the totality or multisensory synthesis) of objects in the environment. For example, if you see an unopened can of a familiar soft drink, you know without touching it just how much it will weigh, how much you will have to open your hand to enclose it, how the aluminum will feel smooth and cool, how much grip strength you will need to hold the can without crushing or dropping it, how fast you can lift it to your lips without spilling it, how fast it will flow when you tip it toward you, and what it will smell and taste like. You can judge its temperature from the presence or absence of condensation on the can. You remember to expect the feeling of bubbles in your nose from the carbonation, so you are not startled into sneezing.

Studies of stroke patients with deficits in a single sensory system reveal that combining information from different senses can help restore the injured system. In patients with impaired tactile sense in the fingers, seeing the touch occur allowed them to actually feel it (Vaishnavi et al., 2001). In patients with visual field defects, an auditory cue spatially coordinated with the visual cue improved visual functioning (Frassinetti, Bolognini, Bottari, Bonora, & Ladavas, 2005). A baby who responds poorly to tactile cues may function better if he can see and smell the nipple in front of him.

Sensory Processing Disorder

Imagine that you have poor sensory processing and some of your "maps" are out of sync with each other, like anaglyphs ("3D" pictures) viewed without colored glasses. If you were trying to pick up that soft drink can, the can might not be exactly where you see it to be, and you might knock it over rather than picking it up. You might grab it too hard and squeeze out some fluid onto your hand, or not hard enough and the can may slip right out of your grip. You might tip it too far, and get a too fast flow and feel as if a fire hose is spraying into your mouth. Even a normal flow might feel that way, as your brain and tongue take longer to communicate about what to do about the liquid in your mouth.

Other abilities would be affected as well. Moving around would be scary. Ladders and stairs might be terrifying, because you would not be confident of locating the steps properly. (We've probably all experienced the jarring sensation of descending a staircase, mistakenly thinking there was another step, and putting a foot down too hard.) This is how the environment seems to someone with a sensory processing disorder. Every behavior takes more effort, because the first attempt is rarely correct. Information coming in is "fuzzy," and provides poor feedback for your efforts. Sensations are poorly modulated, and might overwhelm you. If you were a breastfeeding baby, you might not notice that soft breast nipple in your mouth at all, or it might trigger your gag reflex. Let's look at some of the specific sensory tasks that breastfeeding entails, and how to help infants and mothers who have sensory processing disorders.

The Role of Sensory Integration and Sensory Processing in Breastfeeding

Intact sensation and sensory processing are important for breastfeeding. The infant must be able to tolerate touch and movement through space to be positioned at breast, and must be able to respond to touch and smell cues from the breast to orient to the nipple, gape appropriately, and grasp a sufficient amount of breast tissue to transfer milk. The infant must modulate muscle tone appropriately, and maintain sufficient arousal to facilitate the work of feeding. The infant needs to respond to the tactile and proprioceptive input of the soft breast in the mouth and use this information to cup and groove the tongue to form a teat and stabilize it in the mouth. Sequential activation of small bundles of the genioglossus and the transverse intrinsic tongue muscles are required for wavelike movements of the tongue. The posterior half of the tongue must depress to pull milk from the breast while the soft palate seals the mouth from behind, and the cheek and lip muscles must have sufficient tone to resist the intraoral negative pressure. Tactile and kinesthetic sensory registration and fine control of tongue, velar (soft palate), and pharyngeal muscles is necessary for coordination of swallowing and breathing.

The innate behavioral program (see Chapter 2) helps to provide a template so that feeding behavior does not have to be learned "from scratch," but modifications need to be made "on the fly" to compensate for fit and flow. Variables include infant mandible length and tongue mobility, maternal breast and nipple characteristics, and milk flow dynamics. The relatively low volumes and high viscosity of colostrum reduce the consequences of imperfect ability to coordinate swallowing and breathing in the inexperienced infant. Learning must occur quickly as milk volume increases rapidly over the first week postpartum.

Neuroscience research (Diedrichsen, Verstynen, Hon, Lehman, & Ivry, 2003) demonstrates that for muscle adjustments to be made properly to compensate for a changing load (the removal of a weight from the palm), the participant must perform a muscle action that leads to the load change. Just knowing the weight is going to be lifted is not enough to guide these *anticipatory adjustments*. For breastfeeding infants, this research suggests that the baby must be an active participant in feeding to produce the correct changes in muscle activity to anticipated changes in the feeding task. This is why pushing the infant's head into the breast does not facilitate latch. Being fed passively without sucking (tube feeding) or having a nipple placed in the mouth are not as good for learning fine control of feeding as active practice at sucking and swallowing and grasping the breast are. Likewise, prodding does not help the baby become more skilled at feeding, and may make coordination of swallowing and breathing more difficult (Lefton-Greif, 1994).

Infants have poorer sensory integration than older children by virtue of their immaturity, inexperience, more rapid cycling through states of arousal, and difficulty resisting the disorganizing effects of stress, hunger, and pain. Neurobehavioral organization is vital to the ability to handle all the incoming sensations and plan and execute the necessary motor responses (Als, 1991). Quiet alert and active alert are the most organized infant neurobehavioral states; crying and conservation-withdrawal are the most disorganized. Infants are more likely to have feeding problems in less organized states. In some infants, organization can be improved through vestibular and tactile-proprioceptive input. Preterm, ill, or otherwise stressed infants may need to sleep to allow them to reorganize.

Skin-to-skin contact with mother is the most organizing input for most infants. Some infants respond to rhythmic rocking or swaying while held snuggled firmly against an adult's chest, gentle swinging from head to toe in a gathered up blanket (see **Figure 10-1**), or swaddling with the hands placed near the face (see **Figure 10-2**). Some infants respond to repetitive sound, such as the traditional shushing sound, during these vestibular/tactile stimulation activities. Sucking is organizing for infants, and brief non-nutritive sucking on an adult finger (with appropriate infection control practices) or a pacifier/dummy may be used to help an infant achieve an organized state. Hunger can be disorganizing for

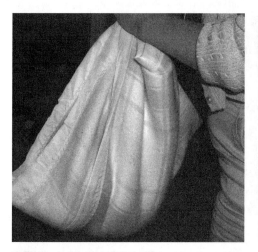

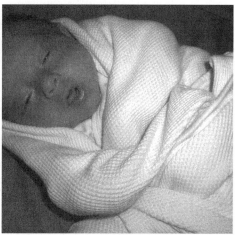

Figure 10-1 Swinging infant from head to toe in a blanket is organizing.

Figure 10-2 Swaddling in flexion—bringing arms across the chest abducts the shoulders—stabilizes neck and jaw.

infants, and giving a small amount of milk in a way that is workable for the infant (spoon, cup, finger feeding, bottle) may allow the baby to settle and work at breastfeeding.

Infants give very clear signs of sensory stress (Als, 1991). Adults working with infants should be aware of these "stop signs" so that stimulation can be reduced to prevent the infant from becoming disorganized. Particularly in preterm or ill infants, stop signs may be subtle: an averted gaze, a single raised finger, or a sign of autonomic instability such as increased respiratory rate, color changes, or yawning. In more vigorous infants, a grimace, finger splaying, or hands held up in a warding off gesture are more easily observed (see **Figure 10-4**). It is important to recognize that infants who are overstimulated can become closed down in an attempt to shut out additional input. A closed down infant holds the eyes shut and is very still, but may display tightened muscles and color changes that distinguish this overaroused state from sleep (see **Figure 10-5**). Alerting activities that are appropriate for sleepy babies just make a closed down infant more stressed. As a general rule, when a baby shows stress cues, stimulation should cease until the baby stops signaling, and a gentler, organizing stimulus should be applied. Environmental alterations such as placing baby skin to skin with mom and perhaps reducing light and noise may be all that are needed to allow the baby to enter a more receptive state for feeding.

Mothers generally respond appropriately to infant stress cues, without necessarily being conscious of them. Acknowledging these interactions when they occur can reinforce the mother's sensitivity to her infant and increase her confidence. If mother is not well integrated

Figure 10-3
Sleeping infant; note the
smooth forehead and
relaxed hand.

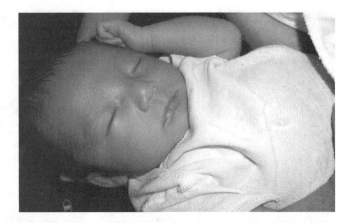

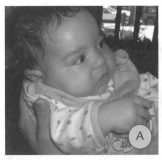 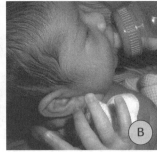 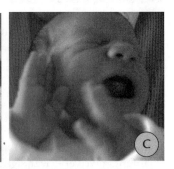

Figure 10-4   Some stress signals in infants are—from left to right—gaze aversion, splayed fingers, and warding off.

Figure 10-5
Closed down infant; note
the muscle tension around
the bridge of the nose and
the tightly closed eyelids.
Compare to Figure 10-3.

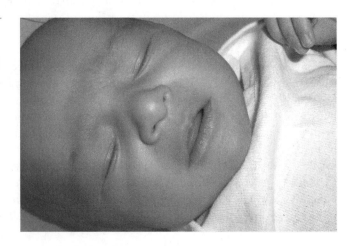

herself, her inability to correctly modulate her responses to her infant can cause feelings of rejection as the infant becomes overwhelmed and cries or closes down (Williamson & Anzalone, 2001). Teaching her how to recognize her own infant's cues and modulate her approach accordingly can improve both the infant's functioning and the maternal-child relationship.

Parents may interpret stress behaviors of their infants in different ways. *Reframing* the infant's behavior by voicing the infant's communication may help the parents to care for their child more appropriately. For example, saying in a high pitched "baby" voice "Mommy, I'm hungry, my hands don't have any milk in them!" when a baby is observed mouthing his hands can be a humorous way to draw parental attention to an important hunger cue. Interpreting frequent infant feeding requests or fussiness as manipulative or spoiled is counterproductive but rampant in Western culture. Brief education about breastfeeding physiology and the ability of maternal adaptation to help compensate for infant feeding deficiencies (Lau & Schanler, 1996) may be helpful, as may a review of infant feeding cues/behaviors (licking and mouthing movements, rooting, hand to mouth, squirming, throwing body down from an adult's shoulder to their chest). Demonstrating ways to help infants reduce arousal levels such as rocking, "colic" hold (see **Figure 10-6**), carrying in a baby sling, swaddling, and so on can help parents to "scaffold" their infant's developing coping skills (see **Figure 10-7**).

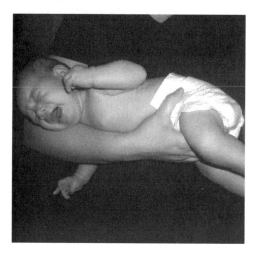

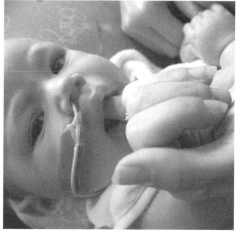

Figure 10-6   Colic hold.

Figure 10-7   Firm pressure to the anterior palate helped this easily disorganized infant with feeding difficulties to reorganize and prepare for breastfeeding. The infant's mother discovered and reinforced this scaffolding technique.

Breastfeeding Infants with Sensory Processing Difficulties

Sensory processing disorders (SPDs) currently are classified as either sensory modulation disorder, sensory discrimination disorder, or sensory-based motor disorder (Lane, Miller, & Hanft, 2000). Sensory modulation disorder has three subtypes:

- Sensory over-responsivity, in which ordinary sensations are overfacilitated and may feel painful and dangerous. Babies who over-respond may have difficulty choosing the important input during feeding attempts, and may be distracted by their clothing, their hands, or other irrelevant stimuli.

- Sensory under-responsivity, in which the threshold is abnormally high.

- Sensory seeking, in which a child who registers sensation poorly seeks strong sensation in order to provide sufficient input to the nervous system.

Sensory discrimination disorder is related to poor processing of sensation. A person with sensory discrimination disorder may be unable to identify an object by feel, or may have difficulty localizing touch sensation on the body. An infant with this disorder may have difficulty responding to touch from the breast and nipple, or may have swallowing difficulties due to poor ability to sense milk in the mouth.

Sensory-based motor disorder is caused by poor sensory processing. *Postural disorders* are an inability to hold the body properly against gravity due to poor integration of vestibular and proprioceptive information. *Dypraxia*, another disorder in this category, is a sensory-based impairment of motor planning and is related to poor tactile processing.

It is rare for infants with SPDs to have difficulty with only one sensory modality. They will likely have difficulty with related sensory systems, such as vestibular/proprioceptive/kinesthetic/visual. The suspicion of a sensory processing disorder is raised when the infant's responses to sensory stimuli are frequently and intensely unusual. These can include avoidance reactions, self-stimulatory behaviors such as head banging, difficulties with arousal, deficient control of autonomic functions including low or variable muscle tone, and irritability. Increased fussing, but not crying, was associated with sensory processing disorder diagnoses in childhood in a prospective study by DeSantis and colleagues (2004).

Early intervention services can improve the infant's ability to function and meet developmental tasks. Breastfeeding usually can't wait for referral, testing, and treatment to be completed, so lactation consultants need to know how to assist infants with sensory processing disorders.

Gravitational Insecurity

Gravity and unrestricted movement can be frightening for newborns, hence the popularity of swaddling. As discussed in Chapter 5, neonates derive all their stability from positional support. Infants vary in their ability to tolerate reduced support and the stimulation of movement when being positioned at breast. An infant with gravitational insecurity will flail, startle, and become disorganized when moved. Firmly containing the baby with the head and shoulders aligned (Creger, 1995), preparing for movement with verbal cues, moving slowly, and allowing him to see where he is going are all helpful interventions for infants with gravitational insecurity. Once the baby is in a breastfeeding position, he will be most secure and better able to attend to feeding if his body is actively snuggled against mom rather than passively resting on a pillow. Alternatively, the baby can be picked up while still asleep, placed skin to skin with mom, and allowed to self-attach to the breast.

Muscle Tone

Muscle tone is a reflection of the level of activation of muscles by the brain to provide the right amount of support for the body against gravity and provide a stable base for movement (see Chapter 11). Decreased activation of muscles (hypotonia) can also be associated with decreased activation of affect, arousal, and attention.

Infants with hypotonia (low muscle tone) can benefit from *alerting* stimulation prior to feeding. Hypotonia and low alertness can be increased by stimulation that requires active postural adjustments by the baby (Lefton-Greif, 1994). Upright rocking while grasping the infant's shoulders, neck, and buttocks (Karl, 2004) or snuggling the infant and bouncing gently in an irregular rhythm both fulfill this requirement. Firm but gentle massage, if the infant tolerates touch, and vibration to low tone areas may also be helpful. Several vibrating teething toys are available; these are useful for increasing oral tone before feeding. Vibration can also be applied by rapidly wiggling a fingertip in place, or a battery-operated vibrator can be held in the palm and a finger used to massage the infant's tongue, cheeks, and lips. Any oral stimulation must be carefully applied, and the infant's consent obtained. The infant consents when he opens his mouth and engages with active attention and wide, "bright" eyes; he withdraws consent by pursing his lips, turning his eyes or head away, or showing stress signs (see **Figures 10-8** and **10-9**).

High tone (*hypertonia*) can be reduced by rhythmic vestibular stimulation, including rocking and swinging from head to toe. A blanket can be used as a low-tech swing, and can provide full body flexion at the same time. The infant is placed diagonally in a strong blanket, and the ends are gathered up in the adult's hand. The infant is swung from head to toe until his muscle tone is reduced and his body flexion increases. Gravitationally insecure infants may not tolerate swinging. As with any intervention, infant stress or distress cues should be respected.

It is important to distinguish hypertonia from both fixing and motoric stress/avoidance behaviors. *Fixing* is abnormal muscle contraction in compensation for low tone. The fixed muscle is tightened and held firmly in place to help provide artificial stability. Fixing interferes with normal range of motion. *Arching*, or extending the head, neck, and trunk backward, can be due to hypertonia if it is part of whole body extension and is the baby's habitual posture, but it can also be a communication that the baby is frustrated and wants to avoid the breastfeeding position, or it can be an attempt to elongate the esophagus in response to the pain of gastroesophageal reflux (Sandifer's sign). A frustrated baby will usually calm when lifted away from the nipple and his face placed on the upper breast. An infant with reflux will show other symptoms, including "cud-chewing" or reswallowing of refluxed milk, preference for low volume feeds, fussiness, and often frequent vomiting or spitting.

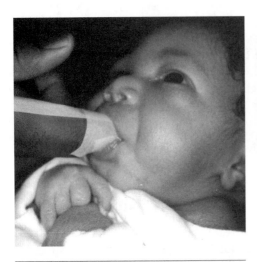

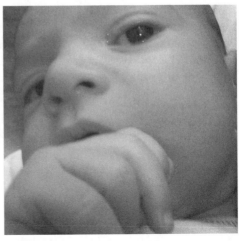

Figure 10-8   En face attention, hands in midline, show this infant is enjoying finger feeding.

Figure 10-9   Babies are most organized if fed when feeding behaviors are first observed.

Tactual Defensiveness

Infants with hyper-registration of tactile input may act as if touch is painful and dangerous. Indeed, the tactile defensive child feels touch more acutely and attempts to avoid it. Generally firmer touch is more tolerable than light touch. Vision predominates over the tactile sense, so touching the infant only where he can see your hands may allow him to modulate the sensation better. Also, self-touch is much more tolerable due to the ability to attenuate sensations when the forward model matches actual input well. Placing a tactually defensive infant prone on mom's trunk so he can self-attach to the breast is sometimes more tolerable for him than all the stimulation of trying to actively latch him on. Soft, smooth-textured cotton clothing may help reduce distractibility and irritation, or the infant may be more comfortable skin to skin. Some tactually defensive infants have only been willing to breastfeed when placed at breast height on a nursing pillow and allowed to approach and self-attach. Some defensive infants prefer the containment of being swaddled in a flexed position for breastfeeding, and some enjoy the firm proprioceptive input of a baby sling.

Oral stimulation should be used cautiously in tactually defensive infants. Providing textured toys for the baby to voluntarily explore may be helpful. Infants with tactile processing issues generally tolerate sensation they apply to themselves much better than sensation that is imposed on them. It is best to place the toy near the baby's lips and invite him to mouth it. Slightly older infants can hold and help control the adult's finger in his mouth.

Infant toothbrushes worn on an adult finger can be used this way. Discontinuous stimuli like tapping are often poorly tolerated because of their unpredictable nature, whereas touch that remains in contact with the infant's body (long or circular massage strokes) may be better accepted. Using a steady rhythm in the massage movements will also help with predictability. The use of a mirror so the infant can see the touch occurring may increase tolerability as well.

Infants with poor tactile processing may also exhibit an elevated sensory threshold. These infants seem not to notice the breast or nipple, and may fail to root well. If firm containment against mom and chin to breast positioning does not trigger rooting, or if the baby attempts to take the breast and pulls away after an abortive attempt to suck as if he has not even noticed the nipple is in his mouth, a nipple shield may amplify the tactile input from the breast. (High-threshold or tongue-tied infants may fail to root when the nipple is already in the mouth. Sliding the baby along the mom's body to bring the tongue tip further from the nipple may allow him to grasp the breast properly.)

Thin, silicone nipple shields with a teat of a sufficient diameter to fit the maternal nipple and some of the surrounding breast but short enough to fit the entire teat and some of the flat portion of the shield in the infant's mouth are best. The shield is shortened (folded back like a turtle's neck) and placed on the nipple, then the mother presses into the fold with two fingers from each hand, and moves the fingers outward slightly so the breast pops into the shield as it everts (see **Figure 10-10**). The shield should be presented as the nipple is, to the philtrum or, at the least, to the upper lip to facilitate the transition to direct breastfeeding (see **Figure 10-11**). It is important not to allow the infant to slide his lips down the shield teat when latching, because this strategy done at the bare breast would push the maternal nipple out of the infant's mouth. When latching on chin to breast, the height of currently manufactured shield teats can be difficult for some infants to clear with their upper lips. Hopefully the development of a variety of teat heights will solve this dilemma. In the meantime, the greater tactile quality of the shield will often allow the infant to latch when it is presented to the lips, even if the chin is not able to contact the breast (see **Figure 10-12**).

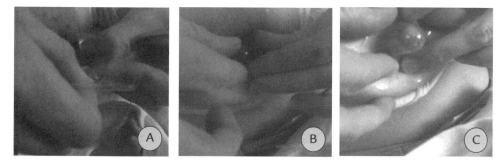

Figure 10-10   Inverting and applying a thin silicone nipple shield.

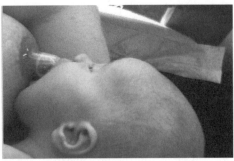
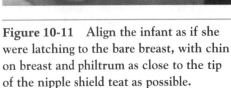
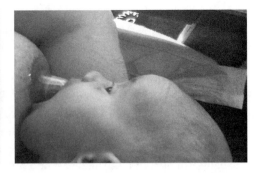

Figure 10-11 Align the infant as if she were latching to the bare breast, with chin on breast and philtrum as close to the tip of the nipple shield teat as possible.

Figure 10-12 Infant grasps both nipple shield teat and some of the breast below it.

Maternal Sensory Processing

Mothers with poor sensory processing are likely to have difficulty with breastfeeding, as with any new skill. Adults also perform better when in an optimal state of neurobehavioral organization than when they are disorganized. Organization is a challenge for individuals with sensory processing problems. A basic assessment of physical organization (which can reflect neurological organization) can be made when you first see a mother or her home. Meeting mom's emotional needs will help improve her organization by lowering unusually strong affect and arousal. She might need empathy about the difficulty of the transition to motherhood, she may need to talk about the birth, or she may need to assess your professional competence by asking some questions.

It is helpful if mom's best sensory modality can be identified and used. Sometimes it is obvious from the language she uses which is her dominant learning modality: "I see what you mean" (visual), "I hear you" (auditory), "That feels right" (kinesthetic). If the dominant modality is not obvious, a brief discussion about how she prefers to learn physical skills is in order. One dyspraxic mom said she felt like she was hopeless in aerobics class, and needed things to be slowed down and repeated in order to not feel like she was three steps behind everyone else. This information allowed the consultation to focus on practicing one feeding position in which the mother could see the baby's face and repeating it in slow motion several times.

If the mother is a visual learner, a small mirror can be placed at her side to allow her to see the baby's approach to the breast, or the baby's body can be tipped so that the lower shoulder and hip are slightly closer to mom's chest than the upper ones, particularly if the nipple points downward at rest. Instant print or digital photos can be provided of the process of latch or the baby positioned at the breast for her to use to consolidate her new skill of providing proper support and alignment for the baby. Visual demonstrations with a doll or a stuffed animal are also helpful to a visual learner.

An auditory learner may prefer to be "talked through" procedures a step at a time, and a kinesthetic learner may appreciate the consultant's hands being placed over hers to guide her movements. For most mothers, a multisensory (cross-modal) approach will lead to the best learning, but when mothers get overwhelmed easily, choosing her one best modality and using it more intensively can reduce overstimulation.

Mothers can be tactually defensive as well. One mother needed to have a thin cloth between her arm and her infant's skin to tolerate feeding. A rules-based approach to breast-feeding management would dictate removing the cloth due to the importance of skin-to-skin contact, but this would have made breastfeeding unworkable for this mother. Creativity and flexibility are needed when assisting mothers with SPDs.

When working with a tactually defensive mother, it is important to avoid accidental touch. The fear of touch will increase physiologic arousal and activate the defense program. (Nils Bergman, MD, reports that defense and feeding are mutually exclusive.)

Staying just out of arms reach from her, remaining within her visual field, and keeping your hands either in her sight or clasped behind your back may help reduce her level of arousal and defensiveness and allow her to attend to feeding her infant. Encouraging her to snuggle her baby closely not only will provide deeper, more tolerable touch, but also will constrain the baby's movements somewhat, and make them feel more predictable. Explaining the tactile cues that baby needs (chin to breast, nipple at philtrum) and movements he uses when attaching (gape, head extension, lunge, and grasp) will help her prepare for them. Swaddling the baby to constrain his movements may be helpful to mom at first. Reiterating baby's competence and discouraging her from fighting with him can also be helpful. For example, allowing him to suck his hands rather than trying to take them away from him, and bringing him closer to the breast when he realizes that hands don't make milk and releases them can reduce everyone's frustration.

Tactually defensive mothers may also have a heightened pain threshold. She might interpret sensations that would be merely annoying to another mother as painful. This does not mean that her pain is not "real" and can be dismissed. She needs help to make the feeding perfect so that she has no discomfort, and she needs to be believed about her degree of pain. If normal management techniques (positioning and latch) are not helpful or are already correct and mom still has discomfort, the infant should be examined for a subtle tongue tie or dysfunctional sucking and any problems addressed.

Dyspraxic moms need simplicity and repetition. Realistic goals should be set for the consultation, such as making feeding comfortable and effective in one position. Minimizing environmental distractions is helpful for moms with any sensory processing disorder, but is particularly important for moms with dyspraxia. Modifying mom's technique to make it workable may be more tolerable for her than doing something completely different. Practice is vital for dyspraxic individuals. Sufficient practice changes breastfeeding from a novel, difficult task to an automatic one, at least in the current environment.

If breastfeeding tools are needed (nipple shields, supplementers, pillows), their effect on the mother's organization and coping skills should be carefully assessed. Mothers with SPD may have more difficulty than neurotypical mothers with these added complications. Good instruction and practice will help moderate the disorganizing effect of new tools, but sometimes not sufficiently to allow the mother to continue efforts to breastfeed. It is better to supplement in a less optimal way than to overwhelm the mother to the point that she weans. A little creativity will usually allow you to come up with an acceptable and effective "plan B."

Parents with SPD may unwittingly disorganize their infants by their poor modulation of stimulation. Infants communicate by their behavior when their ability to maintain homeostasis (a smoothly functioning nervous system) is compromised by overstimulation. These include gaze aversion (looking away), yawning, increased motor activity, or autonomic changes such as color changes or changes in respiratory patterns. When the infant communicates impending overstimulation, the adults need to back off, reduce or eliminate stimulation, allow the baby to recover, then use more gentle stimulation that helps baby organize. Pointing out the baby's cues and reframing the infant's withdrawal as protecting himself rather than rejecting mom is vital. When parents or other caretakers have SPD, merely demonstrating sensitive interactions is usually insufficient; active instruction is necessary.

Occupational and physical therapists with sensory integration training are vital team members when there are sensory processing disorders in the family. Early intervention programs will generally cover these services for infants with feeding problems and regulatory issues. The lactation consultant or feeding specialist should work with the infant's intervention team to advocate for goals that will facilitate normal feeding (i.e., breastfeeding).

Conclusion

Recent neuroscience research has illuminated the processes that human beings use to interact meaningfully with their environment. Consistent interactions help to hone sensory integration over time. Newborns have less developed sensory processing due to inexperience, immaturity, and rapid cycling through neurobehavioral states, and some individuals have sensory processing disorders (SPDs) that disadvantage them further. Promoting neurobehavioral organization, using the sensory modality that functions best, and enhancing predictability of stimulation can improve the breastfeeding abilities of dyads affected by these issues.

References

Als, H. (1991). Neurobehavioral organization of the newborn: Opportunity for assessment and intervention. *NIDA Research Monograph, 114,* 106–116.

Ayres, A. J. (1979). *Sensory integration and the child.* Los Angeles: Western Psychological Services.

Baranek, G. T., Foster, L. G., & Berkson, G. (1997). Tactile defensiveness and stereotyped behaviors. *American Journal of Occupational Therapy, 51*(2), 91–95.

Biel, L., & Peske, N. (2005). *Raising a sensory smart child: The definitive handbook for helping your child with sensory integration issues.* New York: Penguin.

Blakemore, S. J., Wolpert, D., & Frith, C. (2000). Why can't you tickle yourself? *Neuroreport, 11*(11), R11–R16.

Blanche, E., Botticelli, T., & Hallway, M. (1995). *Combining neuro-developmental treatment and sensory integration principles: An approach to pediatric therapy.* San Antonio, TX: Therapy Skill Builders.

Capra, N. F. (1995). Mechanisms of oral sensation. *Dysphagia, 10,* 235–247.

Creger, P. (Ed.). (1995). *Developmental interventions for preterm and high-risk infants.* San Antonio, TX: Therapy Skill Builders.

DeSantis, A., Coster, W., Bigsby, R., & Lester, B. (2004). Colic and fussing in infancy, and sensory processing at 3 to 8 years of age. *Infant Mental Health Journal, 25*(6), 522–539.

Diedrichsen, J., Verstynen, T., Hon, A., Lehman, S. L., & Ivry, R. B. (2003). Anticipatory adjustment in the unloading task: Is an efference copy necessary for learning? *Experimental Brain Research, 148,* 272–276.

Dowling, D., Danner, S., & Coffey, P. (1997). *Breastfeeding the infant with special needs.* New York: March of Dimes Birth Defects Foundation.

Fisher, A., Murray, E., & Bundy, A. (Eds.). (1991). *Sensory integration: Theory and practice.* Philadelphia: F.A. Davis.

Frassinetti, F., Bolognini, N., Bottari, D., Bonora, A., & Ladavas, E. (2005). Audiovisual integration in patients with visual deficit. *Journal of Cognitive Neuroscience, 17*(9), 1442–1452.

Gaebler, C. P., & Hanzlik, J. R. (1996). The effects of a prefeeding stimulation program on preterm infants. *American Journal of Occupational Therapy, 50*(3), 184–192.

Green, A. M., & Angelaki, D. E. (2003). Resolution of sensory ambiguities for gaze stabilization requires a second neural integrator. *The Journal of Neuroscience, 23*(28), 9265–9275.

Karl, D. J. (2004). Using principles of newborn behavioral state organization to facilitate. *The American Journal of Maternal Child Nursing, 29*(5), 292–298.

Lane, S. J., Miller, L. J., & Hanft, B. E. (2000). Towards a consensus in terminology in sensory integration theory and practice: Part 2: Sensory integration patterns of function and dysfunction. *Sensory Integration Special Interest Section, 23*(2), 1–3.

Lau, C., & Schanler, R. J. (1996). Oral motor function in the neonate. *Clinics in Perinatology, 23*(2), 161–178.

Lefton-Greif, M. A. (1994). Diagnosis and management of pediatric feeding and swallowing disorders: Role of the speech-language pathologist. In D. N. Tuchman & R. S. Walter (Eds.), *Disorders of feeding and swallowing in infants and children* (pp. 97–113). San Diego: Singular Publishing Group.

Lewis, R. F., Gaymard, B. M., & Tamargo, R. J. (1998). Efference copy provides the eye position information required for visually guided reaching. *Journal of Neurophysiology, 80,* 1605–1608.

Lundqvist-Persson, C. (2001). Correlation between level of self-regulation in the newborn infant and developmental status at two years of age. *Acta Paediatrica, 90*(3), 345–350.

Palmer, M. M. (1998). Weaning from gastronomy tube feeding: Commentary on oral aversion. *Pediatric Nursing, 23*(5), 475–478.

Palmer, M. M., & VandenBerg, K. A. (1998). A closer look at neonatal sucking. *Neonatal Network, 17*(2), 77–79.

Ro, T., Wallace, R., & Hagedorn, J. (2004). Visual enhancing of tactile perception in the posterior parietal cortex. *Journal of Cognitive Neuroscience, 16*(1), 24–30.

Royeen, C. B. (1986). The development of a touch scale for measuring tactile defensiveness in children. *American Journal of Occupational Therapy, 40*(6), 414–419.

Stevenson, R. D., & Allaire, J. H. (1991). The development of normal feeding and swallowing. *Pediatric Clinics of North America, 38*(6), 1439–1453.

Vaishnavi, S., Calhoun, J., & Chatterjee, A. (2001). Binding personal and peripersonal space: Evidence from tactile extinction. *Journal of Cognitive Neuroscience, 13*(2), 181–189.

Weiss-Salinas, D., & Williams, N. (2001). Sensory defensiveness: A theory of its effect on breastfeeding. *Journal of Human Lactation, 17*(2), 145–151.

Williamson, G. G., & Anzalone, M. E. (2001). *Sensory integration and self regulation in infants and toddlers: Helping very young children interact with their environment.* Washington, DC: Zero To Three.

Wolf, L., & Glass, R. (1992). *Feeding and swallowing disorders in infancy: Assessment and management.* San Antonio, TX: Therapy Skill Builders.

Zeskind, P. S., Marshall, T. R., & Goff, D. M. (1992). Rhythmic organization of heart rate in breast-fed and bottle-fed newborn infants. *Early Development and Parenting, 1,* 79–87.

Zeskind, P. S., Marshall, T. R., & Goff, D. M. (1996). Cry threshold predicts regulatory disorder in newborn infants. *Journal of Pediatric Psychology, 21*(6), 803–819.

Chapter 11

Neurological Issues and Breastfeeding

Catherine Watson Genna

Judy LeVan Fram

Lisa Sandora

The nervous system is the director for other body systems, with stacked layers of control systems that interact in complex ways to help infants meet their needs and maintain homeostasis. Brainstem centers contain central pattern generators for breathing and sucking, providing basic programs for these functions. Chemoreceptors for carbon dioxide regulate respiratory rate; water receptors in the airway provoke apnea to limit aspiration of fluids (Thach, 2001). Higher brain centers modify the basic programming based on input from these receptors, the cranial nerves (particularly the vagus), and the special senses, and also exert control on autonomic functions through feedback loops. Abnormal development of the brain or injury as it develops can have significant consequences on the infant's ability to perform the many movements that need to be coordinated in feeding and swallowing.

Causes of Neurological Disability in Newborns

Brain "Bleeds"

Bleeding or insufficient blood flow in the brain is a common cause of temporary or permanent neurological disability in the fetus or infant. Preterm infants are more vulnerable to cell death from brain bleeds due to:

- Deficient control of cerebral blood flow under conditions of hypoxia or changes in peripheral blood pressure
- Underdevelopment of the vasculature between the main arteries of the brain
- Increased vulnerability of some cell populations (particularly oligodendrocyte precursors, which differentiate into myelin-producing cells) (Volpe, 2001)
- Underdeveloped antioxidant protection against free radical damage due to hemorrhage, ischemia, or infection

Full-term infants are less vulnerable to intracranial bleeds, but these can occur in cases of blood vessel malformations, mutations in clotting factor genes, cardiorespiratory disorders that cause extremes of blood pressure, and cytokine release in response to infection. Though they can also be caused by reduced oxygen transfer through the placenta before or during birth, it is now recognized that a wide variety of mechanisms can disrupt brain blood flow, including intense crying (Ludington-Hoe, Cong, & Hashemi, 2002). The narrow term *hypoxic-ischemic brain injury* has therefore been replaced with *newborn or neonatal encephalopathy.*

Neonatal Encephalopathy

Newborn encephalopathy is defined as depression of the central nervous system as revealed by decreased level of consciousness and impaired control of breathing. Feeding difficulty requiring tube or intravenous feeding is the sign of cerebral depression most likely to correlate with later minor neurological dysfunction. The next most likely correlation is the presence of neonatal seizures, and the need for mechanical ventilation (Moster, Lie, & Markestad, 2002). APGAR scores at 1 and 5 minutes after birth grade infant autonomic functions on a scale of 0–10, providing a simple way to differentiate infants who are making their postbirth physiological transitions well from those who require further observation or immediate intervention. Though APGAR scores have not been shown to have a linear relationship with neurological risk, low 5-minute APGAR scores (less than 5) were associated with increased risk of infant death and cerebral palsy (Moster, Lie, Irgens, Bjerkedal, & Markestad, 2001) in full-term, low risk infants.

Developmental Structural Issues

Neuronal Proliferation Disorders

Brain structure is integrally connected with function. Errors in prenatal development can affect the brain either in isolation or in addition to other organs. An unusually large (macrocephaly) or small (microcephaly) head can be a marker for abnormal brain cell proliferation during gestation. Errors in differentiation and overproliferation are associated with a large brain (megalencephaly, or hemimegalencephaly if mainly one hemisphere is involved) that is poorly organized, with abnormal cells and masses of abnormally placed, disorganized gray matter (heterotopia). Motor, cognitive, and behavioral deficits are noted when the brain is improperly organized. Microencephaly can be caused by reduced brain cell proliferation due to infections during pregnancy, maternal alcohol use (Gohlke, Griffith, & Faustman, 2005), metabolic disorder, or other toxic exposures including drugs of abuse and radiation. Genetic causes can be familial or sporadic. Microencephalic infants usually have below average intelligence, and many have motor difficulties and seizures.

Fetal Alcohol Spectrum Disorders

Alcohol exposure in utero is the most prevalent preventable cause of developmental disability. Fetal alcohol syndrome (FAS) is diagnosed by the cluster of typical facial features, growth restriction, and central nervous system abnormalities (Bertrand, Floyd, & Weber, 2005). In infants with FAS, the severity of the typical facial features (shortness of palpebral [eye] fissures, flatness of the philtrum, and thinness of the upper lip) correlates well with neurological deficits measured by brain imaging and psychometric testing (Astley & Clarren, 2001). However, alcohol-related neurodevelopmental disorder (ARND) can exist without telltale facial features. Even low levels of ethanol (drinking alcohol) exposure during pregnancy can affect neurobehavioral functioning of newborns, decreasing arousal and operant learning, which is important to feeding, and increasing habituation (Streissguth, Barr, & Martin, 1983). Infants with FAS suffer from growth retardation, are frequently hypotonic, have reduced fine and gross motor skills, and may have small upper jaws.

Neuronal Migration Disorders

Abnormal brain structure can occur with or without changes in brain size. The organized, layered, networked structure of the normal brain is due to carefully timed migration of new neurons during fetal development from the center of the brain outward along glial (support cell) pathways to form the layers of the cortex. A minority of neurons travel orthogonally (across the normal radial lines of migration) to become the interneurons that connect different brain structures. Some of these interneurons become GABAergic (using gamma aminobutyric acid as their neurotransmitter; Gressens, 2005, p. 968). GABA is the chief inhibitory neurotransmitter, responsible for modulation of input and responses, and seems important in reducing seizure susceptibility.

Disorders of neuronal migration lead to a variety of structural brain disorders with functional consequences. If the disordered area is small, the disorder may not even be diagnosed until the infant's development begins to lag, or seizures occur. If there is a more extensive area of involvement, the infant may have greater difficulty with the activities of everyday life, such as maintaining appropriate alertness, interacting with mother and the environment, and coordinating sucking, swallowing, and breathing.

Lissencephaly is a severe failure of neuronal migration that reduces gyrus formation, leading to a smooth brain surface. Because neurons do not reach their appropriate destination, brain structure may be very abnormal. Severity can vary from agyria (lack of brain convolutions with immature brain structure) to variable degrees of pachygria (decreased gyrus formation with shallow sulci). Lissencephalic infants usually fail to thrive and have a high risk of pneumonia (Pavone, Rizzo, & Dobyns, 1993), generally from aspiration (Ashwal, 1999, p. 258). Microcephaly and seizures develop during the first year of life, initial hypotonia may give way to spasticity, and mental retardation is moderate to profound. Infants with syndromic forms of lissencephaly have small mandibles, which can further impact feeding ability.

Subcortical band heterotopia is now considered part of the lissencephaly spectrum, and consists of normal to reduced convolutions, with a thickened cortex and a band of white matter just below the cortex and above a layer of misplaced gray matter (Guerrini, 2005, p. 291). Several genes (LIS1, DCX) are responsible for the agyria-pachygyria-band spectrum;

mild (missense) mutations cause less severe cases, whereas deletions or truncating mutations cause more severe lissencephaly with proportional cognitive and motor deficits. Infants with lissencephaly have indentations at the temples, small mandibles (lower jaws), and may have a weak suck. Swallowing difficulties, aspiration, severe reflux, and feeding refusal may become apparent after a few months as hypotonia gives way to spasticity (abnormal muscle stiffness). Human milk is particularly important to these infants, who are at high risk of aspiration pneumonia.

Cortical Dysplasia

Cortical dysplasias are abnormalities of the layered structure of the cerebral cortex that are caused by postmigrational events, possibly genetically based defective cell differentiation or failure of the blood supply of one or more cortical layers. The most common cortical dysplasia is polymicrogyria, or small, closely packed convolutions of the cerebral cortex that can occur in one of several brain areas. Some microgyria have no layering at all; in others, only four of the six cortical layers are present. Bilateral perisylvian polymicrogyria is associated with pseudobulbar palsy, causing weakness or diplegia (bilateral paralysis) of the facial, tongue, masticatory (jaw closing), and palatal muscles, which obviously impacts feeding. Tongue movements, particularly protrusion (extension) and lateralization, were restricted; the orbicularis oris was often weak; and gag reflex was absent in the majority of 31 children studied (Kuzniecky, Andermann, & Guerrini, 1993). Swallowing problems are prominent in this disorder (Kim, Palmini, Choi, Kim, & Lee, 1994), probably due to weakness and poor motor control of the tongue and pharyngeal muscles. Nevertheless, there is a wide range of severity of this disorder, and the author (CWG) is aware of a child with bilateral perisylvian polymicrogyria who was able to breastfeed.

Effect of Seizures and Anticonvulsants

Seizures (abnormal synchronization and proliferation of electrical impulses in the brain) are commonly associated with neurological dysfunction in newborn infants. Seizures can be generated by the brain's attempt to make working connections in the presence of abnormal neural migration or brain injury (symptomatic), or they can be the result of genetically based dysfunction of ion channels involved in the firing of neurons (idiopathic). Seizures can be difficult to identify in young infants, because the well-defined patterns that occur in older children are not usually seen. Any recurrent, stereotyped motor or sensory event that cannot be interrupted by stimulating or distracting the child may be the result of seizure activity. Infants who have been diagnosed with seizures may have special feeding concerns.

Seizures can affect the infant's arousal level, making them functionally unavailable for feeding. Some seizures produce a *post-ictal* (after the seizure) reduced level of consciousness. Auras, or partial seizures that presage a wider spread of abnormal electrical activity in the brain, may be disconcerting or disorienting to the child, reducing their ability to attend to hunger or work at attaching to the breast. Even seizures that remain localized without changes in consciousness (simple partial seizures) can reduce a child's motivation to eat. Seizures can cause perception of a bad taste or smell (parietal lobe), strong unprovoked fear (limbic system), paroxysmal stomach pain, nausea, or the feeling of rising stomach contents (temporal lobe). It is unknown if infants experience these sensory seizures, but careful observation of the infant for behavioral signs of distress may help identify optimal states for feeding.

Anticonvulsant side effects can cause significant feeding issues. Phenobarbital is often the first line medication for newborns because it can be rapidly titrated, but it is very sedating and may contribute to developmental delay. Benzodiazepines are useful for stopping prolonged seizures, but are also sedating and may accumulate in newborns due to reduced breakdown by immature liver enzyme systems (Mandelli, Tognoni, & Garattini, 1978). Anticonvulsants can also greatly increase (valproate) or decrease (topiramate or zonisimide) appetite. Close monitoring of the infant and the presentation of frequent feeding opportunities when the baby seems comfortable and alert can help overcome some of these issues.

Hydrocephaly

The brain is cushioned by cerebrospinal fluid (CSF) that circulates through and around the brain and spinal cord. If there is a blockage in the circulatory path for CSF, it can build up in the ventricles, or if there is oversecretion or reduced absorption, CSF can build up throughout the head. In young infants, the increased pressure in the head causes the fontanels to bulge and/or sutures to separate. Frequent vomiting, irritability, and unusual eye movements are early effects of the increased intracranial pressure (see **Figure 11-1**). The infant's primary physician should be alerted to vomiting that interferes with growth or is associated with infant distress, so that the cause can be sought and treated. Feeding ability deteriorates rapidly as CSF pressure builds. Once the pressure is relieved by surgical installation of a

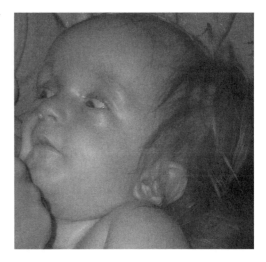

Figure 11-1
Rapid head growth with rotation of eyes downward (sunset sign) increase suspicion of hydrocephalus.

shunt to drain excess CSF into the peritoneum, feeding abilities generally recover. Shunts have a high failure rate in infants under one year of age and those born preterm (McGirt et al., 2002), and require revision if symptoms recur.

Autistic Spectrum Disorders

Children with autism or pervasive developmental disorder have deficits in reciprocal social interactions, nonverbal and verbal communication, and behavioral flexibility. Various theories exist about the reasons for these deficits, including an extreme manifestation of sensory processing disorder, generally disordered information processing, increased testosterone exposure in utero (Knickmeyer & Baron-Cohen, 2006), or, most recently, a defect in mirror neuron function that reduces the ability to empathize and imitate behaviors and cognitive/emotional states (Dapretto et al., 2006). Children with autism seem to extract less information from complex stimuli, and it is possible that differences in memory function prevent autistic children from extracting information from the environment to guide adaptive behavior (Williams, Goldstein, & Minshew, 2006). A case-control study of autistic and neurotypical children showed a more than threefold risk of weaning in the first week of life for the autistic children (Tanoue & Oda, 1989). The study's authors discuss whether this difference is due to a potentially protective effect of breastfeeding, or increased difficulty initiating breastfeeding on the part of autistic infants.

Breastfeeding is a prototypical reciprocal social interaction and depends on consistent infant cueing, maternal response (making the breast available), infant response to the breast by attaching and feeding, and releasing the breast when sated. Although autism is generally not diagnosed until preschool age, examination of home movies generally shows that the reduced facial expression and eye contact, lack of joint attention (looking at what caregivers look at, and later bringing their attention to items of interest), difficulty tolerating environmental change, and stereotypical play are present from early infancy. Infant-related questions on the Pervasive Developmental Disorders Screening Test: Stage 2 include unpredictability in sleep patterns or short sleeping bouts, staring or tuning out, ignoring most toys in favor of a few favorites, disinterest in learning to talk, and enjoyment of chasing and tickling but not interactive lap games such as peek-a-boo and pat-a-cake (Siegel, 1996). Tuning out the unfamiliar often extends to people as well as to objects; the infant may respond to family members and may ignore others.

Symptoms that are most often seen in newborns include reduced facial expression and eye contact, and an increased propensity to shut down and tune out. Newborns in the author's practice who were later diagnosed with autistic spectrum disorders were underresponsive to normal feeding stimuli, and needed to be taught to feed in a step-by-step manner by stimulating individual steps in the feeding sequence with a finger and providing milk upon completion of the sequence, then generalizing the feeding movements to the breast. Sequential stimulation of feeding-related reflex movements is one method of doing this (see oral exercises in the Oral Stimulation section later in this chapter).

Genetic Neurological Conditions

Genetic syndromes can cause neurological dysfunction by interfering with brain structure or function. *Down syndrome* (trisomy 21) is the most common of these, causing variable degrees of cognitive disability, hypotonia (low muscle tone; see **Figure 11-2**), a small mandible, and reduced energy and alertness (see **Figure 11-3**). The frequent presence of cardiac malformations in infants with Down syndrome further impacts their feeding ability. Feeding difficulties include difficulty with attachment due to the relatively large tongue for the small jaw, decreased stability and increased work expended during feeding due to the low muscle tone, and impaired coordination of sucking movements (see **Figure 11-4**). Allowing the infant to learn to breastfeed immediately after birth if stable seems to be important. Stabilizing the head and neck is particularly important in infants with Down syndrome, because there might be malformation or laxity of the ligaments of the first two cervical vertebrae (atlanto-axial instability) that can put pressure on the brainstem or spinal cord with head flexion or excessive extension.

For some genes, a parent of origin effect exists due to differential inactivation according to parental gender. *Prader-Willi syndrome (PWS),* which causes hypotonia and feeding difficulties in the first years of life (see **Figure 11-5**), can be caused by deletion (loss) of the paternal chromosome 15q long arm bands 11–13 (abbreviated 15q11–13⁻), maternal uniparental disomy (two of chromosome 15 from mom, none from dad), or from errors of inactivation in the paternal chromosome 15. Errors of imprinting, where one parent's DNA is not properly inactivated, causing an effective double-dose of the gene's protein product, are becoming

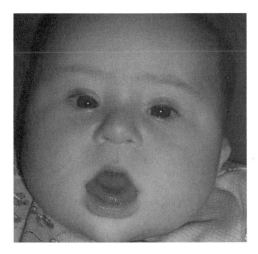

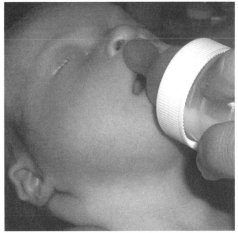

Figure 11-2 Well-nourished breastfed infant with Down syndrome. Note the effects of hypotonia—mouth hangs open, mild tongue protrusion, and reduced facial creases.

Figure 11-3 Presenting a bottle across the lips helps preserve normal gape response. Note the low alertness and energy in this young infant with Down syndrome.

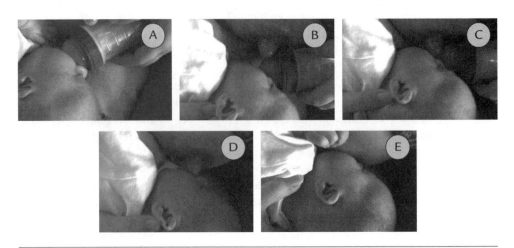

Figure 11-4 Bait and switch technique to move from bottle to breast with nipple shield. Infant is fed from a wide-based bottle near breast, and is moved into alignment for good attachment as the bottle is removed. Baby latches onto breast and continues sucking. Use of the nipple shield can be continued if it helps the infant maintain attachment and transfer milk, or it can be eliminated once breastfeeding becomes familiar.

Figure 11-5 Infant with Prader-Willi syndrome. Note the low muscle tone, small mandible, downturned mouth, and gastrostomy "button." The use of a g-tube allows infants with significant feeding difficulties to get expressed human milk through the tube, allowing unpressured development of oral feeding at breast.

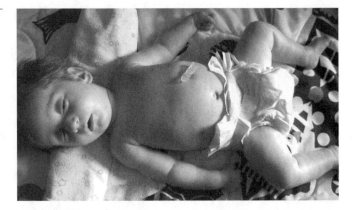

more common due to assisted reproductive technologies (Niemitz & Feinberg, 2004). Feeding difficulties in this syndrome stem from incoordination of oral motor movements, significant hypotonia, and impaired hypothalamic control of satiety (see **Figures 11-6** through **11-9**). There is a high incidence of laryngomalacia/tracheomalacia in infants with PWS, which can further impact feeding. Children with Prader-Willi syndrome require fewer calories for their weight and age and are at extreme risk of obesity. Exclusive human milk feeding and growth hormone supplementation may both be helpful in achieving a healthy weight. Nutritionists may need education about normal intakes of breastfed infants to avoid overfeeding, especially when the infant is fed via gastrostomy tube.

Loss of small bits of DNA from the chromosomes (deletions) can cause significant issues. *Williams syndrome* (7q11.23⁻) causes infants to have feeding difficulties and reduced growth, with cognitive strengths (memory and music) and weaknesses (visual-spatial processing and fine motor delays). Growth retardation is usually greater when the maternal chromosome 7 has the deletion, because the paternal area involved seems to be imprinted. Infants and children with Williams syndrome are reluctant to eat, and may feed better if music is played during their feedings.

Phelan-McDermid syndrome (22q13⁻) causes hypotonia, developmental disability, reduced sleep requirement, and extremely delayed or absent speech (see **Figure 11-10**). The same neurological dysfunction that leads to speech difficulty contributes to feeding difficulties in newborns with this syndrome. Swallowing may be particularly problematic for infants with Phelan-McDermid syndrome, and they should be allowed to self-pace their feedings.

Cri du Chat (cat-cry) Syndrome (5p⁻) causes a malformed larynx and epiglottis that cause a characteristic cry, reduced birth weight with a round face and small head (microcephaly), small jaw (micrognathia), hypotonia, and severe developmental delay. Speech is generally more delayed than receptive language (understanding). Breastfeeding is possible, and therapy should be initiated early if there are sucking or swallowing problems (Cerruti Mainardi, 2006). Distractibility (Clarke & Boer, 1998) may add to the challenge of feeding these infants. Feeding with head extension in prone positions that supply good support can help ease the respiratory symptoms while allowing the infant better jaw contact with the breast.

Kabuki syndrome (genetic cause unknown) causes eyes that resemble those of traditional Japanese Kabuki actors, with long palpebral fissures and a lower lid that is everted at the lateral corner (see **Figure 11-11**). A high arched palate and poor oral motor function, hypotonia and poor growth during infancy, and the persistence of fetal finger pads may be seen in infants with this syndrome. Joint hypermobility is evident in infancy. Tactile defensiveness and dyspraxia may occur, and defects are common in multiple organ systems (Adam & Hudgins, 2005). The use of firm touch during positioning for breastfeeding may help them tolerate touch better, and keeping the feeding position as similar as possible from feeding to feeding may help compensate for the reduced motor planning (see Chapter 10). Holding the baby very close during feeding may help to increase stability and help to maintain latch. Sidelying or upright positioning may be helpful if there are swallowing difficulties, and breast compression can improve the baby's milk transfer. Preparatory oral stimulation immediately before feeding can improve muscle tone and oral motor endurance.

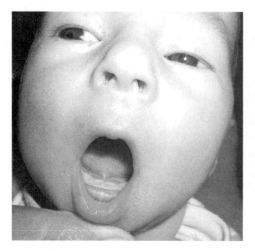

Figure 11-6 This infant with Prader-Willi syndrome has ankyloglossia (tongue-tie) as well as hypotonia, making oral feeding even more problematic.

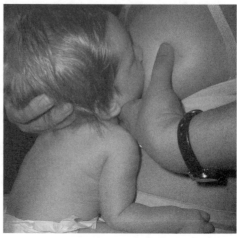

Figure 11-7 Straddle position with jaw support and mild head extension.

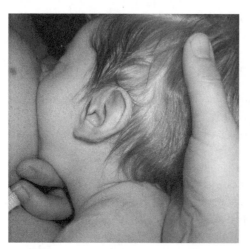

Figure 11-8 Close-up view of jaw support.

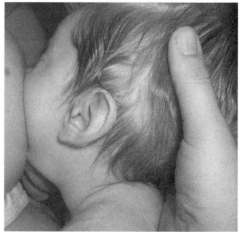

Figure 11-9 Sublingual support and massage can be substituted for jaw support. Light pressure or circular massage is concentrated on the underside of the chin, rather than on the jaw bone, supporting tongue movements during sucking.

Figure 11-10
Low-set prominent ears and an unusual
palate in an infant with Phelan-McDermid
syndrome. This infant's habitual posture was
with one arm held across the body's midline.
Growth had been slow in the early months
(approximately one pound per month),
and hypotonia was diagnosed at birth.
Weight loss at 4–5 months of age was
initially attributed to breastfeeding. The
physician was receptive to the lactation
consultant's suggestion that the problem was
global, and the child was rapidly diagnosed
and provided with a gastrostomy tube and
appropriate therapy.

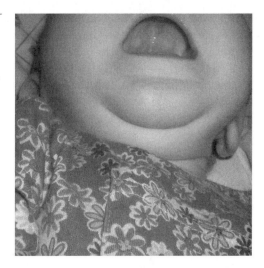

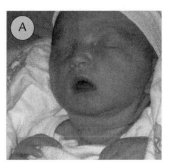 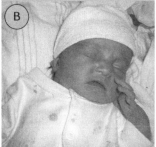 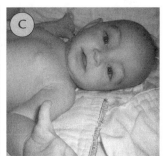

Figure 11-11   Exclusively breastfed infant with Kabuki syndrome. Note the signs of
hypotonia (mouth hanging open, soft facial creases), joint hypermobility (hitchhiker
thumb), long lateral palpebral fissures (eye slits), and arched, sparse eyebrows.

The feeding difficulties in many of these syndromes result from low muscle tone and difficulty coordinating the movements of feeding, swallowing, and breathing. Low muscle tone
makes every feeding movement weaker and more effortful, reducing the amount of milk transferred and increasing fatigue. Less coordinated and skillful tongue movements, weaker jaw
opening and closing, less ability to maintain and increase negative pressure in the mouth
with the tongue and to resist it with the cheeks and lips, and poorer ability to swallow safely
are commonly seen. Nevertheless, the authors have worked with infants with these diagnoses
who breastfed exclusively or partially. Each infant's feeding skills should be assessed and

feeding supported by modifying techniques and expectations while providing facilitative techniques for the improvement of muscle tone and the development of missing skills. A team approach is ideal, with a lactation consultant and a feeding therapist working together.

It is generally helpful to research syndromic conditions to have an idea how the infant may be impacted. The Online Mendelian Inheritance in Man database http://www.ncbi.nlm.nih.gov/omim/ is a database of human genes and genetic disorders that includes clinical synopses. Many disorders have support organizations whose websites contain accurate but less technical information that may be useful in planning a strategy for helping affected infants to feed. General textbooks on newborn diseases or pediatric neurology can provide useful background information, and are often available in libraries or on the Internet. Lactation consultants and therapists should carefully examine materials and websites before referring parents to them for feeding information, because some are unduly dismissive of breastfeeding and others contain outdated or commercially slanted information. It can also be valuable to network with colleagues through local or international professional associations and online networking lists such as Lactnet (http://community.lsoft.com/archives/LACTNET.html) to communicate with peers who have had direct experience with these uncommon disorders.

It is important to note that there is marked variability of severity even within the same diagnosis. Such is the nature of a syndrome. Each infant should be assessed as an individual, and not have breastfeeding arbitrarily ruled out due to their diagnosis. Breastfeeding seems to improve the neurological maturation of infants over time. General movement quality, a sensitive indicator of neurological condition, is significantly improved in infants exclusively breastfed for at least 6 weeks over their own baseline measurements (Bouwstra et al., 2003). Breastfeeding promotes normal development of tongue movements and optimally shapes the oral cavity (Palmer, 1998), provides immune cross-talk between mother and infant from saliva entering the nipple, and is a normalizing experience for both mother and child. Infants with severe feeding difficulties who receive their nutrition by tube can practice oral feeding at the breast. If aspiration is a significant risk, the breast can be expressed before the feeding, to minimize milk flow (Narayanan, Mehta, Choudhury, & Jain, 1991), though there is less risk of aspiration during breastfeeding, and less risk from aspirating human milk. Moreover, safer swallowing occurs during bottle feeding with human milk than with formula or water (Mizuno, Ueda, Kani, & Kawamura, 2002).

Special growth charts are available for several syndromic conditions, including Down syndrome and Cri du Chat syndrome. The use of these special charts allows the infant to be compared with peers, and avoids parental anxiety and excessive supplementation. Infants with very significant feeding problems may benefit from the placement of a gastrostomy tube, allowing human milk to be delivered into the stomach while the infant practices oral feeding at the breast. If a feeding tube is used, the infant should be offered the breast immediately before, during, or just after the tube feeding, to reinforce the relationship between suckling and satiety.

Rare syndromes may not be diagnosed until the infant fails to thrive. Careful monitoring of early growth with early referral to a lactation consultant can help protect maternal milk production. It may be difficult to differentiate between the effects of suboptimal weight gain on the infant's energy and feeding skills and the effects of a neurological condition. Infants who are underfed due to structural, management, or maternal issues are likely to conserve energy by suppressing movement and sleeping more. Their muscle tone may seem low at first, but when the feeding problem is addressed and they begin to gain weight, energy and activity improve markedly. In contrast, children with neurological disorders do not "perk up" the same way. Signs of neurological deficit include rapid fatigue without changes in respiratory pattern or other signs of cardiorespiratory stress; floppiness, especially when combined with unusual positioning of the head, arms, or legs; or poor quality of movements. Dysphagia (difficulty swallowing) is much more common in infants with neurological conditions, and may lead to feeding refusal. Some infants with genetic conditions just look unusual, with subtly *dysmorphic* (unusually shaped) facial features. Areas that are particularly sensitive to genetic influences include:

- The philtrum, or ridge between nose and mouth

- The spacing between the eyes—*hypertelorism* (unusually widely spaced eyes, can be associated with a submucous cleft palate or genetic conditions; see **Figure 11-12**)

- The length of the eye slit (short or long *palpebral fissures*)

- The shape of the skull—*dolichocephaly/scaphocephaly* (disproportionately long, narrow skull) or *brachycephaly* (unusually flat skull)

- The nose (depressed nasal bridge is a common feature of genetic disorders)

- The palate (generally high arched and abnormally shaped)

- The mandible, which may be short due to intrauterine positioning, normal inheritance, or genetic disorder

- The ears, which are generally low-set and unusually shaped, and sometimes pitted (*ear pits*) or have extra fleshy protuberances (*preauricular tags*) near the tragus (ear flap) (see **Figures 11-13** and **11-14**)

Lactation consultants can help determine whether a breastfeeding problem exists, or if there is suspicion of a more global infant feeding problem, and communicate these findings to the infant's health care provider so the infant can be carefully examined. Infants with hypotonia of unknown origin are generally examined by a neurologist and a geneticist. Infants whose feeding skills seem intact but who are failing to gain weight are generally first seen by a gastroenterologist to rule out malabsorption syndromes.

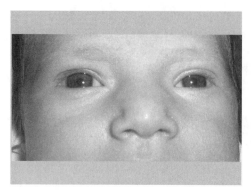

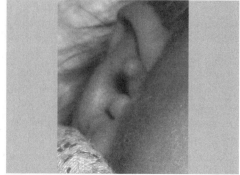

Figure 11-12 Hypertelorism (widely spaced eyes) and paranasal bulging increase suspicion of palate abnormalities.

Figure 11-13 Preauricular tags.

Figure 11-14
Ear pits and small preauricular tag in an infant with Beckwith-Weidemann syndrome.

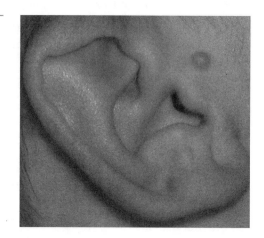

Neuromuscular Junction Issues

Myasthenia gravis (MG) is an autoimmune process in which antibodies attack the acetyl-choline (ACh) receptor, causing skeletal muscle weakness and fatigue, especially with repeated activity. These IgG antibodies transfer through the placenta (Shehata & Okosun, 2004), though only a minority of infants are symptomatic (Tellez-Zenteno, Hernandez-Ronquillo, Salinas, Estanol, & da Silva, 2004). In one large Italian study of mothers with MG, all breastfed their unaffected infants (Batocchi et al., 1999). Although maternal immunosuppressant medications may transfer through milk, several studies have demonstrated no adverse effects of maternal ingestion of cyclosporine on their breastfed infants (Moretti et al., 2003; Munoz-Flores Thiagarajan, Easterling, Davis, & Bond, 2001; Nyberg, Haljamae, Frisenette-Fich, Wennergren, & Kjellmer, 1998).

Signs of neonatal myasthenia gravis evolve over the first few hours of life, and include hypotonia and feeding difficulties, and rarely, ventilator dependence. Anticholinesterase medications improve symptoms in most affected infants (Ciafaloni & Massey, 2004).

Feeding issues for affected infants include rapid muscle fatigue and hypotonia. Gavage (nasogastric or orogastric tube) feeding is generally required until treatment is effective, but the infant may be put to the breast for very short feedings if maternal and infant condition permits.

Effect of Neurological Disorders on Feeding

Some of the issues affecting feeding skills in infants with neurological conditions include muscle tone differences, cognitive deficits that impede learning, coordination difficulties, impeded function of specific nerves or neuromuscular units, and lack of appropriate alertness or energy for feeding.

The brain directs muscle activity and the nerves serve as the messengers of the brain's directions, so any dysfunction in either or both leaves the muscles less able to perform work. Coordination and rhythm are vital to the effectiveness of feeding movements (Lau & Schanler, 1996, p. 164), so even the correct movements performed without proper timing can be ineffective, just as a familiar melody played without regard to the proper duration of each note can become unrecognizable. This is a familiar phenomenon to anyone who has observed a child just learning to play a musical instrument. It takes so long for a beginner to recognize the note on the paper, play that note, and move on to the next one that the timing of the melody becomes distorted, and the song becomes unrecognizable. This is recognized as a problem in feeding; Marjorie Meyer Palmer's Neonatal Oral-Motor Assessment Scale (NOMAS) includes a category for disorganized sucking, which is defined by deficiencies in rate and rhythm (Palmer & VandenBerg, 1998). Moreover, computer modeling of breastfeeding shows that optimal timing in the suction cycle of the wavelike tongue movements increases milk flow (Zoppou, Barry, & Mercer, 1997).

The Reciprocal Nature of Muscle Activity

Muscles work in pairs, flexing (making the angle between two bones smaller) and extending (making the angle between two bones larger). For example, when a baby bends at the hips, the belly muscles will contract while the back muscles extend. If the tone in the back extensors is higher than normal, the baby may have difficulty not only flexing at the hips, but even maintaining the hips at neutral. An extensor pattern may also translate into a feeding difficulty as over-firing extensors call other muscles into the pattern, pulling back the baby's shoulders and upper spine. This makes it difficult for the baby to be in the workable ear/shoulder/hip aligned configuration, and makes attaching to the breast a challenge by retracting (pulling back) the tongue.

Physical and/or occupational therapy can help normalize tone with preparatory handling techniques and by positioning the baby in supportive, pattern-interrupting ways to help reduce the effects of abnormally high tone.

Increased Effort with High/Low Tone

The muscular system is a miracle of balance: flex and extend, contract and release, shorten and lengthen. Moreover, this shortening and lengthening happens in a very controlled manner on either side of a joint. Any time muscle tone is out of balance between reciprocal (antagonist) muscles, or a group of synergistic muscles, the ease of movement is reduced, work increases, and energy expenditure increases. If tone is out of balance toward the high side (*hypertonia*), movement can be restricted as muscle groups are caught ("stuck"), unable to release extension so contraction can occur on the opposite side of the joint.

This is one reason we encourage mothers to be comfortable while they nurse; not only does it feel better to be comfortable, it is also more sustainable because increased tension wastes energy. Ergonomic use of the body reduces the risk of injury and increases ease of movement. Use of large muscles for holding the baby is easier than stressing smaller muscles. Encouraging mothers to use gravity and their trunk to support the baby's weight rather than their relatively weaker wrists can be important in preventing exacerbation of repetitive stress injuries such as carpal tunnel syndrome.

Being out of balance the other way is also challenging. Low tone (*hypotonia*) may mean that muscles lack the power to achieve the necessary range of movement; for example, a baby with low tone in the jaw muscles may be unable to open her or his mouth enough to latch well. In addition, these restrictions of movement range may lead to the baby recruiting other muscles to join in assisting the action. This can be challenging because the muscles joining in may not be efficiently designed for this new role. The effect of this is familiar to most LCs when watching a baby with a structural tongue limitation: A baby with a restrictive lingual frenulum, unable to latch deeply enough to feed with stability and power, compensates for the instability of a shallow latch by using the muscles of the upper lip. This is not only painful for mom, but also tiring for the baby because upper lip muscles are better at the subtle movements of speech than the power movements of repetitive feeding. In similar fashion, muscles recruited to compensate for lack of range of motion caused by neurological limitations can rapidly fatigue.

Early Intervention Referral

Infants with neurological conditions are often diagnosed in the postpartum unit, but sometimes breastfeeding difficulties are the first manifestation of altered development. Early intervention (EI) programs provide free or subsidized evaluation and treatment for infants experiencing, or at high risk for, developmental delay. An Internet search using the keywords "early intervention *county or locality name*" will generally yield local information and contacts. Generally, physicians, parents, and other health care personnel (including lactation consultants) can refer infants by contacting the local coordinator or agency. The family is assigned a case coordinator, the parents are interviewed, and the child is tested by specialists in cognitive, language, and motor development. If therapy is prescribed for a child under 3, it is usually provided in the family home.

Where bottle feeding has been the cultural norm, the lactation consultant may be the first to point out the need to provide therapy or assistance to the infant. Poor recognition of incoordination among sucking, swallowing, and breathing during bottle feeding allows infants with feeding problems to go undiagnosed. If caregivers lay the infant down, actively insert the artificial nipple, and invert the bottle so the milk flows rapidly into the baby's mouth (as recommended in bottle and formula manufacturers' literature and websites), it is possible to miss the baby's inability to initiate and follow through with normal feeding subskills like wide gaping, tongue depression and extension, tongue grooving around the teat, and rhythmic tongue and jaw movements to transfer milk. The more passive, or reactive, nature of standard bottle feeding, and the acceptance of rapid, gulpy feeds with milk loss and/or vomiting as normal, can conspire to mask baby's difficulty with normal, active feeding skills. The physiological challenges presented by bottle feeding, including lack of standardization of nipple flow rates, high flow rates that compromise respirations, and the lack of conformity to the infant's anatomy, may negatively impact acquisition and maintenance of normal feeding skills. Consequently, abnormal compensatory movements may develop and override normal skill development.

The LC may be the first, or only, person to suggest that the baby has a feeding issue. The issue may be temporary or it may have its basis in static or progressive neurological deficits. Parents can be reassured that the recommendation for EI evaluation does not imply a lifelong challenge for the baby. If breastfeeding were the cultural norm, all babies having trouble achieving the norm would be evaluated and supported toward that norm. Because some health care professionals still consider breastfeeding disposable "as long as the baby can bottle feed," even poorly, EI may not have been suggested before. Parents will need extra support as to the simple normalcy of breastfeeding, that they are not following some maternal agenda for a feeding "style," but simply want their baby to achieve normal developmental milestones. Dialogue with parents about the simple normality of feeding at the breast will be critical. They need information and support that their baby is not being asked to work toward something too challenging for some (like marathon running) but simply to the norm (like walking).

Supportive Techniques

For infants with hypotonia, particular attention should be paid to support and alignment at breast. Swaddling in body flexion (with hips and knees flexed, hand brought to midline, and shoulders gently forward) may help floppy infants to use their tongue and jaw more skillfully. Hypotonic infants who have difficulty maintaining attachment or have wide jaw excursions can benefit from chin and jaw support. The *Dancer hand position* (McBride & Danner, 1987) consists of using the webbing between the thumb and first finger to support the infant's jaw while the thumb and first finger support the cheeks. Generally when cheek support is given, forward traction is applied toward the lips. (See photos in Chapter 12.)

Those with weak tongue movements may be assisted by *sublingual support,* where the feeder places a fingertip under the baby's chin on the soft tissue behind the jaw bone (see **Figure 11-15**). Gentle upward pressure is provided to assist tongue movements, and gentle forward traction may help as well. As always, the effect of these interventions needs to be carefully observed. Jaw and cheek support in bottle feeding infants may increase bolus size. Although it is unlikely that the same is true for breastfeeding infants, the infant should be observed for any difficulty coordinating swallowing and breathing.

Positioning

Infants with hypotonia and reduced energy and alertness may feed better in more upright positions (see **Figure 11-16**), such as the straddle or more vertical versions of the clutch hold (**Figure 11-17**). Optimal support is important for stability in these infants with reduced postural stability. When using sidelying, mother may want to lay the infant's head on her upper arm and use her lower arms to keep him snuggled against her body for positional stability (**Figure 11-18**). See Chapter 12 for more on therapeutic positioning.

Head positioning for neurologically impaired infants during feeding is controversial. For healthy, full-term infants, the ideal head position during breastfeeding is one of mild extension to bring the jaw forward, increase tongue and jaw contact with the breast, and open the airway for reduced resistance to air flow for unstressed breathing. Radiological evidence has shown that head extension facilitated correct sucking and swallowing when feeding with a modified bottle in an infant with structural disabilities (Takagi & Bosma, 1960). Therapists have long been taught to use a neutral head position or "chin tuck" in feeding neurologically impaired infants. It is believed that the slight chin tuck mechanically improves the safety of swallowing, because flexion narrows the airway and raises the larynx. There is evidence that chin tuck during swallowing reduces the number of aspirations in adults with surgical or age-related swallowing problems (Rasley et al., 1993; Shanahan, Logemann, Rademaker, Pauloski,

Figure 11-15
Sublingual support.

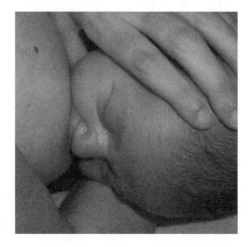

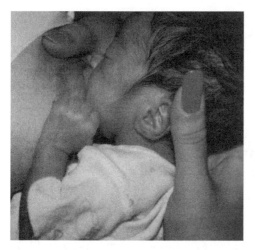

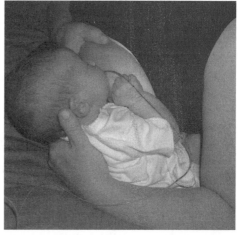

Figure 11-16 Preterm infants with low muscle tone may benefit from upright positioning.

Figure 11-17 Sitting clutch; note that the infant's knees and hips are flexed. If mother reclines, this position becomes more ergonomic. A 5-French feeding tube is providing additional milk.

Figure 11-18
Providing optimal support in sidelying.

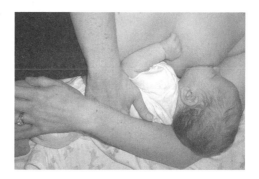

& Kahrila, 1993), but the maneuver was less effective in younger patients and those whose swallowing problems did not stem from overflow from the valeculae. The anatomy of the newborn airway offers protection against aspiration from this mechanism due to the apposition of the soft palate and epiglottis during sucking. Additionally, infants with respiratory instability are less likely to time their swallows appropriately. In newborns, and particularly preterm infants, overflexion of the neck may result in the occlusion of the pharyngeal airway by the larynx (Ardran & Kemp, 1968).

LCs working with neurologically impaired infants need to weigh these competing concerns and observe the results of any intervention particularly carefully. Because aspiration can occur without coughing in young infants (Arvedson, Rogers, Buck, Smart, & Msall, 1994), careful assessment of the coordination of swallowing sounds and observation of the infant's respiratory sounds for wet or congested qualities is necessary when feeding neurologically impaired infants. Cervical auscultation is particularly useful for this purpose (see Chapter 1).

Interaction of Birth Interventions with Neurological Issues

Any motor pattern or state condition that interferes with the baby's ability to be in a quiet alert state, with relaxed but ready musculature and neuromotor responses, can inhibit a baby's ability to successfully go through the instinctive feeding sequence. Some babies have temporary but significant challenges due to labor or delivery medications or procedures. In the first 48 hours, frequency of feeding helps calibrate future milk production, with 13–16 breastfeeding sessions on the second day of life creating a significantly increased milk production even 6 weeks later in multiparous women, versus the commonly recommended 8–12 feedings (Chen, Nommsen-Rivers, Dewey, & Lonnerdal, 1998). Newborn babies need frequent and untimed access to the breast to receive adequate amounts of colostrum, which provides irreplaceable immunological protection and trophic functions to prepare the gut for larger volumes of mature milk. If the baby is either too irritable or too overwhelmed and shuts down, feeding can be difficult. Restoring skin-to-skin positioning with mom is sometimes enough to restore normal feeding behavior within 15–30 minutes. Hospital routines that expect newborns to interval feed like older babies can disrupt the important calibration and learning period of the first few days.

Colostrum's low volume and high viscosity facilitate practice of coordination of sucking, swallowing, and breathing with a low risk of aspiration. This practice is especially important for neurologically impaired infants who may have a greater risk of aspiration when the milk volume and flow increase (Arvedson et al., 1994; Stevenson & Allaire, 1991, p. 1450).

Healthy, unmedicated babies will show interest in and initiate feeding when they are ready and need not be rushed, especially if they have been kept skin to skin with their mother since birth. Neurologically impaired infants who are also under the influences of medications, procedures, or separation from their mother are likely to be more disorganized from these interventions than neurotypical infants.

Preparatory Handling

For disorganized or challenged infants, it can be helpful to position/move them in certain ways before the breast is even presented. Babies with tonal issues can be assisted toward the middle of the tone or state continuum by being in positions that either enhance or calm the effects of tone outside the functional middle of the continuum.

Hypertonia

A baby with high tone might need to be wrapped in a blanket, providing full body support for the head, neck, trunk, and limbs, and rocked gently through the air from head to feet (see **Figure 11-19**). This can be relaxing, lowering higher tone toward the middle norm, and allowing the baby to move the head and neck more independently from the trunk and limbs. It may also calm an overstimulated or overstressed baby.

Babies can also be calmed by placing them in the "colic hold": draped over the forearm with the baby's belly along the forearm muscle of the person holding the baby, with baby's legs and arms allowed to relax around the sides and down around the holder's arm, and the baby's head resting at the side of the widest part of the forearm (see **Figure 11-20**).

By switching arms, the holder has the baby over the other forearm, baby's legs on either side of the palm, and the holder's other hand supporting the baby's forehead. The infant can be offered a finger to suck in this position (charm hold, see Chapter 12), which can help bring the tongue forward in the mouth and give the lactation consultant another perspective on the tongue's tone, range of motion, and strength.

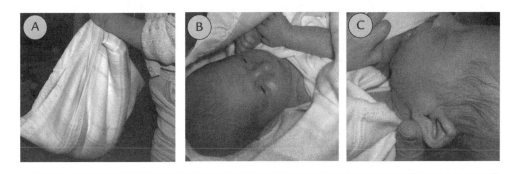

Figure 11-19   Using a blanket swing to relax a stressed, arching infant into flexion, improving neurobehavioral organization and allowing attachment.

Figure 11-20
Colic hold.

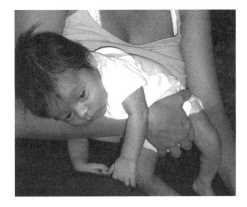

Hypotonia

A baby with lower tone can be assisted to sit on an adult knee and be gently but arrhythmically bounced, or leaned forward and back to stimulate *equilibrium reactions* (righting responses)—attempts to maintain posture despite movement away from a stable center (see **Figure 11-21**). Movements that stimulate equilibrium reactions increase alertness and/or tone so that the baby can better move the neck and jaws in the instinctive feeding initiation sequence pattern. Babies with suitable neck strength can be supported in a standing position with their feet on a sitting adult's thighs. Most infants placed in this position will enjoy repeatedly pushing down with their feet by extending and flexing their knees (see **Figure 11-22**). The proprioceptive input of bouncing or jumping on a slightly resilient surface is believed to improve muscle tone and motor performance in hypotonic children.

These movements and positions are simple, brief, and may help improve readiness and capabilities for normal latching and feeding in babies who are temporarily or mildly affected by tone or state issues. Babies with severe or ongoing issues may benefit from referral to early intervention (occupational, physical, or speech/language therapists) or to private practice speech/feeding therapists, osteopathic physicians, chiropractors, or other bodywork practitioners, in addition to continuing to work with the lactation consultant. Team communication and sharing of perspectives and skills is vital to optimizing normal feeding skills in infancy and beyond.

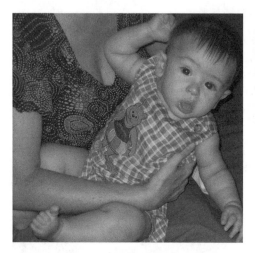

Figure 11-21 Stimulating equilibrium reactions by tilting the baby backward slightly.

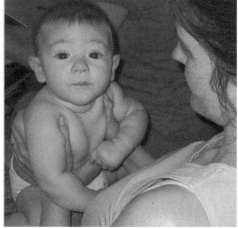

Figure 11-22 Preparatory handling with an infant.

Alertness

Cerebral depression causes reduced alertness and a lower level of consciousness that can range in severity from coma to an increased proportion of the day spent in sleep. As mentioned earlier in the chapter, anticonvulsants prescribed for neonatal seizures can further sedate the infant. In a neonatal intensive care environment, compromised infants may withdraw from the constant overstimulation, increasing their unavailability for feeding.

Removing aversive stimuli as much as possible and providing organizing stimulation (cuddling, skin-to-skin contact, gentle rocking or swaying) may help infants who are shut down to feel safe. It is generally helpful to watch for behavioral signs of light sleep (squirming, mouthing, sucking, rapid eye movements) and place the depressed infant to breast as soon as these occur. Skin-to-skin care (kangaroo mother care) can help to take advantage of briefer periods of alertness by keeping the baby close to the breast and in a more organized state.

In general, arrhythmic vestibular stimulation is alerting, and rhythmic stimulation is organizing. Compromised or preterm infants may find any movement stressful and disorganizing. Skin-to-skin contact with mom without stroking or maternal movement may help a stressed infant become available for feeding. Sensitive observation of the infant will allow stimulation to be withdrawn if the baby shows stress signals.

Sucking Issues in Neurologically Impaired Infants

Infants with neurological deficits may use a disorganized, up and down piston-like movement of the tongue during sucking. Sucking pressure can be absent in infants with severe neurological issues (Mizuno et al., 2006). Infants with neurological challenges generally are able to improve their feeding skills (McBride & Danner, 1987), and depending on the severity of their condition, many will learn to breastfeed. Improvement in feeding skills is a good prognostic indicator for future neurological functioning (Mizuno, 2005). Breastfeeding can be initiated while the infant is still being gavage (tube) fed, and the gavage feedings reduced or eliminated as the baby becomes able to obtain his nutritional needs at breast. Counseling mom to maintain her supply at a higher level than needed can be helpful for her infant with imperfect sucking skills, as long as the rapid milk flow does not compromise coordination of swallowing and breathing. Sometimes stimulating a swallow by introducing a little bit of milk into the mouth by breast compression or with a periodontal syringe, eyedropper, or tube can lead to stimulation of the central pattern generator for sucking and initiate the suck, swallow, breathe sequence (see **Figure 11-23**).

If maternal milk production is low or the infant is weak and requires more reward for his efforts, additional milk can be given through a tube at breast. Several commercial devices exist for this purpose, including the Lact-Aid Nursing Trainer System (LA), the Supply Line, and the Medela Supplemental Nursing System (SNS). (ee **Figures 11-24** and **11-25**.) Getting flow correct is important. Too high a flow can stress the infant's cardiorespiratory system by forcing frequent swallows, suppressing breathing, and reducing blood oxygen levels. Fast

Figure 11-23
Providing an instant reward for mouthing the breast with a curved tip (periodontal) syringe.

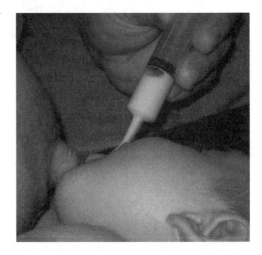

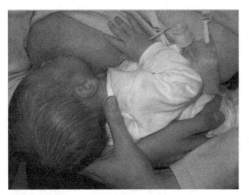

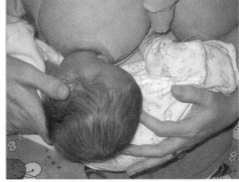

Figure 11-24　The Lact-Aid nursing trainer provides additional milk at breast, and is easy to clean and assemble.

Figure 11-25　The Supplemental Nursing System has two tubes, and can be used with twins as well as singletons.

flow can also stress the ability to coordinate the swallow correctly and increase the risk of aspiration. Too low a flow fails to provide consistent sensory input for continued sucking efforts, and may lead to a spiral of increasing fatigue, poorer feeding, and weight loss.

Except in situations where the feeder is attempting to "jumpstart" the sucking sequence by delivering a small bolus of milk, the infant should ideally be in control of milk delivery, either actively by pulling milk from the device or by feeder coordination of delivery with the infant's sucking efforts (see **Figure 11-26**). In addition to the danger of aspiration, the infant does not learn as well if milk flow is not contingent on his efforts. Infants with cognitive impairments especially require consistency in cueing and oral motor movements required to move milk.

There is a fine balance between rewarding an infant's continued attempts to breastfeed and reinforcing dysfunctional sucking behaviors. Occasionally, motivation may be more important than stimulating correct suckling. Neurologically impaired infants in the author's practice have responded to a nipple shield repeatedly filled with expressed milk with a curved tip syringe or butterfly tubing and syringe. Despite the use of a tongue thrusting pattern, several infants were able to remove milk from the prefilled teat before they were able to transfer milk from the breast (**Figure 11-27**). The experience of obtaining milk from the breast provided positive feedback that led to further attempts at breastfeeding. Tongue movements gradually improved with the use of facilitative techniques and the infants' own experimentation.

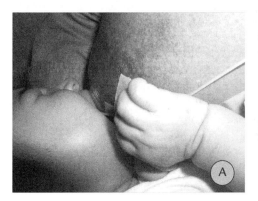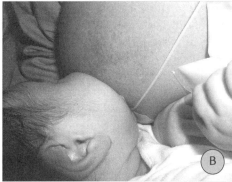

Figure 11-26   Latching on with a Lact-Aid tube. Placing the tube at the center of the lower lip helps ensure proper tube placement without disrupting latch mechanics.

Figure 11-27
Prefilling a nipple shield allowed this infant to transition back to breast after recovery from neonatal encephalopathy.

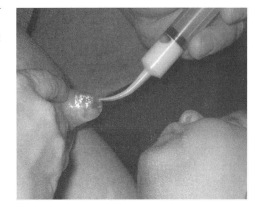

Why Some Babies Need Supplementing, Even Though Mom Is Making Sufficient Milk

Daly, Owens, and Hartmann (1993) found that breastfeeding infants will remove an average of 76% of the stored milk from the breast. Infants with sucking problems, particularly tongue-tied or neurologically impaired infants in the author's (Genna) practice, have been able to remove between 10% and 60% of the milk their mother can subsequently pump. Supplementing at breast generally increases the amount of milk that inefficient infants are able to receive from the breast. This can be demonstrated by weighing the filled supplementer and the baby separately before and after feeding on a scale designed to detect breast milk intake. These scales are generally accurate to a few grams, allowing a good estimation of milk intake. Feeding promptly after weighing, and reweighing immediately after feeding, reduce the impact of *insensible water loss* (water vapor lost through normal metabolism and respiration). If the baby is an ineffective feeder, there may be more milk removed from the breast using the supplementer (the baby will have gained more than the supplementer lost) than without it. If the entire milk intake came from the device, then the infant might have been sucking the tube alone (which is obvious by the sound of air being drawn into the mouth and the baby's pursed lips). If straw drinking was not occurring, and little milk was taken from the breast, maternal milk production may be very low. Efforts should be made to increase milk removal to stimulate increased supply.

Some infants' feeding attempts are particularly flow dependent—when the flow of milk subsides, they seem to give up and stop working. Supplementing at breast with a tube feeding device can provide continuous flow to infants for whom breast compression is insufficient. Infants with limited endurance can benefit from supplementation at breast, allowing them to feed in a reasonable time frame, and allowing their mother time for milk expression to help protect or increase her supply.

There are two types of supplementer devices, those that require suction (negative intra-oral pressure) and those that are active, or feeder controlled. A periodontal syringe or syringe attached to tubing is an example of an active supplementation device. Obviously, active supplementation is required in infants with overt clefts who cannot create negative pressure in their mouths. Active supplementation also works well with infants who lack energy due to underfeeding. Active supplementation must be performed carefully, to avoid exacerbating any underlying condition that led to the infant being unable to feed well. For example, cardiac and respiratory problems that cause an increased respiratory rate or increased work of breathing leave less time for swallowing. Pushing an infant with one of these issues to swallow more frequently can easily reduce their respiratory rate below that needed to maintain oxygenation. The feeder generally waits for the infant to initiate a sucking burst, and then supplies small boluses with each suck. If the baby loses milk from the lips or shows signs of flow intolerance, the bolus size is reduced and/or the flow is slowed; if the baby shows impatience (tugging, squirming, lack of swallowing) the flow is increased. The infant is allowed to pace the feeding; the feeder stops delivering milk during respiratory pauses. If the infant is not self-pacing, the feeder observes for increased respiratory rate or stress signs (see Chapter 10), and the flow is interrupted until recovery occurs.

The Lact-Aid Nursing Trainer, the Supply Line, Medela's Supplemental Nursing System, and devices assembled by placing a feeding tube in a container of milk all require negative intraoral pressure. When the infant sucks, milk is drawn out of the breast. If a full mouthful comes from the breast, little or no milk is removed from the supplementer. If only a partial mouthful is removed from the breast, milk flows through the tube to fill the mouth. Flow from the device can be controlled in several ways—crimping the tube in a slot in the commercial devices, or lifting the tube out of the supplement stops the flow of milk; lifting the container increases gravity's influence and increases speed of flow; a larger diameter tube increases flow; and for a twin tube device like the SNS, venting the device by opening the second tube increases the flow as well. Taping the venting tube to the container with the opening pointing toward the ceiling can help keep air moving in and prevent milk from moving out.

Tube devices can make attachment more challenging. Holding or taping the tube where the center of the baby's lower lip will touch it during latch can improve tube placement, bringing it in midline on the tongue, under the nipple. When the tube is placed at the upper lip, mother may pay attention to ensuring that the upper lip covers the tube, and may allow the lower lip to slide up to the base of the nipple. This is opposite to the optimal latch, which is obtained when the lower lip and tongue tip are as far from the nipple as possible.

Another challenge of tube devices is that some infants will straw-drink and remove milk only from the tube. Withdrawing the tube slightly, so that it no longer extends to the nipple tip or beyond, can reduce this behavior. Infant feeding involves learning, and it is important to provide the right lesson. If supplementation at breast is not leading to correct sucking that removes milk from the breast, it might not be the right intervention. The infant should be assessed again, and other interventions (or a different supplementer device) considered.

If feedings are prolonged even with a supplementer device, tube placement in the infant's mouth should be checked, and the tubing should be examined to ensure there are no crimps or clogs. Powdered formula use is a common cause of clogged tubing, and the Lact-Aid comes with a filter to strain out lumps during filling. Rubbing the tubing between the thumb and forefinger may soften lumps or release crimps and improve flow. If the infant is getting sufficient milk at breast with the supplementer, but the feeding is long (> 30–45 minutes), mother can be counseled to use the device every other feeding, and use a faster alternate feeding method in between, to help preserve the dyad's energy and maintain time for milk expression. Milk removal is vital to continued production, and for some dyads, less time at breast and more time spent pumping is the best use of their energy until the baby's skills improve.

Weaning from Supplementers

As the infant shows improved ability to transfer milk from the breast, the mother can be counseled to gradually reduce either the amount of supplement in the container or the proportion of the feeding times when the device is used. Leaving the tube closed off at the beginning of the feeding when the milk ejection is strongest, or offering the device only with the second breast if *paired feedings* (both breasts) are given are ways to achieve this.

Generally the infant will be able to feed at the breast alone at the first morning feeding or whenever the breast is more full, and will gradually progress to more and more feedings without the device.

Oral Motor Dysfunction and Facilitative Techniques

Specific facilitative techniques are typically used to assist infants with abnormalities in oral motor skills. While these do not necessarily correct the compensatory sucking strategies, they can help the infant achieve more functional feeding. Facilitations should be based on a firm understanding of the normal activity of each structure.

Jaw

The mandible is the moveable part of the jaw. The mandibular gum ridge should be aligned parallel to the maxillary gum ridge; jaw opening should be smooth and symmetrical, and the gape should be large. Impaired nerve transmission can cause unequal jaw opening, as can positional asymmetries from in utero position such as torticollis. Tongue-tie is often associated with an insufficient gape, perhaps due to traction on the hyoid bone.

Excessive jaw excursions during breastfeeding may be the result of hypotonia, in which case *jaw support* may be helpful. Poor control of the jaw in a neurologically impaired infant may result in slippage of the jaw, providing poor stability for tongue movements (Morris & Klein, 2001, p. 125), leading to decreased milk transfer and fatigue.

A more common cause of excessive jaw excursions that interrupt attachment to the breast is *ankyloglossia* (tongue-tie). Failure of the anterior tongue to maintain contact with the breast when the posterior tongue depresses enlarges the oral cavity, and requires a larger jaw excursion to create sufficient negative pressure to pull milk from the nipple. The excessive jaw excursion may overcome the ability of the lips to seal on the breast, causing repeated loss of attachment. The cheeks may not be capable of resisting the negative pressure in the front of the mouth, and may collapse. Dimpling of the cheeks in a full-term infant during breastfeeding is an indication that this may be occurring (see **Figure 11-28**).

Figure 11-28
Excessive jaw excursions cause flattening or dimpling of the cheeks and loss of attachment.

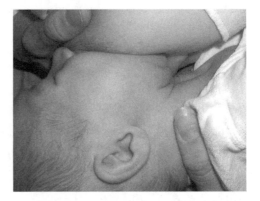

Increasing the depth of attachment will generally improve sucking dynamics by sharing the work of maintaining latch better among the tongue and lips.

Some infants with neurological impairments will move the jaw sideways (lateral *deviations*) or in a circle (*rotary movements*) instead of straight up and down. Lateral deviations may occur in torticollis; rotary movements are normal during chewing, but don't occur developmentally in a younger infant. Rotary movements may be compensatory for poor tongue mobility or coordination. Jaw support might stabilize the jaw sufficiently for these infants to breastfeed while therapy addresses the nerve and/or muscular imbalances behind the abnormal movement pattern.

Tongue

Many healthy infants with abnormal tongue movements are attempting to compensate for tongue-tie. Infants with neurologically based sucking difficulties often display a disorganized, up and down piston-like tongue movement. There is generally poor tone and poor central grooving of the tongue. There may be difficulty organizing and initiating sucking movements, and tremors of the jaw and tongue are typically observed (McBride & Danner, 1987, p. 114). Tremors associated with neurological issues will generally be observed near the beginning of the feed, and will be frequent and persistent, whereas fatigue tremors in tongue-tied infants are more likely to occur later in the course of the feeding.

Specific oral exercises may be helpful to increase tongue grooving, stimulate the sequential wavelike movements of normal sucking, and allow a baby with neurological difficulties to breastfeed.

Lips

The tongue provides most of the anterior seal between the breast and mouth; the lips are more relaxed and the orbicularis oris muscle (the circular muscle surrounding the lips) is much less active than the mentalis muscle during breastfeeding (Jacinto-Goncalves, Gaviao, & Berzin, 2004). Fixing of the orbicularis oris may occur when a hypotonic infant attempts to overuse this muscle to improve stability (**Figure 11-29**).

If significant spilling occurs from the lips (see **Figure 11-30**), perioral tapping or circular massage just outside of the vermillion border of the lips may help improve lip seal. Infants with swallowing difficulties may deliberately spill milk from the lips. As always, the results of any intervention need to be observed before that intervention is repeated or taught to the infant's parent.

Excessive sweeping movements of the lips may be seen as a compensation for tongue-tie, and are usually associated with large sucking blisters and friction calluses along the upper lip. These are often found in midline on the upper lip, but can occur across the skin of both upper and lower lips in infants with extreme difficulties with stability in the author's experience (JLF).

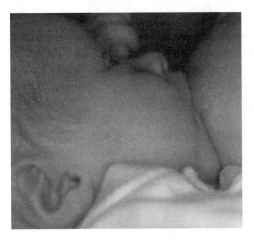

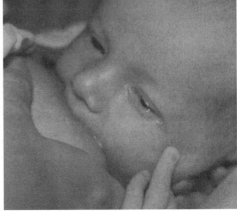

Figure 11-29 Lip fixing at breast.
This is easier to see with the narrower latch on a Haberman feeder teat in Plate 3.

Figure 11-30   Spilling milk from the upper lip.

Cheeks

Full-term infants have a large fat pad in each cheek to form a border for tongue movements that help to keep the tongue in midline during sucking, and help to increase the bulk of the cheeks to help them stay rounded during the negative pressure phase of sucking. In hypotonic infants, the cheek muscles may not have sufficient tone to resist negative pressure of normal jaw opening during sucking and may collapse. Cheek support from a fingertip on each cheek with gentle forward traction (toward the angle of the lips) can be helpful.

Palate, Velum, and Pharynx

The hard palate is immobile and plastic, and is shaped by tongue movements (see **Figure 11-31**). The more abnormal the hard palate shape, the more likely the tongue movements are to be abnormal (see **Figure 11-32**). Interventions should be directed to improving tongue function. A very abnormal palate shape may be the result of a genetic disorder.

Like all bony structures, the palate is subject to *Wolf's Law,* the understanding that bones adapt to the loads placed on them. When muscle power or range are affected by neurological compromise—yielding high, low, or vacillating tone—the bones these muscles attach to adapt to these abnormal stresses. In the case of the palate, tone issues affecting the tongue have an impact on the hard palate. In utero sucking and swallowing movements work to sculpt the palate, but when range of motion, power, or sustained rhythms are compromised, the palate may not be lowered and widened to its most effective feeding configuration. (The same law applies when tongues are mechanically restricted by anky-

Figure 11-31
Normal palate.

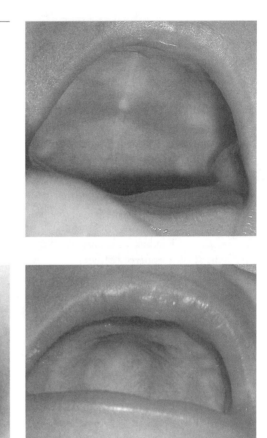

Figure 11-32 High, narrow palate shapes associated with ankyloglossia (tongue-tie).
Note the reduced tongue elevation in part A and the reduced gape in part B.

loglossia.) A limited or weak tongue can cause palatal adaptation towards a higher, narrower palate. The limited tongue movements lead to a constellation of feeding challenges practitioners may have noted. This constellation may include the inability to extend, lateralize, or stabilize the tongue; tongue humping or bunching; tongue asymmetry; and concomitant difficulties with the rhythmic, easy interplay of positive pressure and negative pressure that characterizes efficient, comfortable milk transfer.

The soft palate (*velum*) moves in concert with tongue movements, dropping to seal against the tongue during sucking, and raising to meet the walls of the pharynx to seal the nasal airway during swallowing. Signs of soft palate dysfunction include milk dripping from the nose during sucking, feeding-induced apnea (nasopharyngeal backflow of milk triggers apnea in infants), nasal regurgitation after or between feedings, and short sucking bursts with harsh or wet respiratory sounds during pauses. In infants with neurological issues, velopharyngeal inadequacy can be due to poor coordination and timing between the soft palate and the pharyngeal muscles, so that the nasal cavity is not fully sealed during swallowing, or not sealed at the right time to keep milk out. Severe gastroesophageal reflux can be associated with nasal regurgitation as well.

Upright feeding positions can be helpful for infants with poor swallowing, as can pacing of the feed (see Figure 11-11 earlier in the chapter). Aspiration, penetration, and nasopharyngeal backflow were more likely to occur after several sequential swallows (Newman, Keckley, Petersen, & Hammer, 2001). Therefore, limiting an infant with swallowing problems to a few sucks before briefly interrupting the feeding can reduce the risk of milk entering the airway. Exercises that facilitate tongue grooving may help improve swallowing by increasing bolus control (Morris & Klein, 2001). Information on velopharyngeal inadequacy due to anatomic issues is provided in Chapter 8.

Helping Infants Who Feed Ineffectively

If the infant is unable to feed orally, the mother should be encouraged to express milk for tube feedings. Sufficient milk production is most likely when the pump kit fits well (the nipples have room to expand in the nipple tunnel during pumping), expression is initiated within 6 hours of birth, both breasts are pumped simultaneously (Jones, Dimmock, & Spencer, 2001) about 8 times in 24 hours (Hill, Aldaq, & Chatterton, 2001), and pumping is preceded by very brief breast massage. Manual expression of milk is effective as well, perhaps even more effective than mechanical pumps for the removal of colostrum. Colostrum can be manually expressed into a teaspoon and fed directly to the infant, or it can be expressed into a medicine cup for feeding with a syringe or eyedropper. If an electric pump is used in the first days of life, a very small collection container should be used to avoid wasting colostrum. A spare Ameda silicone diaphragm can be upended in the top of any standard collection bottle, and can be used as a feeding cup (see **Figure 11-33**).

When infants breastfeed ineffectively despite intervention, it may be helpful to provide brief feeds at breast for practice while supplying the bulk of the baby's nutrition another way. Limiting time at breast until the infant can transfer significant amounts of milk helps preserve the energy of both mother and baby and allows time for milk expression to maintain production, but may lead to flow preference and breast refusal. Rather than prescribing a set time limit for breastfeeding, mothers should be taught to recognize effective feeding by the infant's lower suck:swallow ratio, open eyes, and intent expression. *Breast compression* (alternate massage) can help increase milk flow to the infant. When baby stops swallowing, mother gently squeezes the breast (far enough from the baby's mouth to avoid disrupting the latch), holds the compression during sucking bursts, and releases it during respiratory pauses (see **Figure 11-34**). Some inefficient infants respond to having their

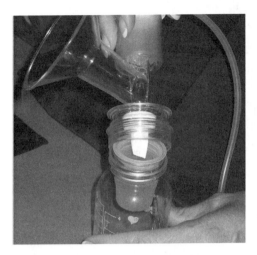

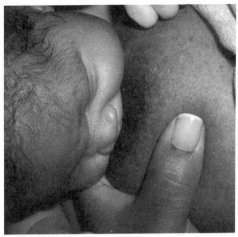

Figure 11-33 Using an Ameda diaphragm as a colostrum collector.

Figure 11-34 When breast compression is used, the fingers should be far enough away from baby's mouth to avoid disrupting the attachment.

cheek or chin tickled to initiate a sucking burst, and others to the delivery of a small bolus of milk through a tube or periodontal syringe, but these techniques must be used judiciously, and with careful observation of the infant's respiratory pattern. They are appropriate for infants with low energy reserves or reduced alertness who have normal cardiorespiratory function. Preterm babies and infants with cardiorespiratory issues are at high risk of hypoxia if their feeding is not self-paced.

Alternative Feeding

Bottle Feeding

Babies are less likely to refuse to breastfeed when they are not frustrated at breast and when alternate feeding maintains active infant participation and as many breastfeeding-appropriate behaviors as possible (see **Figure 11-35**). When using a bottle for a breastfed infant, a nipple with a cylindrical teat and a wider base is usually preferable (Kassing, 2002) (see **Figure 11-36**). A shorter or softer teat may be helpful for infants with a hypersensitive gag reflex, or those who cannot get their lips well back on the wide base of the teat otherwise. It is also helpful to have a bottle design that allows for horizontal holding of the bottle, so flow can be initiated and more directed by the baby (see **Figure 11-37**). Bottles that must be tipped up high for milk to flow, especially ones with anything other than a quite slow flow, can encourage a baby to become a reactive feeder, thus making transition to breast much more difficult as initiating skills and patience are extinguished.

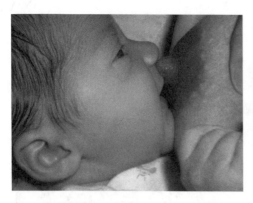

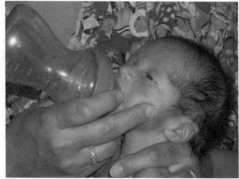

Figure 11-35 Instinctive position for attaching to breast. Note where breast touches infant's face.

Figure 11-36 Providing cheek and jaw support during bottle feeding with a wide-based teat.

Figure 11-37
Horizontal positioning of the bottle reduces flow, but this infant is still having difficulty, indicated by the spillage at the lips.

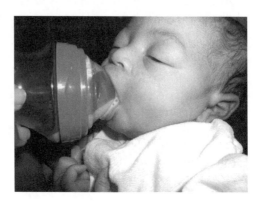

The teat can be held across the infant's upper and lower lips with the tip at the philtrum (the ridge between nose and upper lip) to cue a wide gape, and the infant can be snuggled onto the bottle as it is tipped into his mouth (see **Figures 11-38** and **11-39**). Similar methods can be used for finger feeding—the feeder should stimulate a wide gape and encourage the infant to pull the finger deeply into the mouth and start sucking properly before allowing milk to be transferred. Alternate feeding can be performed against or near the bare breast, to help the infant associate the breast with feeding.

Finger Feeding

There is little published research on finger feeding of newborns, though it is recommended by respected clinicians as an alternative to cup feeding for infants who are unable to breast-feed (Marmet, Shell, & Aldana, 2000; Newman, 1990, 1996). Substitution of finger feeding

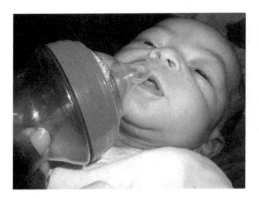

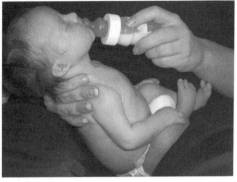

Figure 11-38 **The bottle is removed from the mouth and rested at the philtrum.** The infant will gape when ready to feed again.

Figure 11-39 **Bottle nipple is held across both lips to stimulate maximal gape response.** The infant is supported with hips flexed against the feeder's thighs and hand in a slightly upright position to increase alertness and improve stability and muscle tone.

for bottle feeding in preterm infants with developing or faulty sucking techniques in a hospital in Perth, Australia, increased the rate of breastfeeding on discharge from 44% to 71% (Oddy & Glenn, 2003).

Finger feeding reinforces the contingent nature of feeding (Bovey, Noble, & Noble, 1999). Done properly, it puts the infant in control. The choice of feeding tool is determined first by the infant's capabilities and needs and then the parent's abilities and preferences. A baby with some oral motor competency can use the Hazelbaker Fingerfeeder (Medela, Inc.). The Hazelbaker container rests in the feeder's hand, and a soft, flexible tube can be held to the finger with the thumb or taped to the finger (see **Figure 11-40**). The top of the container is valved, so the infant needs to draw milk from the tube by forming negative pressure in the mouth. The container is soft enough to allow the feeder to squeeze it to supplement the infant's efforts.

Whichever device is chosen, the tube is placed either atop or beside an adult finger. A large finger such as the index finger or middle finger is preferred, for better modeling of the mouth position on the breast. The finger is held pad side up to better conform to the palate. The feeder should stimulate the infant's gape response and encourage a wide gape, to preserve this breastfeeding behavior. To stimulate the gape response, the feeder can cross the nail side of the finger across the infant's lips, with the second knuckle bent and the finger tip at the infant's philtrum. When the infant opens wide, the finger is slid along the palate until it reaches the junction of the hard and soft palates. The infant will quickly learn to assist with the tongue in pulling the finger into the mouth. This skill can later be generalized to breastfeeding.

Figure 11-40
Hazelbaker Fingerfeeder used by the father of a preterm infant. Note the use of a large finger and the position of the finger across the lips to stimulate gape.

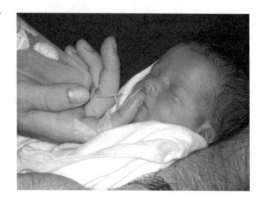

When the infant sucks, a small bolus (0.5–1 cc) is delivered to the infant. If milk spills from the corner of the baby's lips, the respiratory rate increases markedly, or the baby shows any stress signs (splayed fingers or widened eyes), the milk flow is slowed. Ideally, feeding should proceed at a pace that allows a 1:1 suck:swallow ratio during sucking bursts, particularly at the beginning of the feeding. Feeding should follow the normal burst:pause pattern of a 3–5-second respiratory break after a sucking burst of 5–20 sucks, depending on the infant's maturity and aerobic capacity. Devices with which the infant self-paces (Hazelbaker Fingerfeeder) should be used only when the infant has sufficient feeding competence to move milk from the device reliably. Devices that are designed for supplementing at the breast (Lact-Aid, Supply Line, and SNS) are useful for finger feeding if a slow flow is needed, such as for an infant with a respiratory issue that causes reduced aerobic capacity. These devices might not supply sufficient flow or might require too much work for preterm or ill infants. As always, careful assessment of the results of any intervention and its appropriateness for each individual dyad is imperative.

Very fine control of milk delivery can be achieved with a periodontal syringe, a curved tip syringe commonly used by dentists to irrigate the mouth. Fine control is particularly important for very preterm infants or infants with swallowing difficulties who need practice in swallowing tiny boluses presented at longer intervals, because control of swallowing is better during isolated rather than sequential swallows (Chi-Fishman & Sonies, 2000). Curved-tip (periodontal) syringes are not soft and flexible like supplementer tubes and therefore should be introduced against the feeder's finger after the baby has grasped the finger to the junction of the hard and soft palate. The feeder should keep the syringe tip pressed against the finger toward the front of the baby's mouth to avoid poking the oral mucosa with the stiff tip.

Finger Feeding for Oral Motor Facilitation. Finger feeding can be used during oral stimulation to couple milk flow with improved tongue movements. It is especially useful to help reduce tongue tip elevation (the firm tactile input helps the infant realize that food sources go on top of the tongue) and to reduce tongue retraction and posterior elevation.

To reduce tongue retraction, a small amplitude circular massage can be performed on the posterior tongue with the (trimmed) nail side of the finger to stimulate extension. Milk is not delivered while the tongue is retracted, and is delivered when the tongue tip is over the anterior gum ridge.

To reduce posterior elevation, the feeder can angle the fingertip downward against the humped posterior tongue to provide counter-pressure, or can use a gentle forward stroking motion (like smoothing out the humped tongue as if it were a wrinkle in a piece of fabric). Sublingual pressure can be provided at the same time to increase the forward traction on the tongue (see **Figure 11-41**). Some degree of posterior tongue elevation is normal during sucking, so the feeder should not attempt to cause the infant to flatten the tongue completely.

Oral Stimulation

In studies of fetal amniotic fluid swallowing, perioral self-stimulation usually preceded swallowing (Miller, Sonies, & Macedonia, 2003). Hand to mouth movements are part of the newborn breast seeking (self-attachment) behavior (Matthiesen, Ransjo-Arvidson, Nissen, & Uvnas-Moberg, 2001). Preterm infants in incubator NICU care benefit from perioral stimulation and show faster maturation of feeding skills (Fucile, Gisel, & Lau, 2005). Earlier experience with oral feeding (Bromiker et al., 2005) and constant skin-to-skin care (kangaroo mother care) (Cattaneo et al., 1998; Penalva & Schwartzman, 2006) also improve the feeding abilities of preterm infants (see **Figure 11-42**).

For infants with impaired oral reflexes and feeding problems, gentle oral stimulation before feeding decreased oral motor dysfunction and improved milk transfer at breast and bottle in a blinded but uncontrolled experiment (Rendon-Macias et al., 1999). Simply stimulating the infant to open the mouth and suck a clean or gloved adult finger may stimulate the infant's central pattern generator for sucking and promote feeding behaviors. This mechanism may underlie the success of suck training (Marmet & Shell, 1984). Bovey, Noble,

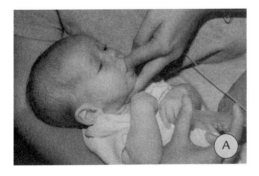
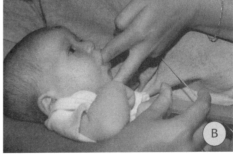

Figure 11-41 Finger feeding with sublingual pressure. When the infant humps the posterior tongue, the feeder provides counter-pressure.

Figure 11-42
Preterm, neurologically impaired infant
receiving gavage feeding after feeding at
breast but transferring little milk.
Sucking on the breast or pacifier during
gavage feedings facilitates the transition
to oral feeding.

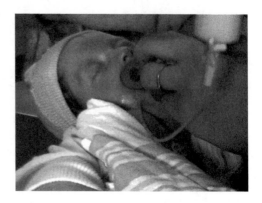

and Noble (1999) recommend observing for specific motor deficits and targeting these rather than using stereotyped interventions.

Infants have a strong drive to suck. In addition to providing food, sucking helps improve neurobehavioral organization and relieves pain. As long as the infant is in control of whether or not a finger enters their mouth and how long it stays, and appropriate infection control is used (hand washing in all cases, and the use of a glove or finger cot if not a member of the infant's household), oral exercises are unlikely to do harm (see **Figure 11-43**). It is important to model sensitivity to and respect for the infant in all interactions, as well as to actively instruct the parents in how to read and respond to the infant's cues. Stress signs in neurologically impaired infants can be far more subtle than in typical infants. Subtly tightening the orbicularis oris muscle to purse the lips, lifting a finger or two, closing the eyes, or subtle changes in respiratory pattern or other autonomic functions mean the infant is overstimulated and needs a break (see **Figures 11-44** and **11-45**).

Books on feeding issues for speech and occupational therapists are fertile sources for oral motor facilitation information, but most are based on the U.S. *cultural* norm of bottle feeding. Lactation consultants and therapists working with breastfeeding infants can modify these exercises to compensate for the differences in muscle activation, movements, and cueing required for the *biological* norm of breastfeeding. Briefly, encouraging a large gape, stimulating the tongue to depress and extend as the mouth opens, increasing midline tongue grooving and wavelike movements from anterior to posterior, decreasing tongue humping, and strengthening lip tone without encouraging pursing are all goals compatible with normal feeding.

Ideally, the infant will be an active participant in the exercise, and it will be enjoyable for both the infant and the adult. Smiling, making eye contact, and making amusing sounds to go along with the touch stimuli can increase enjoyment for infants who tolerate multimodal stimulation. Those who are easily overstimulated may prefer a quieter voice and less eye contact. Infants with low alertness or energy may not respond immediately, and may benefit from being "primed" for oral stimulation by gentle massage near the temporomandibular joint (TMJ) and stroking of the cheeks from the TMJ to the corner of the lips. Low energy infants may not open the mouth spontaneously at first. Gently running a finger across the

Figure 11-43
Infant enjoying finger feeding.

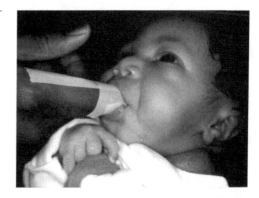

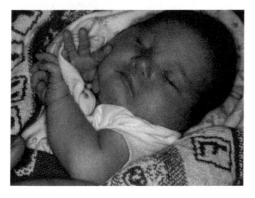

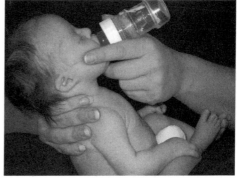

Figure 11-44   Infant with Down syndrome warding off stimulation.

Figure 11-45   Cheek and jaw support during bottle feeding for an infant with Down syndrome and significant hypotonia.

lips until they relax (see **Figure 11-46**), slipping a finger under the lip to massage the outer surfaces of the gums until the baby opens the mouth (see **Figure 11-47**), stroking the hard palate until the tongue makes an attempt to grasp the finger (see **Figure 11-48**), and then presenting the finger to suck may allow a low energy infant to wake up and participate.

The timing of oral exercises needs to be individualized. Cognitively impaired infants may have more difficulty generalizing learning. This may make it more difficult for them to transfer newly learned tongue movements from the finger to the breast if the exercises are not temporally associated with feeding. Neurologically impaired infants are also more likely to become disorganized by stimulation, which negatively impacts feeding skill. Careful observation of the infant for alert times between feedings, starting the exercise before the infant shows feeding behaviors or cues, or doing the exercise after feeding from one breast and before offering the second (for infants who need paired feedings) are all possible timing strategies for infants who do not tolerate a brief facilitation break before feeding.

Figure 11-46
Touch to the lips encourages the infant to
open the mouth.

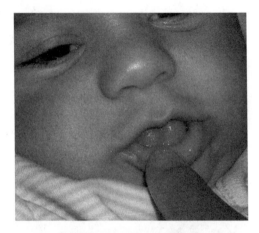

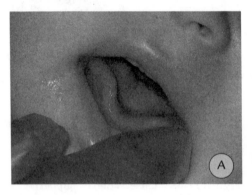

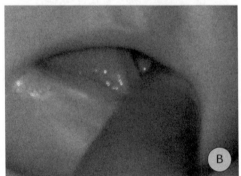

Figure 11-47 Stimulating the transverse tongue reflex, which causes the tongue to
lateralize when the side of the gum is stroked.

Figure 11-48
The finger pad is up and deep in the
mouth, with the fingertip at the junction
of the hard and soft palates.

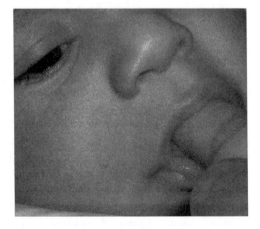

Basic Suck Training

In this method by Marmet and Shell (1984), the rooting reflex is stimulated by stroking the cheek toward the lips with a fingertip, then the lips are brushed to induce the infant to open the mouth. The gums are massaged, first the outside of the lower gums, then the tooth-bearing surfaces, then the outsides of the upper gums and their tooth-bearing surfaces. The finger is slid into the mouth with the pad side up, and alternately rubs the posterior hard palate and tongue, giving downward and forward pressure to the tongue. Alternatively, the finger can be inserted with the pad side toward the tongue and behind the humped posterior tongue, which is gently pulled forward with the fingertip. Milk is supplied when the tongue is correctly positioned over the lower gum. The authors recommend using the suck training technique before each feeding until the infant's suckling pattern is corrected.

The Oral Stimulation Program for Infants with Neurologically and Medically Based Sucking Disabilities

This program, created by Rendon-Macias and colleagues (1999), started with the infant's head extended, and the rooting reflex was gently stimulated by light fingertip touch to the cheeks and lips. The upper lip and anterior surface of the gum was massaged using a small circular motion for 5 minutes, then a 1 cm circular motion was used at the lateral gums and inner surfaces of the cheek. Gentle pressure was applied to the lower lip, and then firm pressure was placed on the hard palate to stimulate sucking. In older infants, a drop of honey was then placed on the palate (human milk should be substituted in infants under one year old, to avoid the risk of botulism), and the infant was given a pacifier continuously between feedings.

The authors reported that "The application of positive oral tactile stimuli with the removal of harmful stimuli, induced the recovery of oral reflexes in the infants in our study" (Rendon-Macias et al., 1999, p. 326).

Oral Motor Preparatory Stimulation for Hypotonic Infants

Babies who do not gape widely can be stroked or massaged in small spirals all along the edge of the jawline starting just in front of the baby's ear and working simultaneously down both sides of the jaw to the tip of the chin. This can cue the baby that these long muscles need to "wake up" and provide the power for a wide gape and the opening and closing of the mouth we see in babies who latch and feed well. This can be repeated two or three times and need not take more than a few seconds.

Speech/language therapists suggest following the jaw massage with several gentle compressions in the middle of each cheek. Gentle compression in the center of each cheek with the thumb and middle finger of one hand provides sensory stimulation to the sides of the tongue as it gently meets the fat pad of each cheek. This can help bring the tongue forward in the mouth in preparation for latching on to the breast. Finally, and also briefly, the baby's lower lip can be gently flipped or stroked downward, providing the baby with the same sensation that initiates seeking as the baby's chin touches mom's breast: gentle neck extension, wide gaping, tongue movement down and forward over the alveolar gum ridge, and overall readiness to draw breast tissue deep into the baby's mouth for effective and comfortable nursing.

Stimulating Central Grooving of the Tongue

Side Sweep. After stimulating the infant to open wide, place the finger flat on the front half of the tongue in midline. Pause. Then sweep the finger along the tongue from center to one side, pause, sweep back to the center, pause, then sweep to the opposite side, pause, then back to center. This stimulates the transverse intrinsic muscle layer that runs from side to side in the tongue, which contracts to form the central groove.

Slide Back. After stimulating mouth opening with a finger to the philtrum, slide the fingertip along the tongue in midline from tip to about halfway back. Repeat several times as tolerated.

Stroking the Tongue. This exercise not only supports central grooving, but also helps reduce tongue retraction. The infant is stimulated to open wide, and a finger is placed on the middle of the tongue in midline. The fingertip is pressed down on the tongue in midline and slides along the tongue as it is withdrawn from the mouth. The infant can be told "tongue down" while the stroke is occurring.

Stimulating Wavelike Tongue Movements

Walking Back on the Tongue. The infant is stimulated to open the mouth by a touch to the philtrum or upper lip. The fingertip is placed on the tongue, just beyond the tongue tip, and wiggled in place to provide vibration to the tongue. The finger slides back a few millimeters, and vibration is repeated. This is repeated all along the front half of the tongue, stopping short of stimulating the gag reflex.

This exercise is meant to stimulate sequential muscle contraction of the tongue from front to back, in the direction of the wavelike movements of normal sucking. If a mechanical vibrator is used, it should be held in the adult's hand so that the vibration is transferred through the finger. The First Years sells vibrating teething toys for infant use; these can be used in this way, or can be given to infants to mouth to increase oral tone.

Wiggle Worm (Joan Dietrich Comrie, CCC-SLP). The infant is stimulated to open the mouth, and the finger pad (up to the second joint) is placed on the tongue in midline, stroking the tongue from anterior to posterior, providing firm but gentle downward pressure, like kneading bread dough. This helps stimulate the wavelike movements of the tongue.

Sequential Stimulation of Feeding-Related Reflex Movements

When infants do not seem to make the correct sequence of movements to attach to the breast, this sequence is sometimes helpful. For infants suspected of autistic spectrum disorders or other infants who are easily overwhelmed by sensations, it is helpful to engineer the environment (lower lights, turn off noise sources, and perhaps undress or swaddle the infant) to reduce the sensory load before using the exercise.

Hold a finger across the infant's lips, with the nail side of the finger at the philtrum, and the second joint right below the center of the lower lip. When the infant opens the mouth (gapes), the fingertip touches the front of the lower gum ridge until the tongue is extended and depressed. The tongue tip is then gently tickled with the fingertip until the tongue grasps the finger and the infant begins to pull the finger into the mouth. The feeder may continue the motion until the finger pad is on the posterior hard palate, at or near the junction of the soft palate. The palate can be stimulated by wiggling the fingertip on the palate to start the sucking reflex. Milk is then delivered from the feeding device as in normal finger feeding. When the infant begins to perform more of the feeding sequence without the individual stimulation steps (searches for the finger with the lips and tongue and draws it in and immediately begins sucking), the infant is placed at breast in the instinctive position and is encouraged to gape by a finger on the philtrum if he does not respond to the breast itself with this behavior. Drops of milk can be expressed onto the nipple for the infant to smell, and a curved tip syringe can be used to deliver a bit of milk to reward any attempt to close the mouth on the areola. These inducements can be withdrawn as the infant becomes more skilled at breastfeeding.

The lactation consultant may encounter infants exhibiting a variety of problems that may interfere with their ability to breastfeed. Interventions that may help the infant to breastfeed can be employed when the basis of the problem is understood and appropriate techniques are chosen. Until oral motor evaluation and facilitation become a standardized part of lactation consultant training, each IBCLC will need to decide which of these techniques fit her expertise and comfort level. Unless the lactation specialist is also a therapist, infants who are having difficulty feeding should be referred for evaluation, particularly when the difficulty occurs during both breastfeeding *and* bottle feeding. The lactation consultant is a specialist in normal feeding, and can provide valuable input to the other members of the feeding team.

Dysphagia and the Neurologically Involved Baby

Infants with neurological deficits are at greater risk for dysphagia. Full-term infants may suffer from neurologically based or structurally based swallowing difficulties, whereas for very low birth weight infants, dysphagia may be among their residual disabilities.

The videofluoroscopic swallow study (VFSS) was developed to study the oropharyngeal phases of the swallow in adults and has been generalized to children (Arvedson & Brodsky, 2002). The VFSS is conducted by a speech-language pathologist (SLP) and radiologist.

In some institutions, an occupational therapist may carry out the study or be present to assist with positioning. A clinical assessment, including a thorough history, is always performed before requesting a VFSS. Postural and flow rate adjustments should be part of the clinical assessment to determine if these will improve feeding safety. Infant endurance, medical condition, cognitive abilities, and level of alertness are prerequisites.

The VFSS allows the therapist to observe the infant/child's oropharyngeal structures during bottle feeding. Health care providers (HCPs) have frequently not evaluated feeding skills at the breast in neurologically impaired infants, nor have they included breastfeeding in therapeutic goals. There have been some reports at feeding conferences that SLPs are including breastfeeding in addition to bottle feeding during VFSS. One SLP has been using barium contrast in breast milk in a supplementer used at breast. The difficulty in performing VFSS during breastfeeding lies in positioning mother and infant in a way that allows imaging without disrupting attachment. A breastfeeding infant evaluated using a bottle does not give an accurate picture of the ability to control flow and transfer milk. Research comparing respiration and heart rate in preterm infants who served as their own controls showed less disruption of either while breastfeeding (Meier, 1988; Meier & Anderson 1987). Furthermore, infants bottle fed different fluids had safer swallowing and better coordination of sucking, swallowing, and breathing with human milk versus formula or water (Mizuno, Ueda, & Takeuchi, 2002). With this information in mind, the infant's breastfeeding abilities deserve evaluation. Ultrasound is becoming an important diagnostic tool to study the oral preparatory and oral phases of the swallow and may provide another modality that is more accurate for breastfeeding infants.

Options when aspiration is diagnosed include positioning changes, pacing the feeding, thickening, and limiting oral feeding and substituting tube feedings. Thickening human milk is problematic due to its enzyme content, and requires that milk come from a container other than the breast. Because infants aspirate least during breastfeeding, and because human milk is less irritating to the human airway than other substances are, the child should not be taken off the breast unless significant sequelae of aspiration are occurring. When the decision is made to thicken liquids, it limits the infant's opportunities for normal feeding skill acquisition at the breast. Limited oral feeding at the freshly expressed breast is an alternative until the infant's coordinating of swallowing improves.

Infants and children with neurologically based feeding problems require periodic monitoring for changes in ability. With a degenerative neurological disorder, swallowing ability will quite probably deteriorate over time. A child with mild cerebral palsy or prematurity may continue to improve. Each infant/child should be approached as an individual with strengths and weaknesses. The mother should be assisted to breastfeed, whether exclusively or in combination with alternative feeding methods.

Postural Support

In addition to swaddling, supportive positioning, and preparatory handling, certain postural modifications may help infants with dysphagia. Some infants handle flow best when sidelying, others when their head is elevated relative to the rest of the body, as in a sitting football hold. Prone positioning with the mother reclining can help an infant pace during breastfeeding. Pacing, or regulating, an infant by breaking the suction when signs of stress occur during feeding can be done at the breast. The mother should be instructed to insert her finger between the gums to break suction. Because breaking the suction and removing the breast from the infant's mouth can make it difficult for the infant to reorganize, it should be carried out when the infant is experiencing a problem, but not on a frequent basis throughout the feeding. One mother sang out "one, two, three" to let her infant know that the pause was temporary. If the preterm or neurologically impaired infant requires frequent pacing at the breast due to incoordination of sucking, swallowing, and breathing, another option would be to have the mother express her breasts until the first (and usually strongest) milk ejection subsides prior to breastfeeding. This reduces the active flow of the breast, when babies typically experience difficulty with bolus control, but can have the unwanted effect of increasing milk production. Signs of difficulty necessitating a break include nasal flaring, rapid respirations, frequent swallows without breathing pauses, gulping, choking, coughing, or stridor. For further suggestions and information on improving flow control issues, see Chapter 6.

Feeding Environment

A quiet feeding environment with low lights may assist the neurologically immature or involved infant by facilitating organization and a quiet alert state. Picking the infant up and maintaining containment by holding him in flexion against the mother's or assistant's body will ease the transition from the sleeping surface to where the feeding will take place (Waitzman, 2002). Some feeding therapists find that rocking a full-term or older infant from head to toe at the rate of one per second helps reinforce the rhythm of suck-swallow-breathe. Other therapists have used classical music that has that same one beat per second rhythm (Morris & Klein, 2001). Rocking and music may be too much stimulation for preterm infants, however, and is generally not recommended.

Gastroesophageal Reflux

Gastroesophageal reflux (GER) is a normal occurrence in infants under one year. According to Rudolf (2006), GER is not a disease in itself, but the consequences of reflux can contribute to disease. Reflux takes place when the strength of the lower esophageal sphincter is overcome by increased abdominal or thoracic pressure (Bibi et al., 2001). Infants who are at greater risk for developing gastroesophageal reflux disease (GERD) have diagnoses of prematurity, congenital heart disease, esophageal atresia, tracheo-esophageal fistula, brainstem tumors, airway anomaly, or neurological impairment. GER affects the esophageal phase of the swallow, and can be present with or without oropharyngeal dysphagia.

GERD can damage the lining of the esophagus and predisposes to aspiration by damaging the recurrent laryngeal nerve (Suskind et al., 2006). GER can be the cause or contribute to the severity of respiratory disease including allergies and asthma. When the infant/child has labored breathing from asthma or bronchopulmonary dysplasia (respiratory disease seen in premature infants), thoracic pressure increases. Some of the signs and symptoms of GERD include: vomiting, gagging, choking, apnea, halitosis, frequent swallowing, burping, stridor, coughing, hiccoughing, gurgly respirations, irritability, torticollis (Sandifer's syndrome), back arching, sleep disturbances, recurrent respiratory infections, feeding refusal, and acute life-threatening events (Arvedson & Brodsky, 2002).

The gastroenterologist uses a variety of tests to diagnose GER. Recent studies report pH testing is more effective when combined with impedance probe monitoring, which has the ability to detect nonacidic refluxate as well as the movement of the bolus through the esophagus (Wenzl, 2003; Wenzl et al., 2001). Endoscopy is another method for evaluating the presence of GERD. Esophagogastroscopy is used for visualizing the mucosa around the esophagus, larynx, and airway, and can be used to determine if esophagitis or other erosive effects of GERD are taking place (Arvedson & Brodsky, 2002).

Gastroenterologists have treated GERD with both surgery and medications. Newer studies report that medications called proton pump inhibitors result in greater healing of the esophageal mucosa and decrease in the GER symptoms in infants/children. Antacids and motility drugs are still being used, but are reported to have more limited effectiveness. Surgical treatment is considered when medications have proven ineffective or there are life-threatening complications. A fundoplication is the procedure commonly performed to treat GERD. This procedure involves wrapping the fundus of the stomach around the distal esophagus. A gastrostomy tube may also be placed to prevent complications sometimes seen with the fundoplication procedure, for non-oral feedings when the infant/child has severe symptoms, or to supplement oral feedings. Outcomes of the surgical procedures have been varied, and selection of patients based on symptoms influences success (Arvedson & Brodsky, 2002; Richards, Milla, Andrews, & Spitz, 2001; Wales et al., 2002).

Feeding therapists have treated GERD in infants by thickening feedings, providing small/frequent feedings, and positioning the infant with the bed elevated after feedings (Arvedson & Brodsky, 2002; Khoshoo, Ross, Brown, & Edell, 2000; Wolf & Glass, 1992). Arvedson and Brodsky report that thickening may worsen symptoms if the patient has delayed gastric emptying from dysmotility.

McPherson, Wright, and Bell (2005) reviewed a number of methods for managing reflux. They summarized the outcomes of studies that employed various methods for treating the symptoms of vomiting and regurgitation. They reported mixed outcomes regarding treatment of symptoms when carob bean gum thickener was used and a decrease in symptoms when rice cereal was used. In studies that measured improvement through pH probe monitoring to test for acidity, thickening with carob bean gum showed mixed improvement and thickening with rice cereal showed no improvement. Regarding positioning, when pH was tested with infants in seats positioned at 60 degrees, their symptoms worsened, and when infants were placed in beds with the head elevated to 30 degrees they showed no improvement. The authors stated that these various studies primarily focused on formula-fed infants, and reported outcomes were insufficient for application to breastfed infants. In addition, they stated that no strategies were offered for supporting breastfeeding while the infant was being treated.

Several studies revealed difficulties with absorption of calcium, iron, and zinc due to the fiber content of many thickeners mixed with formula (Bosscher et al., 2000, 2001; Bosscher, VanCaillie-Bertrand, & Deelstra, 2001; Corvaglia et al., 2006). Breast milk was found to have better bioavailability of those minerals when mixed with starch-based thickeners (Bosscher, Lu et al., 2001; Bosscher, VanCaillie-Bertand et al., 2001); however, a study of preterm infants who were fed breast milk thickened with a starch-based product found no evidence of decrease in reflux episodes (Corvaglia et al., 2006).

Feeding teams should make every effort to maintain breastfeeding infants at breast. In addition to proton pump inhibitors (medications that reduce stomach acid release), strategies that seem useful clinically include short frequent feedings, holding the infant upright for 20 minutes after a feeding, and non-nutritive sucking after feeding to help stimulate esophageal peristalsis.

Conclusion

Infants with neurological deficits may present with significant feeding challenges. A combination of compensatory strategies and gentle facilitation techniques have been covered that can be employed to help infants with neurological problems achieve normal feeding. Each infant should be evaluated as an individual, and not as a diagnosis, though knowledge of the mechanisms of neurological disorders is helpful in creating strategies to assist feeding. Infants with significant impairments benefit from the input of a feeding team and early intervention specialists. Ideally, the lactation consultant will continue to participate on the child's team, to provide expertise in normal feeding.

References

Adam, M. P., & Hudgins, L. (2005). Kabuki syndrome: A review. *Clinical Genetics, 67*(3), 209–219.

Ardran, G. M., & Kemp, F. H. (1968). The mechanism of changes in form of the cervical airway in infancy. *Medical Radiography and Photography, 44*(2), 26–38.

Arvedson, J., Rogers, B., Buck, G., Smart, P., & Msall, M. (1994). Silent aspiration prominent in children with dysphagia. *International Journal of Pediatric Otorhinolaryngology, 28*(2–3), 173–181.

Arvedson, J. C., & Brodsky, L. (2002). *Pediatric swallowing and feeding: Assessment and management* (2nd ed.). Albany, NY: Singular Thomson Learning.

Ashwal, S. (1999). Congenital structural defects. In K. F. Swaiman & S. Ashwal (Eds.), *Pediatric neurology: Principles and practice* (3rd ed., pp. 234–300). St. Louis: Mosby.

Astley, S. J., & Clarren, S. K. (2001). Measuring the facial phenotype of individuals with prenatal alcohol exposure: Correlations with brain dysfunction. *Alcohol and Alcoholism, 36*(2), 147–159.

Batocchi, A. P., Majolini, L., Evoli, A., Lino, M. M., Minisci, C., & Tonali, P. (1999). Course and treatment of myasthenia gravis during pregnancy. *Neurology, 52*(3), 447–452.

Bertrand, J., Floyd, L. L., & Weber, M. K. (2005). Guidelines for identifying and referring persons with fetal alcohol syndrome. *Morbidity and Mortality Weekly Report, Recommended Reports, 54*(RR-11), 1–14.

Bibi, H., Khvolis, E., Shoseyov, D., Ohaly, M., Ben Dor, D., London, D., et al. (2001). The prevalence of gastroesophageal reflux in children with tracheomalacia and laryngomalacia. *Chest, 119*(2), 409–413.

Bosscher, D., Lu, Z., VanCaillie-Bertrand, M., Robberecht, H., & Deelstra, H. (2001). A method for in vitro determination of calcium, iron and zinc availability from first-age infant formula and human milk. *International Journal of Food Science and Nutrition, 52*(2), 173–182.

Bosscher, D., VanCaillie-Bertrand, M., & Deelstra, H. (2001). Effect of thickening agents, based on soluble dietary fiber, on the availability of calcium, iron, and zinc from infant formulas. *Nutrition, 17*(7–8), 614–618.

Bosscher, D., VanCaillie-Bertrand, M., Van Dyck, K., Robberecht, H., Van Cauwenberg, R., & Deelstra, H. (2000). Thickening infant formula with digestible and indigestible carbohydrate: Availability of calcium, iron, and zinc in vitro. *Journal of Pediatric Gastroenterology and Nutrition, 30*(4), 373–378.

Bosscher, D., Van Dyck, K., Van Cauwenberg, R., & Deelstra, H. (2001). In vitro availability of calcium, iron, and zinc from first-age infant formulae and human milk. *Journal of Pediatric Gastroenterology and Nutrition, 32*(1), 54–58.

Bouwstra, H., Boersma, E. R., Boehm, G., Dijck-Brouwer, D. A., Muskiet, F. A., & Hadders-Algra, M. (2003). Exclusive breastfeeding of healthy term infants for at least 6 weeks improves neurological condition. *Journal of Nutrition, 133*(12), 4243–4245.

Bovey, A., Noble, R., & Noble, M. (1999). Orofacial exercises for babies with breastfeeding problems? *Breastfeeding Review, 7*(1), 23–28.

Bromiker, R., Arad, I., Loughran, B., Netzer, D., Kaplan, M., & Medoff-Cooper, B. (2005). Comparison of sucking patterns at introduction of oral feeding and at term. *Acta Paediatrica, 94*(2), 201–204.

Cattaneo, A., Davanzo, R., Worku, B., Surjono, A., Echeverria, M., Bedri, A., et al. (1998). Kangaroo mother care for low birthweight infants: A randomized controlled trial in different settings. *Acta Paediatrica, 87*(9), 976–985.

Cerruti Mainardi, P. (2006). Cri du chat syndrome. *Orphanet Journal of Rare Diseases, 1,* 33.

Chen, D. C., Nommsen-Rivers, L., Dewey, K. G., & Lonnerdal, B. (1998). Stress during labor and delivery and early lactation performance. *American Journal of Clinical Nutrition, 68*(2), 335–344.

Chi-Fishman, G., & Sonies, B. C. (2000). Motor strategy in rapid sequential swallowing: New insights. *Journal of Speech, Language, and Hearing Research, 43*(6), 1481–1492.

Ciafaloni, E., & Massey, J. M. (2004). The management of myasthenia gravis in pregnancy. *Seminars in Neurology, 24*(1), 95–100.

Clarke, D. J., & Boer, H. (1998). Problem behaviors associated with deletion Prader-Willi, Smith-Magenis, and cri du chat syndromes. *American Journal of Mental Retardation, 103*(3), 264–271.

Corvaglia, L., Ferlini, M., Rotatori, R., Paoletti, V., Alessandroni, R., Cocchi, G., et al. (2006). Starch thickening of human milk is ineffective in reducing the gastroesophageal reflux in preterm infants: A crossover study using intraluminal impedance. *Journal of Pediatrics, 148*(2), 265–268.

Daly, S. E., Owens, R. A., & Hartmann, P. E. (1993). The short-term synthesis and infant-regulated removal of milk in lactating women. *Experimental Physiology, 78*(2), 209–220.

Dapretto, M., Davies, M. S., Pfiefer, J. H., Scott, A. A., Sigman, M., Bookheimer, S. Y., et al. (2006). Understanding emotions in others: Mirror neuron dysfunction in children with autism spectrum disorders. *Nature Neuroscience, 9*(1), 28–30.

Fucile, S., Gisel, E. G., & Lau, C. (2005). Effect of an oral stimulation program on sucking skill maturation of preterm infants. *Developmental Medicine and Child Neurology, 47*(3), 158–162.

Gohlke, J. M., Griffith, W. C., & Faustman, E. M. (2005). A systems-based computational model for dose-response comparisons of two modes of action hypotheses for ethanol-induced neurodevelopmental toxicity. *Toxicological Sciences, 86*(2), 470–484.

Gressens, P. (2005). Neuronal migration disorders. *Journal of Child Neurology, 20*(12), 969–971.

Guerrini, R. (2005). Genetic malformations of the cerebral cortex and epilepsy. *Epilepsia, 46*(Suppl. 1), 32–37.

Hill, P. D., Aldaq, J. C., & Chatterton, R. T. (2001). Initiation and frequency of pumping and milk production in mothers of non-nursing preterm infants. *Journal of Human Lactation, 17*(1), 9–13.

Jacinto-Goncalves, S., Gaviao, M. B., & Berzin, F. (2004). Electromyographic activity of perioral muscle in breastfed and non-breastfed children. *Journal of Clinical Pediatric Dentistry, 29*(1), 57–62.

Jones, E., Dimmock, P. W., & Spencer, S. A. (2001). A randomised controlled trial to compare methods of milk expression after preterm delivery. *Archives of Disease in Childhood, Fetal Neonatal Edition, 85,* F91–F95.

Kassing, D. (2002). Bottle-feeding as a tool to reinforce breastfeeding. *Journal of Human Lactation, 18*(1), 56–60.

Khoshoo, V., Ross, G., Brown, S., & Edell, D. (2000). Smaller volume, thickened formulas in the management of gastroesophageal reflux in thriving infants. *Journal of Pediatric Gastroenterology and Nutrition, 31*(5), 554–556.

Kim, H. I., Palmini, A., Choi, H. Y., Kim, Y. H., & Lee, J. C. (1994). Congenital bilateral perisylvian syndrome: Analysis of the first four reported Korean patients. *Journal of Korean Medical Science, 9*(4), 335–340.

Knickmeyer, R. C., & Baron-Cohen, S. (2006). Fetal testosterone and sex differences in typical social development and in autism. *Journal of Child Neurology, 21*(10), 825–845.

Kuzniecky, R., Andermann, F., & Guerrini, R. (1993). Congenital bilateral perisylvian syndrome: Study of 31 patients. The CBPS Multicenter Collaborative Study. *Lancet, 341*(8845), 608–612.

Lau, C., & Schanler, R. J. (1996). Oral motor function in the neonate. *Neonatal Gastroenterology, 23*(2), 161–178.

Ludington-Hoe, S. M., Cong, X., & Hashemi, F. (2002). Infant crying: Nature, physiologic consequences, and select interventions. *Neonatal Network, 21*(2), 29–36.

Mandelli, M., Tognoni, G., & Garattini, S. (1978). Clinical pharmacokinetics of diazepam. *Clinical Pharmacokinetics, 3*(1), 72–91.

Marmet, C., & Shell, E. (1984). Training neonates to suck correctly. *The American Journal of Maternal Child Nursing, 9*(6), 401–407.

Marmet, C., Shell, E., & Aldana, S. (2000). Assessing infant suck dysfunction: Case management. *Journal of Human Lactation, 16*(4), 332–336.

Matthiesen, A. S., Ransjo-Arvidson, A. B., Nissen, E., & Uvnas-Moberg, K. (2001). Postpartum maternal oxytocin release by newborns: Effects of infant hand massage and sucking. *Birth, 28*(1), 13–19.

McBride, M. C., & Danner, S. C. (1987). Sucking disorders in neurologically impaired infants: Assessment and management. *Clinical Perinatology, 14*(1), 109–130.

McGirt, M. J., Leveque, J. C., Wellons 3rd, J. C., Villavicencio, A. T., Hopkins, J. S., Fuchs, H. E., et al. (2002). Cerebrospinal fluid shunt survival and etiology of failures: A seven-year institutional experience. *Pediatric Neurosurgery, 36*(5), 248–255.

McPherson, V., Wright, S. T., & Bell, A. D. (2005). Clinical inquiries. What is the best treatment for gastroesophageal reflux and vomiting in infants? *Journal of Family Practice, 54*(4), 372–375.

Meier, P., (1988). Bottle- and breast-feeding: Effects on transcutaneous oxygen pressure and temperature in preterm infants. *Nursing Research, 37*(1), 36–41.

Meier, P., & Anderson, G. C. (1987). Responses of small preterm infants to bottle and breast-feeding. *American Journal of Maternal Child Nursing, 12*(2), 97–105.

Miller, J. L., Sonies, B. C., & Macedonia, C. (2003). Emergence of oropharyngeal, laryngeal and swallowing activity in the developing fetal upper aerodigestive tract: An ultrasound evaluation. *Early Human Development, 71*(1), 61–87.

Mizuno, K., Aizawa, M., Saito, S., Kani, K., Tanaka, S., Kawamura, H., et al. (2006). Analysis of feeding behavior with direct linear transformation. *Early Human Development, 82*(3), 199–204.

Mizuno, K., Ueda, A., & Takeuchi, T. (2002). Effects of different fluids on the relationship between swallowing and breathing during nutritive sucking in neonates. *Biology of the Neonate, 81*(1), 45–50.

Mizuno, K., Ueda, A., Kani, K., & Kawamura, H. (2002). Feeding behaviour of infants with cleft lip and palate. *Acta Paediatrica, 91*(11), 1227–1232.

Moretti, M. E., Sgro, M., Johnson, D. W., Sauve, R. S., Woolgar, M. J., Taddio, A., et al. (2003). Cyclosporine excretion into breast milk. *Transplantation, 75*(12), 2144–2146.

Morris, S. E., & Klein, M. D. (2001). *Prefeeding skills.* (2nd ed.). San Diego, CA: Academic Press.

Moster, D., Lie, R. T., Irgens, L. M., Bjerkedal, T., & Markestad, L. (2001). The association of Apgar score with subsequent death and cerebral palsy: A population based study in term infants. *Journal of Pediatrics, 138*(6), 798–803.

Moster, D., Lie, R. T., & Markestad, L. (2002). Joint association of Apgar scores and early neonatal symptoms with minor disabilities at school age. *Archives of Disease in Childhood, Fetal and Neonatal Edition, 86*(1), 16–21.

Munoz-Flores Thiagarajan, K. D., Easterling, T., Davis, C., & Bond, E. F. (2001). Breast-feeding by a cyclosporine-treated mother. *Obstetrics and Gynecology, 97*(5 Pt. 2), 816–818.

Narayanan, I., Mehta, R., Choudhury, D. K., & Jain, B. K. (1991). Sucking on the "emptied" breast: Non-nutritive sucking with a difference. *Archives of Disease in Childhood, 66*(2), 241–244.

Newman, J. (1990). Breastfeeding problems associated with the early introduction of bottles and pacifiers. *Journal of Human Lactation, 6*(2), 59–63.

Newman, J. (1996). Decision tree and postpartum management for preventing dehydration in the "breastfed" baby. *Journal of Human Lactation, 12*(2), 129–135.

Newman, L. A., Keckley, C., Petersen, M. C., & Hamner, A. (2001). Swallowing function and medical diagnoses in infants suspected of dysphagia. *Pediatrics, 108*(6), 106.

Niemitz, E. L., & Feinberg, A. P. (2004). Epigenetics and assisted reproductive technology: A call for investigation. *American Journal of Human Genetics, 74*(4), 599–609.

Nyberg, G., Haljamae, U., Frisenette-Fich, C., Wennergren, M., & Kjellmer, I. (1998). Breast-feeding during treatment with cyclosporine. *Transplantation, 65*(2), 253–255.

Oddy, W. H., & Glenn, K. (2003). Implementing the Baby Friendly Hospital Initiative: The role of finger feeding. *Breastfeeding Review, 11*(1), 5–10.

Palmer, B. (1998). The influence of breastfeeding on the development of the oral cavity: A commentary. *Journal of Human Lactation, 14*(2), 93–98.

Palmer, M. M., & VandenBerg, K. A. (1998). A closer look at neonatal sucking. *Neonatal Network, 17*(2), 77–79.

Pavone, L., Rizzo, R., & Dobyns, W. B. (1993). Clinical manifestations and evaluation of isolated lissencephaly. *Child's Nervous System, 9*(7), 387–390.

Penalva, O., & Schwartzman, J. S. (2006). Descriptive study of the clinical and nutritional profile and follow-up of premature babies in a kangaroo mother care program. *Jornal de Pediatria, 82*(1), 33–39.

Rasley, A., Logemann, J. A., Kahrilas, P. J., Rademaker, A. W., Pauloski, B. R., & Dodds, W. J. (1993). Prevention of barium aspiration during videofluoroscopic swallowing studies: Value of change in posture. *American Journal of Roentgenology, 160*(5), 1005–1009.

Rendon-Macias, M. E., Cruz-Perez, L. A., Mosco-Peralta, M. R., Saraiba-Russell, M. M., Levi-Tajfeld, S., & Morales-Lopez, M. G. (1999). Assessment of sensorial oral stimulation in infants with suck feeding disabilities. *Indian Journal of Pediatrics, 66*(3), 319–329.

Richards, C. A., Milla, P. J., Andrews, P. L., & Spitz, L. (2001). Retching and vomiting in neurologically impaired children after fundoplication: Predictive preoperative factors. *Journal of Pediatric Surgery, 36*(9), 1401–1404.

Rudolf, C. D. (2006). The impact of GERD on feeding in infants with neurodevelopmental disorders. Presented at Pediatric Dysphagia Series: Exploring the Brain-Gut Feeding Connection, Conference session, Cincinnati Children's Hospital Medical Center.

Shanahan, T. K., Logemann, J. A., Rademaker, A. W., Pauloski, B. R., & Kahrila, P. J. (1993). Chin-down posture effect on aspiration in dysphagic patients. *Archives of Physical Medicine and Rehabilitation, 74*(7), 736–739.

Shehata, H. A., & Okosun, H. (2004). Neurological disorders in pregnancy. *Current Opinions in Obstetrics and Gynecology, 16*(2), 117–122.

Siegel, B. (1996). *World of the autistic child: Understanding and treating autistic spectrum disorders.* New York: Oxford University Press.

Stevenson, R. D., & Allaire, J. H. (1991). The development of normal feeding and swallowing. *Pediatric Clinics of North America, 38*(6), 1439–1453.

Streissguth, A. P., Barr, H. M., & Martin, D. C. (1983). Maternal alcohol use and neonatal habituation assessed with the Brazelton scale. *Child Development, 54*(5), 1109–1118.

Suskind, D. L., Thompson, D. M., Gulati, M., Huddleston, P., Liu, D. C., & Baroody, F. M. (2006). Improved infant swallowing after gastroesophageal reflux disease treatment: A function of improved laryngeal sensation? *Laryngoscope, 116*(8), 1397–1403.

Takagi, Y., & Bosma, J. F. (1960). Disability of oral function in an infant associated with displacement of the tongue: Therapy by feeding in the prone position. *Acta Paediatrica Supplementum, 49*(Suppl. 123), 62–69.

Tanoue, Y., & Oda, S. (1989). Weaning time of children with infantile autism. *Journal of Autism and Developmental Disorders, 19*(3), 425–434.

Tellez-Zenteno, J. F., Hernandez-Ronquillo, L., Salinas, V., Estanol, B., & da Silva, O. (2004). Myasthenia gravis and pregnancy: Clinical implications and neonatal outcome. *BMC Musculoskeletal Disorders, 5,* 42.

Thach, B. T. (2001). Maturation and transformation of reflexes that protect the laryngeal airway from liquid aspiration from fetal to adult life. *American Journal of Medicine, 111*(Suppl. 8A), 69–77.

Volpe, J. J. (2001). Neurobiology of periventricular leukomalacia in the premature infant. *Pediatric Research, 50*(5), 553–562.

Waitzman, K. A. (2002). Developmental care/feeding readiness. Presented at Neonatal CORE, TriHealth Hospitals, Cincinnati, Ohio.

Wales, P. W., Diamond, I. R., Dutta, S., Muraca, S., Chait, P., Connolly, B., et al. (2002). Fundoplication and gastrostomy versus image-guided gastrojejunal tube for enteral feeding in neurologically impaired children with gastroesophageal reflux. *Journal of Pediatric Surgery, 37*(3), 407–412.

Wenzl, T. G. (2003). Evaluation of gastroesophageal reflux events in children using multichannel intraluminal electrical impedance. *American Journal of Medicine, 115*(Suppl. 3A), 161–165.

Wenzl, T. G., Schenke, S., Peschgens, T., Silny, J., Heimann, G., & Skopnik, H. (2001). Association of apnea and nonacid gastroesophageal reflux in infants: Investigations with the intraluminal impedance technique. *Pediatric Pulmonology, 31*(2), 144–149.

Williams, D. L., Goldstein, G., & Minshew, N. J. (2006). The profile of memory function in children with autism. *Neuropsychology, 20*(1), 21–29.

Wolf, L. S., & Glass, R. P. (1992). *Feeding and swallowing disorders in infancy: Assessment and management.* Austin, TX: Pro-Ed.

Zoppou, C., Barry, S. I., & Mercer, G. N. (1997). Comparing breastfeeding and breast pumps using a computer model. *Journal of Human Lactation, 13*(3), 195–202.

Chapter 12

Therapeutic Positioning for Breastfeeding

Chele Marmet

Ellen Shell

The Importance of Positioning

Supportive positioning facilitates breastfeeding and when necessary helps to compensate for special problems. Although older, healthy babies can breastfeed in a variety of positions of their own invention, including practically standing on their heads, young babies and those with special problems need positional stability. Mothers and babies instinctively adopt a great variety of positions, but common to all effective positions is stability.

A newborn's natural posture is physiologic flexion. He is the most stable in a prone position on a supportive surface, and can even move forward in a coordinated pattern (Widstrom et al., 1987). When supine, limb movements often elicit a startle reflex, interfering with controlled mobility. Normal neuromuscular development increases stability in the *proximal* (central) parts of the body (hips and trunk). Once this proximal base of stability is established, the baby has greater mobility and more refined distal control, including of the mouth and tongue (Morris & Klein, 1987). Refined oral-motor skills rely on a proximal base of stability from the neck and shoulder girdle, which in turn are dependent on trunk and pelvic stability (Wolf & Glass, 1992). Even the structures of the face and oral cavity need stability in order to function. Bosma (1972) describes the tongue's contact with the cheeks, hard and soft palate, alveolar ridge, and lips as providing stability for the tongue. He posits that the buccal fat pads and other subcutaneous oral fat deposits provide a functional "exoskeleton" to support oral, pharyngeal, and temporomandibular joint stabilization for refined mandibular movement.

It is vital to have a basic understanding of neonatal neuromotor development and the relationships between proximal stability and distal mobility in order to be able to analyze which position(s) will be therapeutic for a complex breastfeeding situation.

Neuromotor and physiologic relationships are complex; however, the key to these concepts is simple. What begins at the hips ends at the lips (stability), so that what begins at the lips (breastfeeding) ends up on the hips (weight gain).

Achieving optimal *latch* and *positioning* is usually the first and often the only treatment needed to facilitate suck and correct most breastfeeding problems. *Therapeutic positioning* is often an important piece of the treatment plan for sore nipples, breast refusal, milk supply issues, or anatomical variations of mother or baby. Additionally, therapeutic positions assist in correcting or compensating for suckling problems (Marmet & Shell, 1993; Snyder, 1995).

Regardless of the breastfeeding position chosen, if the baby is gaining weight and thriving, and breastfeeding is comfortable for mother and infant, no intervention is needed. Because of variations in the size, shape, physical abilities, and preferences of mothers and infants, no *one* position is correct for all breastfeeding couples (Cioni, Ferrari, & Prechtl, 1989). Likewise, Blair and colleagues (2003) found that no one group of attributes (head position, body position, or breastfeeding dynamic) was more related to the level of pain experienced by the mother than another. The researchers concluded that no one aspect of positioning is more crucial than another. Successful intervention requires recognition of the need for special positioning as well as the ability to create dyad-specific positions when required.

Naming Positions

Names chosen for positions in this chapter most frequently describe the baby's position in space, but some were chosen because they reflect the mother's relationship to the baby (Marmet & Shell, 1993). Descriptive names with universal appeal have been selected so that they are easy to remember and are translatable to other cultures and languages. Standardized naming of positions creates a common vocabulary so that verbal and written information can readily be exchanged. The intention is not to create a body of jargon, but to facilitate clear and accurate communication between professionals, with parents, and in charting. In some cases, both descriptive and medical names are available for positions (e.g. top-breast-lying-down vs. Sims; reclining vs. modified-semi-Fowlers). When working with a mother, however, descriptive terms are easier for her to understand and remember.

The Importance of Skin-to-Skin Contact

Mammals are preprogrammed with neurobehaviors to expect a specific habitat or place during the newborn period (Alberts, 1958). For humans this habitat is skin-to-skin, heart-to-heart with their mothers—warm, safe, and close to the breast for feeding. Harlow's (1958, pp. 1–25) famous primate studies of attachment describe the infant as "actively seeking to adhere to as much skin surface on the mother's body as possible." This is the basis of healthy development (Schore, 2001a, p. 32). Likewise, when a human baby is in his habitat, skin-to-skin with his mother, preprogrammed neurobehaviors naturally play out in breastfeeding, which stimulates mother's milk release and production. Hector Martinez and Edgar Rey reported in 1983 that kangaroo mother care (continuous skin-to-skin contact) was superior to incubator care for stable preterm infants, and hundreds of research articles have since validated their findings (Anderson, Marks, & Wahlberg, 1986; Anderson, Moore, Hepworth, & Bergman, 2003; Browne, 2004; Charpak, de Calume, & Ruiz, 2000; World Health Organization, 2003).

On the other hand, animal and human research reveals protest-despair behavior as a universal mammalian response to separation from the correct habitat (mother). When a newborn is separated from his habitat/mother, he exhibits a hyper-arousal response. His sympathetic autonomic nervous system is suddenly and significantly activated, increasing the heart rate, blood pressure. The newborn's distress "is expressed in crying, then screaming" (Schore, 2001b, p. 210) (Christensson, Cabrera, Christensson, Uvnas-Moberg, & Winberg, 1995). Human babies separated from their mothers make 10 times as many cry signals as babies in skin-to-skin care (Rosenblum & Andrews, 1994). G. C. Anderson's (1988) research has led her to suggest that the crying of protest is detrimental for the infant, because it impairs lung functioning, jeopardizes the closure of the foramen ovale in the heart, increases intracranial pressure, and initiates a cascade of stress reactions that puts the infant at risk for poor adaptation to extrauterine life. If there is prolonged separation and the crying of protest fails to elicit maternal care, despair occurs. Then the baby exhibits disassociation, conserves energy and, to foster survival, will feign death, a passive state of profound detachment where blunting endogenous opiates are elevated and the heart rate and blood pressure are decreased. Human MRI research of the developing brain provides evidence of "toxic neurochemistry" caused by abuse and neglect (Schore, 2001b, p. 210).

The beginning of all positioning is ideally skin-to-skin. Harlow (1958), in discussing his cloth vs. wire mother monkey studies, said,

> We were not surprised to discover that contact comfort was an important basic affectional variable but we did not expect it to overshadow so completely the variable of nursing; indeed, the disparity is so great as to suggest that primary function of nursing is that of insuring frequent and intimate body contact of the infant with the mother. (p. 36)

Similarly, Montegue (1971) stated that the skin is the largest organ system of the body and perhaps, other than the brain, the most important. Of all of the human organs, the skin is the most sensitive organ and also the first medium of communication (pp. 1–25). The sense of touch is essential not only to the baby, but also for the mother, so it is critical to foster skin-to-skin contact between the mother and infant.

Some breastfeeding experts have reported when helping mothers with breastfeeding problems that just placing the mother and baby in unclothed chest-to-chest contact and allowing time for them to relax together leads to the baby self-attaching and breastfeeding well. When infants are stressed, they cannot access their feeding and growth responses. Difficulty latching to the breast and disorganized sucking behavior may result. Is it possible that continuous skin-to-skin contact of the baby and mother may reboot the neurobehavioral programming into the feeding mode and remove the negative stress patterns that had been interfering with breastfeeding? Though skin-to-skin contact will not correct all breastfeeding problems, it is certainly the correct habitat for babies and provides a strong foundation during the process of correcting whatever problems exist.

It seems prudent to extrapolate that regardless of the variety of positions utilized, keeping the mother and young baby skin-to-skin as much of the time as possible is ideal. A carrier that keeps the baby skin-to-skin with mother, except for changing, bathing, and occasional attention from other family members, such as the one used traditionally by the Basque community in Spain (Crawford, 1994), may be an ideal tool for universal use.

If skin-to-skin care cures breastfeeding problems, then we may ask why it is necessary to labor over specific positions. The answer is that even with an all-natural birth, and no separation, breastfeeding difficulties still occur in a small percentage of term babies.

Therapeutic Positions for Treatment

Alteration in positioning for breastfeeding can be an effective compensatory strategy for sucking problems, anatomical variations, and neurological deficits. Consider the following issues when choosing a therapeutic position: the mother's and baby's general anatomy and health status, the relationship of the breast and baby in space, and the specific breastfeeding issues involved. For example, a mother with long forearms, carpal tunnel syndrome, and large breasts with a 35-week premature baby might need very different modifications than a reference-sized mother with reference-sized breasts and a term infant with a bubble palate (Marmet & Shell, 1993; Snyder, 1995, 1997). As with all interventions, careful evaluation of the effectiveness of positioning suggestions is required.

Hand Position on the Base of the Baby's Head

If the position requires the mother's hand to hold the baby's head, her thumb and first finger wrap around the base of the skull (occiput) just under the ears (see **Figure 12-1**). Placing the hand higher on the back of the baby's head can interfere with the baby's ability to latch, especially when the baby is experiencing problems. The heel of the mother's hand and her pinky and ring fingers rest on the shoulders, supporting the back and neck. By providing support for the head, stability is achieved in the back, neck, and shoulders, thus protecting the neck.

Figure 12-1
Thumb and first finger wrap around the neck at or just under the ears, giving support at the base of the occiput.

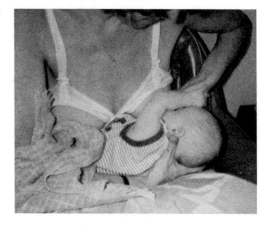

Baby Sitting (Mother Sitting)

It is possible that sitting/upright positions might be a good choice for many compromised babies. Research indicates that premature babies in kangaroo mother care (KMC) are best kept in upright positions (World Health Organization, 2003). Clinical experience has provided evidence that an upright position helps correct some breastfeeding problems.

Straddle Sit, Side Saddle Sit, and Clutch-V Position

Maternal comfort and infant muscle tone determine which of these three positions is chosen though the Straddle Sit and Side Saddle Sit require tone that is typically not found until a baby is over six weeks old. Some mothers like to use a combination of these at different feedings. The most common reasons for selecting sitting positions are:

- To assist babies with consistent tongue elevation; upright positions may work with gravity to bring the tongue down.
- For a baby with a cleft palate, velopharyngeal inadequacy, or repeated ear infections, especially if on artificial infant milk supplements, vertical positions help prevent milk from entering the nasopharynx and Eustachian tubes.
- Bringing the baby into a more upright position can help improve alertness and give support for improved sucking in some neurologically impaired infants.

Straddle Sit. In a straddle sit position (**Figure 12-2**) the baby's legs straddle one of the mother's legs. If needed, a pillow or rolled blanket can be used to prevent excessive head extension in the infant.

Figure 12-2
Straddle sit.

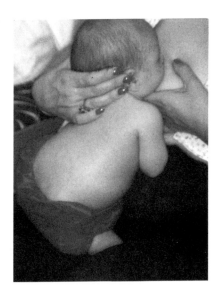

Side Saddle Sit. The baby sits on the mother's leg in a side-saddle position, with his chest to her chest (see **Figure 12-3**). Neurotypical babies approximately 4 months and older can rotate at the hips to face the mother while maintaining shoulder and ear alignment. A younger baby's whole body must be angled to face its mother and maintain alignment of the ears, shoulders, and hips.

Clutch-V Position. This position provides physiologic flexion along with vertical positioning. Starting from a clutch position (where the baby's body and legs form an L at the mother's side), elevate the baby's shoulders so that the baby is flexed at the hips into a V position (see **Figure 12-4**). Depending on issues such as the size and the shape of the mother and baby, the baby's legs may either be flexed as in the fetal position or extended up the back of the chair.

Mother Sitting (Baby in Other Positions)

Physiologic Flex

When to use: Physiologic flexion is helpful for calming an extremely fussy baby and reducing arching in hypertonic infants.

Description: The baby's arms and legs are placed in physiologic flexion and held in this curled up position against the mother's trunk (**Figure 12-5**).

"Fake Position"

When to use: This position is helpful for a baby who is having difficulty breastfeeding on one breast, but does well on the other. This position "tricks" the baby into thinking he is on his preferred side, and can accommodate an ear infection or a unilateral structural problem such as torticollis, vocal fold paralysis, or respiratory malformations that are more severe on one side.

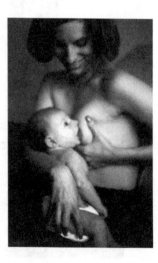

Figure 12-3
Side-saddle
sit.

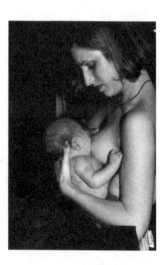

Figure 12-4
Clutch-V
position.

Description: After breastfeeding the baby on his preferred breast in the preferred position, slide the baby across to the other breast, keeping the baby's head and body in the same position and plane (**Figure 12-6**). If the baby has difficulty with skin contact, the baby's body may need to rest on pillows rather than across the mother's lap. It is relatively easy to slide a pillow with the baby on it to the other breast.

Baby Prone Positions (Mother Supine)

Robin's 1934 study indicated immediate improvement in oral and pharyngeal function, including reduced symptoms of upper respiratory obstruction, with prone or partially upright ("orthostatic") feeding positions. Sick babies bottle feeding in prone position showed better oxygenation and higher sucking pressures than when supine (Mizuno, Inoue, & Takeuchi, 2000). Prone positions seem helpful for breastfeeding compromised babies. Breastfed preterm babies had better oxygenation than when they bottle-fed (Meier & Anderson, 1987). Breastfeeding in any position is likely better for compromised babies than bottle feeding.

Vertical, Horizontal and Diagonal Prone Positions

When to use: The vertical, horizontal, and diagonal prone positions can be used interchangeably.

- Prone positioning works with gravity to bring the tongue forward.
- A baby with a short tongue, tongue held retracted or a tongue-tie can improve tongue contact with the breast using gravity.
- Prone positions may help infants who have difficulty handling milk flow.

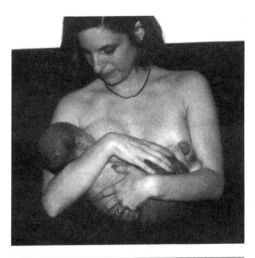 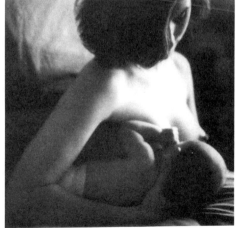

Figure 12-5 Physiologic flex.   **Figure 12-6** "Fake position."

Description: In all prone positions the mother is supine and the baby is prone and they are chest to chest. The mother can control the baby's head with her hand at the forehead or at the base of the skull. If desired, a rolling latch can also be employed, but it is often not as effective in this position (Curley et al., 2005). Well-placed firm pillows facilitate the mother's comfort and her ability to assist the baby with latch. A pillow or two under the mother's head, but not her shoulders, allows her to see the baby. A pillow along each of the mother's sides provides elevation and support for her arms and pillows under her bent knees helps avoid a backache.

Vertical Prone. The baby is prone and vertical to the mother (see **Figure 12-7**).

Horizontal Prone. The baby is prone and horizontal to the mother (see **Figure 12-8**).

Diagonal Prone. The baby is prone and diagonal to the mother (see **Figure 12-9**).

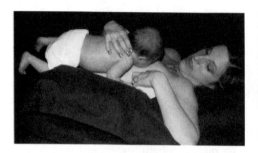

Figure 12-7 Vertical prone.

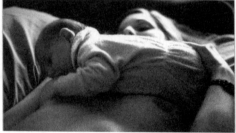

Figure 12-8 Horizontal prone.

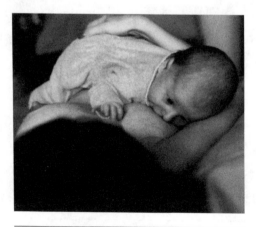

Figure 12-9 Diagonal prone.

Other Prone Positions

Prone Suck Training/Finger-Feeding Charm Hold. Suck training in prone position is also beneficial for babies with a retracted tongue, a short tongue, or a tight frenulum. The chest is supported by the mother's arm or hand while her other hand supports the forehead so her first or second finger can reach the mouth for suck training (Marmet & Shell, 1984). The hand is curved, giving the baby an air pocket for breathing (see **Figure 12-10**). It works like a charm!

Over-the-Shoulder Prone Position

When to use: This position is especially useful when the mother has nipple or areolar injury or infection, and the pressure points from suckling need to be changed dramatically to allow healing to occur.

Description: The baby kneels on the bed and leans over the mother's shoulder to reach the breast (**Figure 12-11**). Older babies may prefer sitting at the mother's shoulder and bending over it to reach the breast.

Floating Prone Position

When to use: This is particularly helpful when repeated unsuccessful breastfeeding attempts have left the baby frustrated and refusing to try again. If the sucking problem has been corrected and the baby is still rejecting the breast, this position often does the trick because the baby does not have the same negative associations in this position—away from the mother's body except for his head. It often helps to explain to the mother that the baby is not rejecting her, but only the method of feeding that he could not make work. Once the baby is successfully breastfeeding, the breast will become the baby's favorite "food delivery system" as designed, and the baby then is usually willing to use other positions.

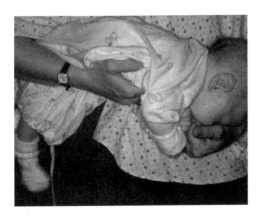

Figure 12-10 Prone suck training/finger-feeding charm hold.

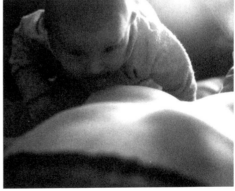

Figure 12-11 Over-the-shoulder prone position.

Description: The baby is placed prone on a pillow that is next to the mother's side so that the baby's body "floats" on the pillow while only his head rests on the mother's breast (**Figure 12-12**). It may be necessary to place a cloth on the mother's breast so the baby's face touches cloth, not skin. Only mouth to breast contact is mandatory. The mother can support the baby's head at the base of the skull (occiput) with her hand, but she may need to use a cloth between her hand and the baby's head.

Lateral Prone Position

When to use: Although it is especially useful for a baby with a receding chin, this position is particularly comfortable when resting or sleeping for dyads with or without breastfeeding problems.

Description: The baby is lateral to the mother and in an angled prone position. For the mother's right breast, the baby is placed on his left side on the mother's right arm, which is on a pillow. Then the whole baby is rolled forward against the mother's body so that he is no longer perpendicular to the bed but is at a 30–45° angle in an angled-prone position. The baby's head is at breast level and his mouth is just below the nipple so that latch can occur. The mother's right arm cradles her baby while pillows cradle her (see **Figure 12-13**).

Kneeling Prone Position

When to use: This position is useful for infants with a receding chin or a mother with abdominal surgery.

Description: The baby is placed kneeling at the mother's side facing her, next to her breast. Once kneeling, the baby's chest is brought forward to latch so that the chest and head are almost prone. The mother needs to be sure the baby's knees don't slip away from her body. With the baby kneeling next to the mother's left breast and the baby's mouth centered just above her nipple, the mother controls her baby's head with her left hand at the base of the baby's occiput while her left arm supports the baby's back, thus keeping the baby tucked tightly next to her. The mother's right hand is free to control the left breast. Initially the mother can "drop" the head onto her breast as soon as the baby is ready to latch. Within a few tries, the baby often latches by himself. The ease with which babies adapt to this position amazes mothers and health professionals alike, but the baby feels right at home in this almost fetal position. Placing a small pillow to the side of the baby's head, once the baby is breastfeeding well, will usually allow the mother to relax her hold on the baby's head and rest her hand (see **Figure 12-14**).

Mother Reclining Positions (Modified Semi-Fowlers)

If mother scoops up baby's buttocks with her elbow and reclines to allow gravity to hold baby against her, she may not need pillows to support her arm.

The reclining angle for these positions is approximately 45°, but may vary depending on the amount of compensation that is needed. It is easy to help a mother into a reclining position in an adjustable hospital bed. This is known as a semi-Fowlers position when the patient is using a hospital bed position. The mother is semi-reclining with bent knees so that her body, upper and lower legs, and feet form a W. When using a standard bed, pillows support the mother's lower back and bent knees. It also helps to brace the mother's feet against a pillow or rolled blanket so they don't slide. In a recliner chair, the mother's knees may need to be bent and supported with pillows depending on the shape of the chair. In a regular chair or sofa, the mother sits nearer the edge and leans back onto sufficient pillows behind her pelvis to support her reclining position. Her shoulders then rest on the chair

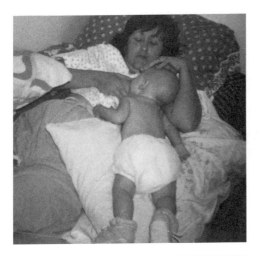

Figure 12-12   Floating prone position.

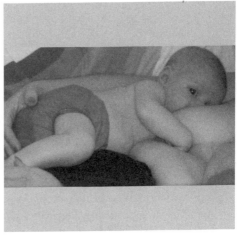

Figure 12-13   Lateral prone position.

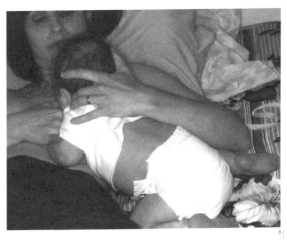

Figure 12-14   Kneeling prone position.

back and her feet rest on a footstool that is nearly chair height so her knees are bent. A very tall mother may find a lower footstool sufficient. Pillows can be used under her knees if desired, but this usually is not necessary; however, arm support is often helpful. In all of these variations, pillows can be used to support the mother's arms.

Reclining Straddle Sit (Baby Semi-Prone)

When to use: This is used for infants with receding chins when the mother needs or wants to sit.

Description: For the right breast, the baby is placed facing the mother straddling her right leg, and is leaned forward into a semi-prone position. A small rolled towel is placed between the baby's chest and the mother to keep the baby's head from overextension (see **Figure 12-15**).

Reclining Cradle

When to use: This is a very comfortable position after a cesarean birth because a pillow can cover the incision area to protect it.

Description: The baby is in a cradle position (**Figure 12-16**).

Reclining Sit

When to use: This is for temporary use as sore nipples heal, especially with older infants.

Description: The baby is sitting next to the mother's side, facing the mother, in a semi-prone position by leaning forward (**Figure 12-17**). Care must be taken to ensure good alignment of the baby's ears, shoulders, and hips.

Dancer Hand Positions

All three dancer hand positions make the oral cavity smaller to help increase intraoral (negative) pressure (Marmet & Shell, 1993; see Chapter 11). This is helpful for infants with a poor seal, weak suck, babies who fall off the breast if not held in place or neuromotor problems including high tone or low tone, e.g., Down Syndrome.

Classic Dancer Hand Position

When to use: This is for infants with excessive jaw excursions in addition to low intraoral pressure (**Figure 12-18**; Danner & Cerutti, 1989).

Description: The hand provides a sling to support the baby's mandible while simultaneously putting pressure with the index finger and thumb into the baby's buccal muscle (check cavities).

Three-Finger Dancer Suck Training Position

When to use: This is used for suck training with or without supplementation when a baby needs jaw support as well as an increase in the intraoral pressure.

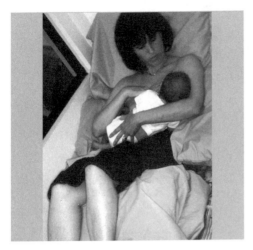

Figure 12-15   Reclining straddle sit.

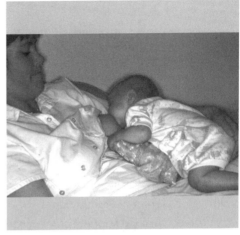

Figure 12-16   Reclining cradle.

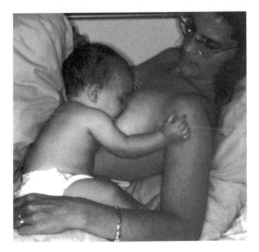

Figure 12-17   Reclining sit.

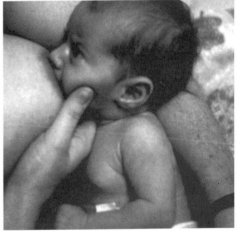

Figure 12-18   Classic dancer hand position.

Description: It can be done in two ways: either using a thumb and two fingers or using three fingers (see **Figure 12-19**). Mother's hand size, finger length, and manual dexterity will determine which digits she uses to apply pressure to baby's cheeks over the buccinators and to support the mandible (chin). An additional finger is used in the baby's mouth for the suck training.

Figure 12-19
Three-finger dancer supplementation
with a periodontal syringe.

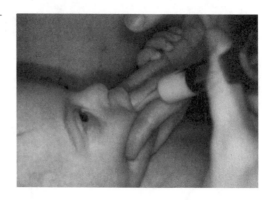

Two-Finger Dancer Hand Position

When to use: When jaw support is not needed, two fingers can be used to decrease intraoral space.

Description: When suck training, eliminate the finger on the chin, leaving two fingers for pressure points on the buccal muscles. When at the breast, two hands are used to provide the pressure points (see **Figure 12-20**).

Modifications for Specific Problems

Receding Chin Prone Positions

A baby with a receding chin (overbite or retrognathia) is easily identified by looking at the baby in profile (see **Figures 12-21** and **12-22**). If his mandible is significantly less prominent than his maxilla, then the baby has a receding chin. Restoring maternal nipple comfort and promoting effective infant milk transfer are goals of positioning strategies. Lateral Prone, Kneeling Prone, and mother reclining with the baby in a Straddle Sit Semi-Prone position are particularly effective.

The mandible grows quickly during the first 3 months of life so that most retrognathic babies can breastfeed in basic positions by 3 months of age.

Note: Another, very rare, malalignment of the mandible is a protruding chin (underbite or prognathic mandible). Positional treatment is the opposite of the treatment for the receding chin, placing the baby in a semi-supine position with the mother sitting and leaning forward.

Cradle Prone (Pierre Robin Position)

When to use: This position is particularly helpful for a baby with Pierre Robin sequence. It helps bring the tongue forward while using pillows to position the baby, thus freeing the mother's hands to support her breasts and manipulate feeding tools used at the breast (e.g., periodontal syringe). It may also be useful for situations other than Pierre Robin that require a mother's hands free while feeding the baby. The semi-prone position helps keep the baby latched during this process.

Description: The mother sits upright or very slightly reclining (no more than 70°) to bring the baby partially prone. The baby is propped on pillows on his side as if in a cradle position, but is not cradled in mother's arms (**Figure 12-23**). Instead, the baby is leaned forward so his chest is supported by the mother's chest, halfway between prone and perpendicular in a spatial sense. If the baby is being supplemented at breast with a periodontal syringe or feeding tube device, the mother may angle him slightly away from her body temporarily to be able to view the mouth for supplementation.

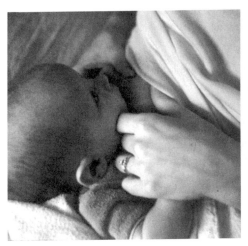

Figure 12-20   Two-finger dancer.

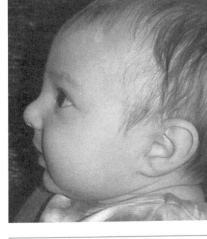

Figure 12-21   Normal chin.

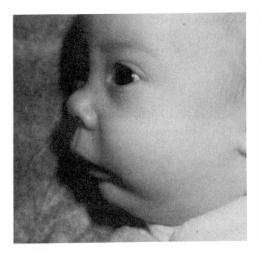

Figure 12-22   Receding chin.

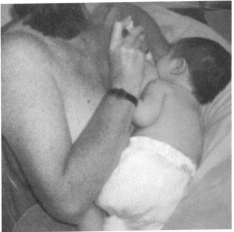

Figure 12-23   Cradle prone.

All Fours Position (Hands and Knees)

When to use: This is an awkward and uncomfortable position, though it is excellent for temporary use to clear plugged ducts, and may help the rare baby who cannot tolerate skin-to-skin contact.

Description: The baby is supine on a supportive surface. The mother is on her hands and knees with her breast hanging down to the baby's mouth (**Figure 12-24**).

Upside Down

When to use: Like the kneeling prone position, this unusual position is terrific if a mother has sore nipples.

Description: Both the mother and baby lie on their sides, but the baby is upside down in relation to the mother, with his feet pointing towards the mother's head (**Figure 12-25**).

Hip Dysplasia Positions

Infants who have hip dysplasia, and are consequently put into a cast or brace, breastfeed well in a straddle-sit position (see **Figure 12-26**). A cradle or transition hold can also be utilized with pillow support between the legs to blunt the weight and the awkwardness of the cast or brace. Because these babies cannot mold their bodies to their mothers' bodies the mother usually has to compress her breast with her finger to make an air pocket.

Modified Cradle Position to Accommodate Large Breasts

If a mother's breasts are too large to allow her arm to support her baby in front of her body, it may be helpful to approximate the position of the baby in the cradle hold using pillows to support and control the baby's head and body (**Figure 12-27**). If the breast is so pendulous that the baby cannot access the nipple while on the mother's lap, a rolled hand towel or cloth diaper can lift the breast to improve access. Variations in mother's or baby's anatomy may require adaptation in position. The infant's body can be pressed against the mother's breast to provide stability (body part to body part) (Morris & Klein, 1987). Other positions can also be modified with these principles.

Positions for Multiples

Breastfeeding twins simultaneously can allow substantial savings of maternal time and energy. With more than two babies, most mothers find planning and record keeping is necessary to be sure each baby gets fed. With triplets, she may feed the first two together, each on one breast for their full feeding, then offer the third both breasts. The babies are rotated at each feeding so that they change breasts and each has a turn at solitary, two-breasted feedings. Mothers of multiples usually need a great deal of help in the early days. Learning to "dance" with more than one partner requires extra time and extra practice.

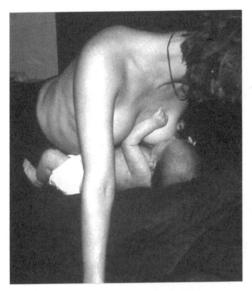

Figure 12-24 All fours position (hands and knees).

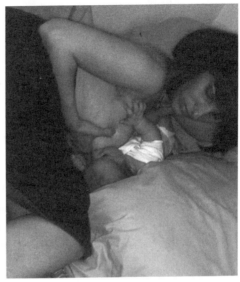

Figure 12-25 Upside down.

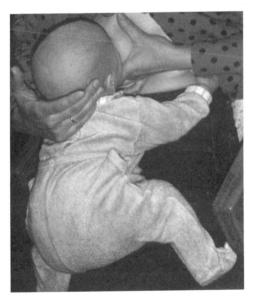

Figure 12-26 Hip dysplasia.

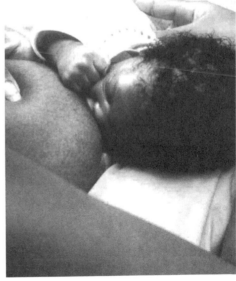

Figure 12-27 Modified cradle position for large breasts.

Double Cradle Position

The mother places the first twin across her trunk, supporting the infant on the same side arm. Then the second baby is cradled in the other arm lying on top of or behind his sibling. The baby in the mother's right arm latches to her right breast, and in her left arm to her left breast (**Figure 12-28**).

Double Clutch Position

For this position, both babies are in a clutch position, each under one of his mother's arms (see **Figure 12-29**).

Parallel Position (Also Called the Cradle/Clutch Position)

When the twins are young, one twin can be placed in a cradle position and the other in a clutch position (**Figure 12-30**). As the babies get bigger, the baby in the clutch position has his legs wrapped around his mother or off to the side, so the twins' legs are parallel to each other.

Double V Hold

This position works especially well for mothers with long torsos. The babies' bodies each are a side of the V they form together in their mother's arms and lap (**Figure 12-31**).

Conclusion

Once the lactation consultant has a firm understanding of normal suckling, the infant's feeding neurobehavior and instinctive feeding position, and issues that can make feeding difficult, therapeutic positions can be developed to help compensate. This chapter reviews therapeutic positions developed by the authors from their long experience working with infants with feeding challenges.

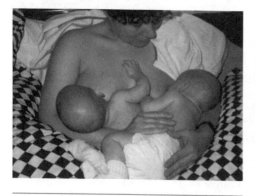

Figure 12-28   Double cradle position.

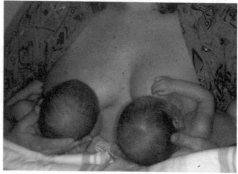

Figure 12-29   Double clutch position.

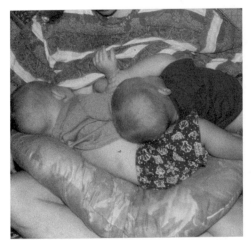

Figure 12-30   Parallel position.

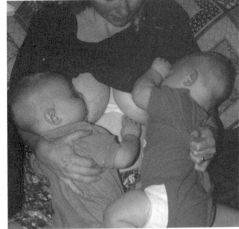

Figure 12-31   Double V hold.

References

Alberts, J. R. (1958). Learning as adaption of the infant. *Acta Paediatrica, 397*(Suppl.), 77–85.

Anderson, G. C. (1988). Crying, foramen ovale shunting, and cerebral volume. *Journal of Pediatrics, 113*(2), 411–412.

Anderson, G. C., Marks, E. A., & Wahlberg, V. (1986). Kangaroo care for premature infants. *American Journal of Nursing, 86*(7), 807–809.

Anderson, G. C., Moore, E., Hepworth, J., & Bergman, N. J. (2003). Early skin-to-skin contact for mothers and their healthy newborn infants. *Cochrane Collaboration Systematic Review.* Oxford: Update Software.

Blair, A., Cadwell, K., Turner-Maffei, C., & Brimdyr, K. (2003). The relationship between positioning, breastfeeding dynamic, the latching process and pain in breastfeeding mothers with sore nipples. *Breastfeeding Review, 11*(2), 5–10.

Bosma, J. F. (1972). Form and function in the infant's mouth and pharynx. In J. F. Bosma (Ed.). *Oral sensations and perceptions in the mouth of the infant* (pp. 3–29). Springfield, IL: Charles C Thomas.

Browne, J. V. (2004). Early relationship environments: Physiology of skin-to-skin contact for parents and their preterm infants. *Clinics in Perinatology, 31*(2), 287–298.

Charpak, N., de Calume, Z. F., & Ruiz, J. G. (2000). The Bogota declaration on kangaroo mother care: Conclusions at the second international workshop on the method. Second International Workshop of Kangaroo Mother Care. *Acta Paediatrica, 89,* 1137–1140.

Christensson, K., Cabrera, T., Christensson, E., Uvnas-Moberg, K., & Winberg, J. (1995). Separation distress call in the human infant in the absence of maternal body contact. *Acta Paediatrica, 84,* 468–473.

Cioni, G., Ferrari, F., & Prechtl, H. F. (1989). Posture and spontaneous motility in full-term infants. *Early Human Development, 18*(4), 247–262.

Crawford, C. J. (1994). Parenting practices in the Basque country: Implications of infant and childhood sleeping location for personality development. *Ethos, 22*(1), 42–84.

Curley, M. A. Q., Arnold, J. H., Thompson, J. E., Fackler, J. C., Grant, M. J., Fineman, L. D., et al. (2005). Effect of prone positioning on clinical outcomes in children with acute lung injury. *Journal of the American Medical Association, 294*(2), 229–237.

Danner, S., & Cerutti, E. R. (1989). *Nursing your baby with Downs syndrome.* Rochester, NY: Childbirth Graphics.

Harlow, H. F. (1958). The nature of love. *The American Psychologist, 13,* 673–685. In Montegue, A. (Ed.). (1971). *Touching: The human significance of skin* (pp. 1–25). New York: Harper & Row.

Henderson, A., Stamp, G., Pincombe, J. (2001). Postpartum positioning and attachment education for increasing breastfeeding: A randomized trial. *Birth, 28*(4), 236–242.

Kroeger M., & Smith, L. J. (2004). *Impact of birthing practices on breastfeeding: Protecting the mother and baby continuum.* Sudbury, MA: Jones and Bartlett.

McKenna, J., Thoman, E. B., Anders, T. F., Sadeh, A., Schechtman, V. L., et al. (1993). Infant-parent co-sleeping in an evolutionary perspective: Implications for understanding infant sleep development and the sudden infant death syndrome. *Sleep, 16*(3), 263–282.

Marmet, C., & Shell, E. (1984). Training neonates to suck correctly. *MCN. The American Journal of Maternal Child Nursing, 9*(6), 401–407.

Marmet, C., & Shell, E. (1993). *Lactation forms: A guide to lactation consultant charting.* Encino, CA: Lactation Institute.

Marmet, C., Shell, E., & Aldana, S. (2000). Assessing infant suck dysfunction: Case management. *Journal of Human Lactation, 16*(4), 332–336.

Meier, P., & Anderson, G. (1987). Responses of small preterm infants to bottle- and breast-feeding. *MCN. The American Journal of Maternal Child Nursing, 12,* 97–105.

Mizuno, K., Inoue, M., & Takeuchi, T. (2000). The effects of body positioning on sucking behaviour in sick neonates. *European Journal of Pediatrics, 159*(11), 827–831.

Montegue, A. (1971). *Touching: The human significance of skin.* New York: Harper & Row.

Morris, S. E., & Klein, M. D. (1987). *Pre-feeding skills.* Tucson, AZ: Therapeutic Skill Builders.

Ransjö-Arvidson, A. B., Matthiesen, A. S., Lilja, G., Nissen, E., Widström, A. M., et al. (2001). Maternal analgesia during labor disturbs newborn behavior: Effects on breastfeeding, temperature, and crying. *Birth, 28,* 5.

Rey, E. S., & Martinez, H. G. (1983). *Manejo racional del niño prematuro.* In: *Curso de Medicina Fetal* (pp. 137–151). Bogotá, Colombia: Universidad Nacional.

Righard, L., & Alade, M. O. (1990). Effect of delivery room routines on success of first breastfeed. *Lancet, 336,* 1105–1107.

Robin, P. (1934). Glossoptosis due to atresia and hypotrophy of the mandible. *American Journal of Diseases of Children, 48,* 541.

Rosenblum, L. A., & Andrews, M. W. (1994). Influences of environmental demand on maternal behavior and infant development. *Acta Paediatrica, 397*(Suppl.), 57–63.

Schore, A. N. (2001a). Effects of a secure attachment relationship on right brain development, affect regulation, and infant mental health. *Infant Mental Health Journal, 22,* 7–66.

Schore, A. N. (2001b). The effects of early relational trauma on right brain development, affect regulation, and infant mental health. *Infant Mental Health Journal, 22*(1–2), 201–269.

Snyder, J. (1995). *Variation in infant palatal structure.* Encino, CA: Lactation Institute.

Snyder, J. B. (1997). Bubble palate and failure to thrive: A case report. *Journal of Human Lactation, 13*(2), 139–143.

Widstrom, A. M., Ransjo-Arvidson, A. B., Christensson, K., Mathieson, A. S., Winberg, J., & Uvnas-Moberg, K. (1987). Gastric suction in healthy newborn infants: Effects on the circulation and developing feeding behavior. *Acta Paediatrica Scandinavica, 76,* 566–572.

Wolf, L. S., & Glass, R. P. (1992). *Feeding and swallowing disorders in infancy.* Tucson, AZ: Therapy Skills Builders.

World Health Organization. (2003). *Kangaroo mother care: A practical guide.* Geneva, Switzerland: Author.

Chapter 13

Counseling Mothers of Infants with Feeding Difficulties

Nancy Williams

Parenting, and perhaps mothering in particular, is generally experienced as both more joyous and more complicated and overwhelming than the parent imagined, expected, or could possibly have anticipated. This is true even for the experienced parent who adds to her or his family, because each baby is a unique individual who must teach his mother and father how to parent him. For the parent who faces feeding difficulties, prematurity, disabilities, and the like, the most intense experience of their lifetime may be encompassed in caring for this child. Few parents are prepared in advance for the unique challenges incurred by a baby with special needs, even if they are relatively simple feeding problems that are time-limited. How much more so for the family whose baby has a myriad of problems or whose feeding difficulties will not be easily resolved with time and a bit of creativity and patience!

Bringing a new child into the family is often an enormous opportunity for marital bonding, and fortunately so, because with this child comes increased stress on the marital unit as well. For an unmarried mother, these stresses may spill over into whatever relationships exist within her home. If she is alone, she will also be faced with isolation and little or no respite from the demands of her infant. The tasks before her are daunting.

Westerners live in a world that is fast-paced, driven by material need and a desire to achieve. This is often not conducive to the demands of motherhood, especially where an infant is demanding special attention, even above the expected. This adds to the complexity of the new roles and tasks before the parents. It is important for the lactation consultant to have some understanding of the maternal context for this baby in order to provide optimum care to each dyad.

As lactation care providers we must realize that some of our prescriptions involve a great deal of time and energy. Depending upon the baby's capabilities, it may be that feeding takes up such a large portion of the day that there isn't time for anything else. Our plan may simply be impossible for a given mother, depending on her resources and support, maturity, experience, obligations to other children or work outside the home, and so on. It is important for us to continually check in with her and to devise our care plan in conjunction with her stated goals, desires, and capabilities. The likelihood of success is much higher when she "buys in" by helping to create the plan.

It may also be appropriate in some instances to help her to sort through exactly where her stressors lie. Commonly, those around her may offer confusing information that point to her attempts to breastfeed as the reason why she is tired, overwhelmed, and so forth. In reality, it is often the normal demands of mothering a small child (or children) coupled with the feeding difficulties that exist apart from breastfeeding. For women who are also trying to juggle jobs, partner issues, or other problems, it may be necessary to assist her in assessing what can be let go or put on hold during this most intense time of need on the part of her little one. It's not unusual to discover that her stress becomes compounded, emotionally as well as physically, following weaning—particularly a weaning that was imposed on the mother by either subtle or overt pressure. This would be true even in the case of an older baby. Weaning—complete or partial—should only take place when the mother and baby are ready. With feeding disorders, readiness on either or both parts may come early out of exhaustion, resignation, or a whole host of reasons not truly associated with lactation problems.

Adult Development

Clearly, a woman experiences monumental psychological upheaval as she makes the transition into motherhood. Many of these changes are positive and may be capitalized on by lactation consultants and others who care for the dyad. Recent animal studies suggest that, rather than diminished cognitive abilities in the period following birth, instead women may be at a lifetime peak in problem-solving abilities. Researchers have suggested that comparing a brain of a nonmother to that of a new mother is comparing apples to oranges (Kinsley & Lamber, 2006). It is important to note that the process of birth and the transformation of becoming a mother results in profound changes in brain function. Erik Erikson, in his classic work on psychosocial development, *Identity, Youth and Crisis* (1968), described stages of change through crisis throughout the lifespan. His model helps us to understand the psychological tasks a woman is undertaking concurrent with assuming her new role as a mother. When motherhood arrives, a woman biologically will be in one of three Eriksonian developmental stages. If she is still an adolescent, she will be in the throes of learning her Identity vs. Role Confusion. If a young adult, she will be struggling with Intimacy vs. Isolation. For an older primipara, the challenge lies in Generativity vs. Self-Absorption/Stagnation. Each of these stages offers ample opportunity to embrace this motherhood experience and to experience great emotional and cognitive growth as a result. Failure to do so often results in a stunting of development and a state of being somewhat "stuck" in an unnecessarily immature state. Recognition by health care providers of the differing needs in each developmental state may help to provide optimal care.

Having some grasp of this can be helpful for the lactation consultant as she assesses how best to teach and plan for her care. Acknowledging that her own developmental experiences may be implicit in the situation to which she is called may also be important. For example, a lactation consultant who is working on Generativity may find herself tempted to inappropriately "mother" the mother in ways that are not productive.

Maternal Adequacy

Very few experiences serve to facilitate adult development as thoroughly and profoundly as becoming a parent. We learn to live outside of ourselves, find a stronger voice, care about the world differently, and mature quickly. This author conducted a survey while preparing for a presentation several years ago, asking men and women both how parenthood had changed them. Although many ideas were brought forth, the one answer given by each and every respondent was, "I'm not as selfish."

If feeding difficulties arrive with the first baby, she has yet to begin this process, identity change, and new lesson in stepping outside of herself. In their seminal work on the acquisition of the parental role, authors Bocar and Moore (1987) describe a predictable sequence of behaviors and internal states that define the development of an emerging new identity with the advent of the first baby. Initially, parents find themselves in what has been called the Formal Stage, where they want rules and proscriptions for everything involved in baby care. Given that feeding or other difficulties add several levels of complexity to the situation, first-time parents may need assistance with opposing tasks: learning what needs to be done while at the same time learning to take command of their situation and become their child's advocate. They may find themselves clinging to the Formal Stage, finding comfort in the promises given by books and professionals, yet being forced to move quickly to more maturity as parents as they seek to understand the needs of this child and possibly be called upon to advocate for him within the complicated context of the medical system.

It would stand to reason that if feeding difficulties first present with a second or subsequent baby, the mother may have already developed a depth of maturity and comfort with her role. In terms of acquiring her parental role, it's likely that she will have arrived at Bocar and Moore's Personal Stage, that is assuming "Mother" as her identity by developing a unique set of behaviors and attitudes that are appropriate for her, leading to confidence and competence. However, she also has a conflict in the fact that her other child(ren) are in need of her energies, obligating her to perform a juggling act with her time and attention. Understanding the mountain of demands being placed on this mother is vital while developing interventions and care plans.

In most normal situations, the mother is encouraged to bond primarily through the baby's attaching behaviors and cues. It is the infant who teaches parents how to care for him and engage his unique personality and needs. Occasionally this may go awry as the baby not only doesn't elicit the usual cues, but also may seem to overtly reject her. Many mothers whose babies arch their back, scream, and push away from the breast (or arms and cradling) are perceived as "not liking" the mother. Persistent and patient parents learn how to help the baby settle into the arms or at breast, but sometimes may need some teaching and encouragement from the lactation consultant. Educating them on the relative cognitive immaturity that would preclude a choice such as rejection can be helpful. Above all, health care providers should not participate in negative interpretations of baby's behavior with comments about his stubbornness, anger, laziness, being a "bad baby," and the like.

Understanding differing stages and experiences allows the lactation consultant to modify her teaching and support in a way that individualizes and makes relevant what she is trying to accomplish. Each mother and her needs are unique, and she needs to be cared for with understanding and creativity that acknowledges a given situation.

Resistance

It is very rewarding to offer educational support to the new dyad and to watch them succeed. It is equally or more discouraging when things don't go well. One possible reason that often leaves medical personnel scratching their heads is resistance.

Resistance can be a compensatory protective means of coping with something that is beyond us. It allows us to feel some modicum of control in an otherwise out-of-control situation. An important thing to remember in the presence of this resistance is that we need to take great care in including parents in the decisions, rather than telling them what to do. This allows them to feel more control.

Understanding the normal course of a crisis may be helpful. Although Kübler-Ross's (1969) model was intended for the dying patient, many have applied it to grief, loss, and crisis in general. One often observes the parents of babies with special needs exhibiting these predictable patterns, which include denial, anger, bargaining, depression, and finally acceptance. It is noteworthy to add that these may not manifest themselves in any linear fashion. It is also possible to return to a state, such as denial, long after one believes it to have resolved. Due to the intensity of the emotional response to crisis, it is often difficult for the parent(s) to think clearly and make rational decisions. Hence it is all the more important that the lactation consultant offer information and guidance gently but firmly as parents sort through advice and directions that seemingly come from all sides. It is also helpful to explain to parents that they won't always feel the way they do right now and to normalize their reaction to such a difficult experience. Our job as caring helpers is to support them in ways that leave them stronger as a result of their crisis, rather than in a more dependent or weakened state.

Therefore, when there is a problem or some deviation from the expectation of the parents, it becomes difficult, at best, to move towards acceptance of the situation. Many levels of resistance and confusion may be at play. The mother may have brought baggage to this experience from previous births, losses, or parenting, not to mention her own childhood.

Other common components to crisis include *ambivalence* and *detachment*. The parents are a bundle of tangled, unnamed negative emotions. This often causes them to swing back and forth in their thoughts, feelings, plans, and decisions. Lactation consultants may use this to their advantage in recognizing that a decision to give up breastfeeding may indeed be immediately reversible or be changed in the near future. Gentle, respectful sharing of information on the ramifications of a decision to wean can be helpful. Detachment is a defense mechanism often seen in the wake of shock, similar to denial. This protects one from the searing pain of feeling the totality of whatever loss is occurring. Sometimes the parent(s) may present with a very flat affect while in the process of some detaching from the situation. The danger lies in parents not being able to move back to engagement, which health care providers can help to guard against. When parents are detached, it may be somewhat more difficult for the health care providers to enter into a caring relationship. Recognizing this phenomenon for what it is may allow the lactation consultant to carefully confront it a bit and move forward.

Attachment

The primary psychological task of any newborn, according to Erik Erickson (1968), is to learn to trust. The baby is "hard-wired" to engage in all manner of attachment-seeking behaviors. It is he who will inspire the parent to respond with bonding behaviors. He smells nice, and she pulls him closer for a whiff. He is soft, and she runs her hands along his skin. He scans his horizon, and she responds with a gaze that he can lock into. He smiles, and she returns his happy countenance. He whimpers, and she picks him up. He mouths his hands, and she feeds him. He cries, and she relieves his discomfort.

The attachment that forms during the first 3 years, with great emphasis placed on the foundational first year, will serve as the basis for the relationships formed by this baby throughout his lifespan. Mary Ainsworth's classic work, *Patterns of Attachment: A Psychological Study of the Strange Situation* (1978), clearly demonstrated that whatever "attachment style" formed in the first year was still being evidenced decades later as spouses and other adult relationships were sought and constructed. John Bowlby (1982) was able to demonstrate the need for young children to have continual access to the primary caretaker, absent of significant separations. Recent work by Nils Bergman (2001) admonishes us to "never separate a mother and baby."

Consequently, the mother-baby relationship being forged is exceedingly important. Additionally, we know that a secure attachment is responsible for helping the child to learn empathy and general social skills (including language) and for helping to build proper synaptic structures in the brain, particularly to develop the orbitofrontal area of the brain that connects thought and emotion, allowing us to make thoughtful responses to a situation, rather than to simply react. A poorly attached child fails to learn emotional regulation—that is, the ability to calm and soothe himself—and be able to cope and move forward when things aren't going well. In short, the emotional abilities seen in babies who fail to attach are so limited as to be crippling throughout life.

In the case of an infant who is not able to cue correctly, eliciting proper responses, there is some risk that the normal course of attachment and bonding may be disrupted. This will likely result in one of two dysfunctional extremes: overcompensating in the form of enmeshment and overprotection, or parental self-protection and withdrawal resulting in disengagement. Parents who fail to bond experience deficits in their parenting abilities as well as in the relationship itself. It is not only the infant who loses when bonding and attachment fail.

When dealing with problems of any kind during the newborn period, some parents find themselves at a loss as to how to bond with the baby, particularly if the baby's attaching behaviors are somehow compromised. It's not unusual for the parent to globalize and feel incompetent and inadequate to the whole of parenting. The converse may also be true wherein parents understand that this particular child will need something from them that they hadn't imagined and they step up to fulfill that need, adding to their feeling of parental power.

Fostering Attachment

Many parents may be appreciative of encouragement and instruction for deliberately engaging in reparative attachment behaviors. Because it is the baby who usually drives this process, when the process is short-circuited it will likely require some compensatory effort on the part of the parents. Soliciting the parents' responses in this way will have the added bonus of creating a feeling of importance in an otherwise powerless situation.

It would be a mistake to assume that because "bonding" got off to a slow start, or even experienced complete disruption in the early days, that all is lost. Although there is a very real risk that the family could continue down a path of disconnection, it is likely that with good support the family can make up for lost time and develop solid attachments. For parents who themselves demonstrate secure attachment styles (Ainsworth, 1978) this task will likely be an easy transition with a bit of reassurance from the health care team.

When working with families who are not as fortunate in their own upbringing and backgrounds, didactic instruction on basics such as the important of eye contact, skin-to-skin contact, availability, engaging facial animation, and so forth are important. Parents can be taught to be deliberately compensatory in their own bonding behaviors to assist the baby. Maybe even more important are referrals to support groups such as La Leche League, where the mother has ample opportunity to observe mother-baby interactions, as well as to "vent" when she feels frustration, fear, or other unexpected emotions.

Birth Resolution

In the last decade, it has become increasingly common for women to experience a myriad of birth interventions. A woman may often find herself without knowledge or power in making the decisions and choices about her baby's birth. The overall effect of this may be that she misses out on the empowerment inherent in a birth of her design as she takes on her new role as mother. If she is to advocate for her child within the medical establishment, this may have disastrous consequences.

If she has had a cesarean or other highly medicalized birth, it is also likely that she will be experiencing pain or psychological discomfort that will make it more difficult to meet the needs of a difficult-to-feed infant. Surely she will benefit from our best helping skills and is likely to experience breastfeeding success, despite obstacles in initiation.

Oxytocin, the hormone responsible for bonding, milk ejection, and satisfaction, may have been inhibited at crucial times. Normally, there is a significant burst at the time of birth. This is initiated as the baby's head creates pressure on the vaginal walls, obviously absent during a cesarean delivery. Additionally, epidural anesthesia is known to inhibit oxytocin release. There is evidence that the pain of labor, which causes endorphin release, also contributes to attachment. Attachment researchers are continuing to question the ramifications of violating the design of biology in this regard.

Many women find their birth experiences to be singularly dissatisfying, even to the point of mourning plans that went awry. A mother may be puzzled about "what went wrong" or she may experience feelings of failure and inadequacy that threaten to invade her perception of her newly developing mothering skills. It's possible that she feels bitter disappointment as she contemplates the reality of her experience alongside her hopes and dreams for birth.

Conversely, it's possible that given her approaches to life in general that she is perfectly happy with allowing others to make decisions about her birth, which follows into her mothering. She may then have difficulty following through, thinking that caring for this baby might better be performed by experts. A passive style such as this can be challenging for the lactation consultant who may be encouraging her to come into a more empowered place. The consultant must realize that for some, this process is substantially protracted.

Imperfect Baby

First responses to birth anomalies often create yet another mix of confusing emotions. It is normal to see parents swing from one emotional extreme to another as they navigate this aspect of the situation. Unfortunately, they may also be subject to the unhelpful advice and opinions of people around them.

During the immediate crisis, it is crucial for health care providers to be as clear and repetitive as possible, in anticipation of the likelihood that the parents cannot take in everything that is being shared. A simplified explanation of all things medical allows the parents to grasp the situation more thoroughly. Having a written summary of care plans, referrals, and the like will be most helpful. It may also be advantageous to include other family members/support people in teaching times so that others can help relay information later, as well as encouraging them to share tasks when appropriate.

Teen Mothers

Although in many respects teen mothers have the same needs and goals as any mother, there are some unique needs within this population that must be considered during teaching and development of care plans.

It is common to note that the average teen mother has both high energy and multitasking abilities. This is fortunate because it is also generally true that she is under a great deal of both internal and external pressure to accomplish several roles at once. She is now a mother, student, family member, girlfriend or wife, social teen, and possibly an employee. She has not been given any extra hours in her day, yet often finds herself trying to accomplish more than is possible.

Often one observes that not only are her financial resources quite limited—an important consideration when advising on pumps, supplementers, and the like—but also due to her immaturity she may simply not have the patience for a difficult feeding regimen. She may also be expected to return to school by 2 weeks postpartum, regardless of the baby's status. Because mother-baby attachment issues are potentially more critical for this dyad, it is important to weigh these aspects and to try and simplify her tasks as much as possible. A back-to-basics approach may be the best, limiting interventions as much as possible. Utilizing peers and adult mentors are both creative ways to provide ongoing support for breastfeeding.

It would likely be a significant mistake to assume that because the mother is young that she would be incapable of learning about the care of her baby. Allison was barely 16 when her son was born, aspirating meconium during birth.

> I checked the machines he was hooked up to, making sure his oxygen saturation levels and heart and breathing rates were what the nurses expected them to be. They were. I would pad down the hallway, back into my room, rubbing my soft, wrinkled tummy and pull out my new breast pump. (Crews, 1999)

Teens are more likely to birth by cesarean and statistically more likely to give birth to premature or anomalous infants. They are also more likely to bottle feed, theoretically because of the multitude of barriers against obtaining help and information regarding breastfeeding. The genuine caring assistance of a lactation consultant may be exactly what she needs to defy the statistics and become a successful breastfeeder, despite any problems getting started.

One potentially positive aspect of working with teens is that they may be exquisitely aware of their need for teaching and support. They usually respond well to adults who do not condescend to them but rather offer genuine caring. Including grandparents in teaching time is often best, in order to enlist their support and to detour incorrect information. Additionally, the lactation consultant can model an attitude that promotes the new young mother's need to occupy her new role.

Advice of Outsiders

Under the best of circumstances new parents find themselves bombarded with advice and suggestions. Usually this is well-intended, though sometimes family members attempt to exert control over the new parent(s) or the situation. Although advice-givers are sometimes knowledgeable and can offer positive suggestions, this is not always the case. Add to that the fact that some personality styles are more susceptible to advice, possibly seeking out multiple opinions, and it can be a very frustrating situation for the health care providers. Bear in mind that if this is a first baby, parents are looking for the rules that will help them to succeed. It can be very positive to include extended family members in care-plan formation and discussion and to validate their concerns and ideas when possible, while at the same time empowering the parents to do what they think is best.

It is also an unfortunate possibility that family and friends will withdraw in the face of a disabled or critically ill infant. Such an event exacerbates the pain of parents who are already struggling to cope. Encouragement, comfort, and referrals to support groups can be very helpful.

Family of Origin Issues

During times of stress, families may be tempted to revert to unhealthy patterns of communicating and interacting. Long-buried wounds may once again rise to the surface. Inabilities to work together, "pushing buttons," and other problems may add to an already difficult situation. Due to the emotional vulnerability of the parents, hypersensitivity may cause new conflicts to erupt.

Conversely, many families find new strengths when stressed. Abilities to share time, energy, and even monetary resources are often discovered for possibly the first time. A new bonding among extended family members tends to take place if the members allow it. The lactation consultant may find herself in a unique role as facilitator as the family looks to her for help, information, and support.

Grief and Coping Skills

Feeding problems are generally perceived as crisis situations, even in the mildest of circumstances. Inherent in any crisis is a feeling of loss, leading to grief. Grief is among the most complex of experiences, with tangled webs of emotion. It is important to note that grief also provides a rich opportunity for personal growth and development. When one survives a crisis with the support of caring people, one often comes out the other side with greater knowledge, strength, compassion, and a multitude of positive developments.

Further, as previously mentioned, grief has a somewhat predictable course, including the roller-coaster ride of emotions that are a conglomerate of positives (hope) and negatives (despair). Old losses may reassert their presence in the form of newly provoked pain. Over time, the intensity that the mother may be feeling this week will diminish. Educating her about this fact will give her something to cling to on her bad days and something to look forward to overall. Bear in mind that the unfolding of grief cannot be hurried, and the parents should expect it to take time. Health care providers will sometimes confuse normal, healthy grieving with the abnormal state of depression. It is important to encourage the parents to allow the grieving process to proceed, and let them know that it has its own pace, and that there is nothing wrong with them. Encouraging the use of antidepressants or other medications to alleviate "symptoms" of normal sadness may be in error and may, in fact, prolong the natural course of mourning.

Healthy acceptance of whatever situation the parents are facing is not to be confused with resignation. Acceptance includes an embracing of the baby, celebration of the positive aspects of the situation, and a powerful moving forward. In the event of the death of the infant, acceptance is still the goal. Resignation connotes a loss of power as well as an inability to see anything worth celebrating.

In the case of a baby with feeding difficulties, the parents will most likely experience what is referred to as ambiguous grief. On the one hand, they have a surviving baby, with many capabilities and lovable qualities. Well-meaning people will often point this out, claiming that there is nothing to be sad about. The reality, however, is that the mother may indeed experience strong grief for the loss of her expectations, whatever they may have been. Disappointing birth experiences or, worse, traumatic births, as well as any fears for her baby's future may accompany such grief, intensifying it. Add to that exhaustion, hormonal shifts, confusing medical advice, and so forth and the potential for a negative state becomes significant.

Grief is a multi-faceted complex experience. In addition to sadness about the situation, many people find themselves isolated in misunderstanding. Well-meaning people may suggest that there is everything to be thankful for, nothing to complain about, and that it's time to move on. After all, the baby is alive, healthy, beautiful, or some other positive adjective. The fact that the mother may be mourning the loss of her expectation of a warm, smooth breastfeeding experience is minimized by those who are telling her what to be thankful for.

It will be important for health care providers and other caring people to encourage the parents to take care of each other and themselves. This may be very challenging if feeding regimens call for little time away. The requirements of constant pumping, feeding, washing of equipment, and so forth all while healing from birth seemingly do not allow for self-care. The reality is that if this isn't built into the care plan, most parents will not manage the long haul. Extended family members and friends may be recruited for help with the mundane: cooking, cleaning, taking care of the car, caring for other children, and so forth. Although this is a gift to any new parents, it becomes crucial with parents who have more than their share of challenges. Religious groups can be called upon to offer such assistance, as well. The added benefit of eliciting help from others is that it is often an opportunity for re-establishing or strengthening important emotional ties with the parents. This will support the grieving process as well as provide practical care and help.

Substance Abuse

In some instances, the feeding difficulties presented in the infant are a result of substance use in one or both parents. Or there may be no direct relationship, yet the baby is born to a parent with addictive patterns already in place.

Lactation consultants have many resources to turn to for their own education, and would do well to have handouts or other information available for clients. Although there may be room for professional disagreement about minimal use of some substances such as alcohol or nicotine, there is consensus that most street drugs are generally incompatible with breastfeeding. Still, some mothers may be able to use "pump and dump" information or, better still, be encouraged towards sobriety on behalf of their baby.

Possibly a more immediate concern with these families would be whether the parents are functioning well enough to care for a baby. This can be explored with the help of the lactation consultant, including reviewing the facts of safe co-sleeping and other issues about which there may be concerns. Note that the lactation consultant may not be hearing the entire accurate picture from a family that has substance abuse in its center, and the LC may want to carefully offer information based on her hunches, even if those hunches are not verbally validated.

Substance users will many times increase patterns of usage in times of stress and crisis. Lactation consultants would be wise to be alert to this possibility. Good referrals for programs, therapy, or other positive support would be in order.

Lactation Consultants' Feelings and Responsibilities

Lactation consultants may also have very strong emotions in situations where breastfeeding goals are not met. Many consultants entered this profession because of the great satisfaction we know when we watch a successfully nursing dyad, accompanied by joy when we observe the relieved look of the mother as the baby finally latches nicely. Consequently, when our best efforts fail to yield the desired result, we may wonder what we could have done differently as we feel frustration, anger, confusion, puzzlement, and much more. Out of our own pain, we may be tempted to withdraw from her or try to affix inappropriate blame. If we are clear and aware of our own process, allowing us to stay connected, we may be invited to enter into the mother's grief, providing support and walking with her down a lonely road. It is not an easy one for the consultant to walk either, despite its privilege. In the end, we may find that we have grown personally and developed new counseling skills as well!

These counseling skills—active listening and reflecting feelings as the mother explores her situation, asking good open-ended questions leading to choices and decision making, and educating her about real options and possibilities—will all help to see the mother through the immediate future as well as down the road. This is time consuming, involving a commitment to the well-being of the family that transcends what we often are doing for breastfeeding support. The rewards to everyone are well worth the cost, however.

The Importance of Listening

Developing listening skills brings many benefits to professional helpers. Active listening (i.e., restating and rephrasing the client's statements) can sometimes feel so simplistic as to be questionable. The client shares that she "has to wean the baby." We reply "You have to wean the baby." As we do so, we have time to gather ourselves from what may be an unexpected remark, we make sure that we are on the same page with the client and that we stay on it if she goes in an unexpected direction, and it encourages her to elaborate. Her next statement may be, "Well, yes, because my husband says my breasts are his."

(continued)

The Importance of Listening (*continued*)

Reflective listening, wherein we explore with her the emotional aspects of her experience, is optimum for creating a connection with her. She states, "I've had it with pumping 10 times a day, then feeding, cleaning parts, and then starting over." We may reply, "It sounds like you are feeling overwhelmed, exhausted, and frustrated." The client then experiences us as understanding her situation more fully and trusts us enough to move to a deeper place of communication. Further, she begins to understand her own tangled mass of feelings that are driving her to making a possibly regrettable decision. Making the effort to understand another person on this level is a true gift.

One of the best ways to help someone to grasp concepts is by asking them to think it through in the form of an open-ended question. Closed-ended questions such as "Do you want to breastfeed?" don't necessarily elicit much information and actually have a tendency to shut down further discussion. Asking "Why don't you want to breastfeed?" implies judgment, puts the client on the defensive, and probably doesn't have a good answer anyway. All of these nonproductive ways of asking can be developed into good questions that make her think. "What are the factors that are causing you to want to wean?" "How did you reach this decision?" "Where do you imagine yourself in the future?" As she formulates responses to these questions she is obligated to weigh her positions in a new way, often leading to a different conclusion.

Finally, once trust has been established and we've developed a caring relationship with her, a tall order to be sure given the time constraints, we may be able to confront her with new information that she hasn't factored in to her decision-making.

> Client: My baby has had so much to deal with since the surgery. My family all think that it would just be easier to wean so the baby and I would both be less stressed.
>
> Lactation Consultant: I've heard you talk about the pressure you are feeling. I'm so impressed at the skills you've already developed as Andrew's mother. I'm wondering what you think about your family's advice. Perhaps you would like to hear about some of the long-term effects of weaning a baby of this age. May I share that with you?

Notice that the information is presented in a way that respects the mother's autonomy and is sandwiched in with praise and validation.

Of course it is also the responsibility of the lactation consultant to do her best to see to it that the milk supply is protected during the period when the baby is unable to feed at breast. Keeping up to date on promoting and maintaining a good supply is crucial, especially as reproductive technology helps mothers with hormonal issues to have babies that they then wish to breastfeed. Clearly we need some counseling abilities as well as the ability to problem-solve milk production issues and help the mother and infant breastfeed. **Figure 13-1** provides an overview of the hierarchy of feeding choices.

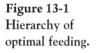

Figure 13-1
Hierarchy of
optimal feeding.

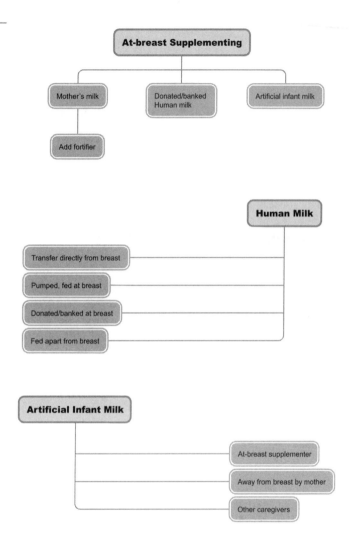

These families are truly in need of the gift of time. Many lactation consultants, especially when working in the context of a hospital or clinic, find themselves feeling pushed and harried to see every client, finish paperwork, and so forth. Yet grief can't and won't be hurried. These special circumstances will require that the lactation consultant set aside the other demands being required of her and give this family as much as they need.

Sometimes we become uncomfortable with a developing dependence on us as the parents look more and more to us beyond the scope of breastfeeding assistance. Some dependence is normal during a crisis. If lactation consultants can accept this without fostering an unhealthy growth of neediness, this can be a positive experience, opening the door to more teaching and help. We may become quite bonded to this mother, which is rewarding in and of itself.

Helping the Bottle-Feeding Mother Nurse Her Baby

There are times when, despite the best efforts of parents, health care providers, and other support people, breastfeeding is deemed to be impossible. Fortunately, this is largely avoidable with skilled help and good information. Nonetheless it does occur, to the dismay of all involved.

The process of breastfeeding is a complex, multilevel experience. It is much more than simply a way of getting nutrition from the mother to the baby, though often it is simplified to terms such as that. In addition to feeding, however, mother and baby will provide mutual comfort and cuddling, entertainment, relational behaviors, warmth, and immunological and hormonal support appropriate for each of them. Consequently, with the loss of breastfeeding comes the threat of much more than compromised nutrition.

Many mothers are able to give pumped milk in a bottle, by cup, or using some other method, even if transfer directly from the breast is impossible. Although this is far from ideal, it is also far from the least favorable option, which is to feed artificial infant milk from a bottle.

Much of this can be ameliorated by assisting the mother in learning to "nurse" her bottle-fed baby. Educating her on the importance of skin-to-breast contact, holding baby for the entirety of each and every feeding, allowing him to pacify at breast if he's able, and so forth can restore some of what might otherwise be lost.

This teaching will promote the bonding and attachment needs of the dyad. So much is now known about the critical need for mother and baby to be together, to spend time skin-to-skin, and to have the time and supportive context for "falling in love." With these challenging situations, such a necessary experience can potentially short-circuit. Therefore, it is incumbent on us to do our best to provide the necessary teaching and support to restore these relational abilities.

Conclusion

The lactation consultant who is faced with assisting families who include babies with feeding difficulties has her work cut out for her! This may be the most time-consuming, sometimes painful, and challenging work that she may be fortunate enough to be engaged in. If she is able to open herself up to the possibilities of both sadness and fear as well as being a conduit for hope and healing, she may also experience more joy in these situations than any other.

References

Ainsworth, M. (1967). *Infancy in Uganda: Infant care and the growth of love.* Baltimore: Johns Hopkins University Press.

Ainsworth, M., Blehar, M., Waters, E., & Wall, S. (1978). *Patterns of Attachment: A psychological study of the strange situation.* Hillsdale, NJ: Erlbaum.

Bergman, Nils (Producer). (2001). *Kangaroo mother care II: Restoring the original paradigm* [Motion picture]. (Available from Nils Bergman, 8 Francis Rd., Pinelands 7405, South Africa, or http://www.kangaroomothercare.com)

Bowlby, J. (1982). *Attachment and loss* (Rev. ed., Vol. 1). New York: Basic.

Bartlik, B., Greene, K., Graf, M., Sharma, G., & Melnick, H. (1999). *Examining PTSD as a complication of infertility.* Retrieved June 20, 2007, from http://www.medscape.com/viewarticle/408851

Bocar, D., & Moore, K. (1987). *Acquiring the parental role: A theoretical perspective.* La Leche League International, Lactation Consultant Series, Unit 16. Garden City Park, NY: Avery.

Crain, W. (2005). Erikson and the eight stages of life. In: *Theories of development: Concepts and applications* (5th ed.). New York: Prentice Hall.

Crews, A. (1999). *When I was garbage.* Retrieved June 15, 2005, from http://www.girl-mom.com

Erikson, E. (1968). *Identity: Youth and crisis.* New York: Norton.

Good Mojab, C. (2002). Helping breastfeeding mothers grieve. Retrieved February 1, 2006, from http://home.comcast.net/~ammawell/helping_mothers_grieve.html

Herforth, D. (1986). *Counseling grieving families.* La Leche League International, Lactation Consultant Series, Unit 12. Garden City Park, NY: Avery.

Hummel, P. (2003). Parenting the high-risk infant. *Newborn and Infant Nursing Reviews, 3*(3), 88–92.

Kinsley, C., & Lamber, K. (2006). The maternal brain. *Scientific American,* January, 72–79.

Kluger-Bell, K. (1998). *Unspeakable losses: Understanding the experience of pregnancy loss, miscarriage, and abortion.* New York: W.W. Norton & Co.

Kohn, I., Moffitt, P.-L., & Wilkins, I. A. (2000). *A silent sorrow: Pregnancy loss—Guidance and support for you and your family.* London: Routledge.

Kübler-Ross, E. (1969). *On death and dying.* New York: Touchstone.

Parker, D., & Williams, N. (2006). *Teens and breastfeeding* (2nd ed.). La Leche League International, Lactation Consultant Series Two, Unit 3. Garden City Park, NY: Avery.

Tagliaferre, L. (2001). *Recovery from loss: A personalized guide to the grieving process.* Gainesville, FL: Center for Applications of Psychological Type.

Vidyashanker, C. (2003). Postnatal depression linked to poor growth of infants. *Archives of Disease in Childhood, 88,* 34–37.

Williams, N. (1997). Maternal psychological issues in the experience of breastfeeding. *Journal of Human Lactation, 13,* 57–60.

Williams, N. (2002). Supporting the mother coming to terms with persistent insufficient milk supply: The role of the lactation consultant. *Journal of Human Lactation, 18,* 262–263.

Williams, N. (2004). When the blues arrive with baby. *New Beginnings, 21*(3), 84–88.

Worden, J. W. (2002). *Grief counseling and therapy: A guide for the mental health professional.* New York: Springer.

Wright, H. N. (1993). *Recovering from the losses of life.* Grand Rapids, MI: Fleming H. Revell.

Wright, H. N. (2003). *The new guide to crisis and trauma counseling.* Ventura, CA: Regal Books.

Index

A

ABC protocol (Smith), 66–73
acceptance vs. resignation, 335–336
active listening, 337–338
active supplementation devices, 278
    See also supplementation
ad libitum (semi-demand) feeding, 172–173
adequacy, mother, 329–330
adult development, understanding, 328
advice from outsiders, counseling about, 334–335
affect, 238
affective synchrony, 86–87
air flow
    anatomy of, 4
    swallowing and, 6–7
airway abnormalities, congenital, 216–220
airway protection, 133–135. *See also* aspiration
    oral-facial anomalies and, 146
alcohol exposure in utero, 254–255
alerting stimulation, 245
alertness, 275
alignment. *See* attachment; positioning
All Fours position, 320
alternative feeding methods, 284–289
ambivalence, 330
amygdala, 47–48
anatomy of infant mouth, 2–5
    congenital airway abnormalities, 216–220
    flow rate and, 146
    hemangioma, 203
    macroglossia (large tongue), 206
    micrognathia and mandibular hypoplasia, 203–206
    oral clefts, 206–216
    tongue-tie. *See* ankyloglossia
    torticollis and, 19–20, 26, 221–222
anesthetics during pregnancy or labor, 60
angling baby against mother, 121–122
. animal newborn feeding behaviors, 80–81

ankyloglossia (tongue-tie), 22–25, 32–33, 72, 181–203
    classification of, 188–194
    effect on breastfeeding, 187
    facilitative strategies, 280
    family history, 228
    finger feeding, 186, 197–198
    latch, improving, 195–197
    management without frenotomy, 194–195
    nipple shields, using, 201–202
    superior labial frenulum, 203
    tongue exercises, 199–201
    treatment of, 194. *See also* frenotomy
anticipatory adjustments, 240
anticonvulsants, side-effects of, 257
APGAR score, 60, 254
apnea, feeding-induced, 142, 146
    See also breathing during feeding
    decreasing milk flow for, 149
arching (body extension), 245
ARND (alcohol-related neurodevelopmental disorder), 255
arousal, infant, 21, 238
    hyperarousal dissociation, 53–54, 65
    state organization (state regulation), 50, 86
        sensory integration and, 240–241
        social interaction and, 86–88
artificial rupture of membranes, 58
artificial teats, 70, 71
aspiration, 11
    See also coordination of infant feeding
    high flow and swallow integrity, 138
    preterm infants, 155
    videofluoroscopic swallow study (VFSS), 295–296
assessment, breast, 28–31
    tongue-tie and, 187
assessment, feeding. *See* breastfeeding assessment
assessment tools, 14–15, 31
    ATLFF tool, 186–187

preterm infants, 163–164
reflexive control of, 7–9. *See also* reflexes, infant
sounds of, 12
swallowing centers (brain), 7
swallowing disorder. *See* dysphagia
sweeping movements of lips, 281
symmetry of infant, 19–20
Syndrome X, 54
syringe, 124, 211, 278
neurologically impaired infants, 277

T

tactile system, 236–237
defensiveness, 246–247, 249
talking to infant, 93. *See also* interaction,
maternal-infant
teen mothers, counseling, 333–334
temporalis muscle, 4
test weights, 144
preterm infants, 172, 173
therapeutic position. *See* positioning
Three-Finger Dancer Suck Training position,
316–317
timetables in infant brain development, 46–47
tone, infant, 18–20, 245, 268
tongue (infant)
anatomy of, 4
assessment of, 22–25, 31–34
exercising (with ankyloglossia), 199–201
function of (sucking vs. suckling), 5
large (macroglossia), 206
motor dysfunction, facilitation for, 281
range of motion, 22–25, 188
See also ankyloglossia
wavelike motion (stripping), 5, 10
tongue massage, 199–200
tongue protrusion, 7, 8
tongue-tie. *See* ankyloglossia
tongue tip elevation, 22, 33, 34, 183
torticollis, 19–20, 26, 221–222
touch. *See* attachment; sensory stimuli; skin-to-
skin contact
tracheomalacia, 218–219
transverse muscle (tongue), 4
transverse tongue reflex, 7, 8
treatment, assessment and, 17

tremors of tongue or mandible, 25
trigeminal nerve, 4
triplets, breastfeeding positions and, 320–322
trust (by infant), reestablishing, 92
tube feeding. *See* feeding tube devices
twins, breastfeeding positions for, 320–322
Two-Finger Dancer Suck Training position, 318

U

under-responsivity to sensory input, 244
upper lip. *See* lips, infant
Upside Down position, 320

V

vacuum vaginal delivery, 63, 72
vagus nerve (X), 63
vagus nerve fibers, 7
velopharyngeal inadequacy, 215–216
velum. *See* soft palate
vertical muscles (tongue), 4
vertical prone position, 311–312
vestibular senses, 236, 244–245
VFP (vocal fold paralysis), 219–220
VFSS (videofluoroscopic swallow study), 295–296
videofluoroscopic swallow study (VFSS), 295–296
visual input, body schema and, 236–237
visual learners, mothers as, 248–249
vocal fold paralysis, 219–220
voicing infant communication, 243
volume, milk. *See* milk; milk flow

W

waking baby for feeding, 148
walking back on the tongue, 294
warn baths, 55
wavelike tongue motion, 5, 10
stimulating, 294
weaning from breastfeeding, 328
weaning from supplementation, 174, 279–280
WHO/UNICEF Baby-Friendly Hospital Initiative,
66, 74
Mother-Friendly Module, 74
wiggle worm stimulation, 294
Williams syndrome, 261
Wolf's law, 282